Traces of the Infantile in Psychoanalytic Therapy with Adults

This book applies parent-infant-therapy techniques to allow therapists to work effectively with adult patients on their earliest traumas.

There is an increased awareness among therapists, parents, and stakeholders that attempts to address psychological challenges in the first year of life could diminish the risk of later non-optimal development. Furthermore, a deeper understanding of such challenges and distress in parent-infant dyads can influence therapeutic work with adult patients by helping them discern "the traces of the Infantile" within. Drawing on his extensive clinical experience and application of the parent-infant psychotherapy (PIP) technique, Salomonsson offers a clear guide to how therapists can tie together experiences from adulthood and childhood, memory and family myth, and verbal and non-verbal communication from the patient to tease out the origin of the adult patient's trauma and to allow for more informed and targeted treatment. The author argues that moving between PIP and adult therapeutic work is compatible with psychoanalytic theory and emphasises the importance of its inclusion in therapy training, Enriched with clinical vignettes and a focus on practical work, this is an essential read for all psychoanalysts and psychotherapists.

Björn Salomonsson is a psychiatrist and member of the Swedish Psychoanalytical Association, working in private practice. He is an Associate Professor at the Karolinska Institute and his research focuses on parent-infant therapies, child and adult analysis, and the 'weaving thoughts' presentation method. This is his fourth book published in English. In 2024, he received the Sigourney award for his contributions to psychoanalytic parent-infant psychotherapy.

Traces of the Infantile in Psychoanalytic Therapy with Adults

Björn Salomonsson

Routledge
Taylor & Francis Group

LONDON AND NEW YORK

Designed cover image: © Getty Images

First published 2026
by Routledge
4 Park Square, Milton Park, Abingdon, Oxon OX14 4RN

and by Routledge
605 Third Avenue, New York, NY 10158

Routledge is an imprint of the Taylor & Francis Group, an informa business

© 2026 Björn Salomonsson

British Library Cataloguing-in-Publication Data
A catalogue record for this book is available from the British Library

ISBN: 978-1-041-07406-9 (hbk)
ISBN: 978-1-041-07034-4 (pbk)
ISBN: 978-1-003-64036-3 (ebk)

DOI: 10.4324/9781003640363

Typeset in Sabon
by SPi Technologies India Pvt Ltd (Straive)

'What do psychoanalysis and astronomy have in common? As surprising as this question may seem, after reading this book every reader will recognize the fascinating equation: both sciences deal with the traces of events that occurred long ago but are effective in the present. Björn Salomonsson not only reminds us of the light shining from afar in the starry sky, but also uses sensitive empathy combined with conceptual diversity to highlight the traces and radiations of the Infantile in the lives of adults. At the same time, he emphasises a crucial difference, because in psychoanalysis, the subjectivity of the analyst and their connection to their own Infantile are of central importance to grasp the Infantile of patients. On the basis of distinct conceptual knowledge and his expertise in parent-infant psychotherapy, Salomonsson formulates the Infantile as a concept: as a source of emotional vitality, but also as a backdrop for later mental conflicts. The clinical examples are full of Salomonsson's clinical-analytical competence in dealing with the Infantile in its various forms. A deeply thoughtful, clinically stimulating and wise book at the same time.'

Heribert Blass, Dr. med. resident elect of the International Psychoanalytical Association

'Page after page, with sure expertise and descriptive mastery, in this fascinating book Bjorn Salomonsson builds a bridge between two territories that the individual psyche, culture, and sometimes even science, often risk separating in an unrealistic and defensive way: the area of the Infantile and that of the adult mind.

Thanks to its clear and effectively integrative style, 'Traces of the Infantile' is an invaluable working tool for connecting theory to clinical practice, but also for encouraging each reader to make intimate contact with their own inner infantile Self, in a humanising process of reconnecting with their deepest experiences.'

Stefano Bolognini, Past President of the International Psychoanalytical Association

'Drawing on his extensive experience in Parent-Infant Psychotherapy, Salomonsson offers new insights into how early relationships influence who we become as adults. He uses the interesting analogy of an astronomer exploring the infinite night sky and the analyst examining the mind's earliest workings, thereby elucidating complex processes and making them more accessible. The session transcripts that are provided illustrate how links to infancy can be made with sensitivity and empathy. The author engages in critical self-reflection, an example of best practice when working in this field. Also included is the latest research and the historical background to many of our theories, making this a valuable and essential addition to the existing psychoanalytic literature.'

Astrid Berg, Cape Town, President of the World Association for Infant Mental Health

In memory of my colleague Johan Norman, who first sparked my interest in applying psychoanalytic practice and theory to distressed babies and parents and, consequently, to my adult patients as well.

Contents

    Clinical epilogue   207

    References   *212*
    Index   *233*

Author's preface

A century ago, astronomers believed that the Milky Way constituted the entire Universe, and that so-called nebulae in the night sky were gas clouds. But in 1924, an American astronomer, Edwin Hubble, claimed that the Andromeda "nebula" is actually a galaxy of its own and way beyond our Milky Way. Many astronomers scoffed at his ideas, but today they agree that Andromeda is indeed an entire galaxy, 2½ million light years away from Earth. On the book cover, you see it as the disc-shaped blue object halfway up. Some years later, Hubble relied on previous discoveries of a redshift in the light of the Universe, a phenomenon that is due to an increased wavelength of the light emitted from distant celestial bodies. Hubble argued that the redshift implied that they are actually moving away from each other and concluded that the Universe is expanding.

Why begin a psychoanalytic book with astronomy? To respond, what I will call "the Infantile" covers experiences and events that seem remote and intricate to discern, similar to what we may feel when we look at the night sky. The Infantile is an almost – but not entirely – unreachable part in our psyche that can affect us profoundly, momentarily, or at length. It is rooted in the prime of our lives but continues blinking forever in the background. It is this omnipresence, sometimes vague and sometimes glaring, and the strange blend of events occurring now and a long time ago, that I wish to cover by the astronomy metaphor. Moreover, Andromeda and its neighbouring constellation Cassiopeia are Greek mythological characters. Andromeda was the daughter of Cassiopeia and her husband Cepheus. Their story is a sad portrait of early object relations that created distress between parents and children. More about this later in the book.

Some decades before Hubble's discoveries, Sigmund Freud began studying the arcane meanings of his Viennese patients' psychiatric disorders. His "telescope" was the psychoanalytic method. His predecessors had viewed psychic aberrations as caused by genetic, chemical, microbial, or degenerative factors. When Freud involved himself in dialogues with his patients, he discovered that their disorders had a meaning, though unconscious to be true.

His key to helping them overcome their ailments was to inspire them to investigate, that is, reflect on their inner universe. Other analysts followed suit by including other groups of patients, such as psychotics, adolescents, children, and psychosomatic cases. Inviting babies and mothers to psychotherapy is a late extension of our psychoanalytic "telescope". The universe of clinical psychoanalysis, and thus of clinical psychiatry, is expanding. The cases that support the book's ideas and arguments are drawn from my psychoanalytically inspired therapies with adults and parent-infant psychotherapies (PIPs). As we will see, the two periods of life have more traits in common than we tend to think.

I will now use the astronomy metaphor to address the question of how we gain empirical knowledge in various disciplines. This is especially important when we as psychoanalysts construe how babies perceive the world and communicate with it. Since they do not talk with us we need, as far as possible, to be clear about our concepts and astute in our observations. This is even more important when we surmise, as I will do in this book, that a part of our personality, *the Infantile*, can cause severe suffering in the adult. Evidently, this concept has to do with infancy – though it is not identical with it.

Returning to our epistemological quest, astronomers use empirical methods to understand the Universe. Likewise, we psychoanalysts use our clinical findings to expand knowledge of the human universe; the mind. Yet, empirical approaches in natural and hermeneutic disciplines have many differences. We need only to think of the diverging *Weltanschauungen* in the mostly Anglo-Saxon tradition of empiricism (Locke, Hume, Mill) and the *Geisteswissenschaften* in German idealism and its many branches. As psychoanalysts, we do apply an empirical perspective as we observe and address our patients. But we do not measure them, as does an astronomer. Instead, we are interested in what occurs in their *Geist*, a German word combining mind and spirit. We seek to find about what happens when *das Ich* (Fichte) of the patient meets with *das Nicht-Ich* of the analyst, and what is going on in the patient's *das Unbewusste* (Schelling) or *das Bewußlose* (Hegel). Our intent is not to *erklären* or explain why the patient feels or thinks in certain ways. Explanations pertain to natural science, for example, "the patient's depression is linked with/caused by a drop of the serotonin level in the brain's synapses". As analysts, we want to *verstehen* or understand the patient, as suggested by Dilthey. To do this, we involve ourselves in a dialogue with him/her, a perspective elaborated further by Gadamer. In other words, one of the analyst's most important tools for understanding the patient is his understanding of himself. I suggest the following works for the interested reader (Gadamer, 1975/1989; Lessing, 2011; Mills, 2002; Nelson, 2019; Palmer, 1969).

Although psychoanalysis is rarely called an empirical science – a claim that astronomy has every right to uphold – there is a similarity between the two disciplines. To exemplify, Hubble discovered that the Universe is expanding by *observing* the celestial bodies through a telescope and calculating his data. When Freud formulated his "rational theory of irrationality" (Whitebook, 2017, 146), he used a "psychoanalytic instrument" to *observe* his patients' words and behaviours, from which he deduced the interplay of their conscious and unconscious layers. He also discovered, albeit reluctantly at times, that he must study the interaction between the patient and himself. Thus, he did not only use conjectures and reflections but also listened to and looked at the patient and himself. There are thus similarities in the empirical approach in astronomy and psychoanalysis, but there are essential differences as well. I will soon return to this topic.

If this book's focus were on the epistemology of psychoanalysis and natural sciences, I could have exemplified with many other sciences than astronomy. After all, it seems so divergent from our discipline! To answer, the astronomy metaphor will hopefully invoke a feel in the reader that our mind is a universe ranging from the here and now to the far away and ancient. As for our troubles, joys, and sorrows of today, they can also relate to events and experiences that occurred ages ago. We all harbour such *traces of the Infantile* that can affect our present lives. As babies, we lived through moments that were happy and pleasant, or scary and unpleasant. Many were perhaps never registered – or they were buried through a mechanism called primal repression, more infrequently written "primary repression". I will address the concept in Chapters 1 and 12. Anyone who is unfamiliar with it could think of a term such as "implicit registration" to get an idea of what it is about. Some may never re-emerge; others will flare up as a recall of a pleasant scent, a tune, an atmosphere. They can also clasp one's entire life and turn into a compulsion, a psychosomatic symptom, or an urge to act destructively. When this happens to patients in psychoanalytically oriented therapies, we can turn our analytic "telescope" to them and investigate their passions as being traces of their Infantile.

At this point, I must qualify the astronomy metaphor and my play with the term "analytic telescope". I just argued that both astronomers and psychoanalysts are empiricists. But importantly, they also need a lot of intuition to grasp what goes on in space and in patients, respectively. The difference is this; astronomers must tame their intuitions through observations that are objective and unaffected by feelings. Their findings must also be accessible to other scientists to be studied in repeated experiments. In contrast, analysts' observations contain a considerable amount of subjectivity. The analyst's person is deeply involved in his or her work. He needs to be constantly attentive to what he thinks happens in the patient – and what he perceives in himself. To emphasise this bidirectional aspect of analytic work I will later, in Chapter 2, try replacing the metaphor "the analytic telescope" to that of an "endoscope".

Another difference between psychoanalysis and astronomy is that one analyst's finding about a clinical situation cannot be rerun experimentally with other analysts or patients. Thus, if the astronomy metaphor would lead anybody to conceive of analysts as sitting behind their patients and looking objectively at them, this would be a serious misunderstanding. I hope the book and its case examples will disconfirm any such notions.

Notwithstanding the caveat I just broached, another factor connects astronomers and analysts. Astronomers will never arrive at Andromeda. They must content themselves with studying *après-coup* the light it emitted some million years ago. Likewise, analysts will of course never arrive at the patient's Infantile in the concrete sense of meeting him or her as a baby. We involve ourselves with his or her memories, feelings, and ideas that we may construe as "emissions" from ancient experiences. Astronomers assume that what they see in the telescope is an unaltered rendition of past events. But they know that actually, they are looking at traces of objects very far away in distance and time. As for us analysts, we know that the patient's story of what happened then and there is *not* an unaltered version of the truth. It has been filtered and re-elaborated through decades of experiences and is now presented to us with a plea for help. We can subsume some of those accounts under the concept of the Infantile. But importantly, it does not refer to any specific calendar time or event in an objective sense. Rather, it refers to events and experiences viewed through an individual's emotional experience (Bion, 1962) or *Erlebnis*, a word meaning "what we have lived". We will work with these distinctions throughout the book.

The conflict between objective truth and subjective experience has been vibrating in psychoanalysis ever since Freud discovered in disappointment that he could no longer believe in the veracity of his patients' childhood accounts (S. Freud, 1897, 259). "There are no indications of reality in the unconscious, so that one cannot distinguish between the truth and fiction that is cathected with affect". The contrast between factual traumas in childhood, such as illness, separation, death of a parent – and our subjective interpretations of them today is a recurrent and contentious theme in psychoanalytic practice and theory. Nowhere is this opposition as evident as in the events and experiences of infancy. This will be shown in many case stories of the book. Some patients had been struck in infancy by medical traumas, early separations, and mothers' depressions. Even so, they must also understand how they have interpreted these events until now and find out if they can construe and handle them differently in the future. If analysts were unable to help patients change perspectives on their early traumas, analytic therapy would be meaningless, futile and simply amiss.

One final comparison between the starry sky and the Infantile: We can lead an entire life without ever knowing about, or being affected by, the Andromeda or other celestial bodies. But no one can lead a life without being affected by the Infantile. It may yield joy, love, and creativity to an individual. But in cases of emotional suffering, we may discern that his Infantile is haunting him. This makes the analyst's and the patient's tasks delicate, painstaking, but in the end also rewarding.

This book aims to accompany therapists who want to refine their knowledge about, and skills in handling, the Infantile of their patients. An equally important intention is to awaken analysts' curiosity about how their own Infantile can obstruct – or promote – empathy with their patients' challenges. Whereas my previous books and papers focused on child analysis and parent-infant psychotherapy (PIP), this book uses examples that are mainly, but not exclusively, drawn from adult work. It addresses therapists who wish to know more about the Infantile as it emerges in their work with adult patients.

I became engaged in PIP a quarter of a century ago. Apart from the satisfaction it offered helping families in profound crises, I became more aware of how the Infantile emerges in adult patients and more versed in talking with them about it. This led to papers focusing on when and how the Infantile emerges in adult therapies (Salomonsson, 2020, 2022) and now to this book. Half of it consists of newly written clinical material and theoretical ideas, the other half of published papers that I have reworked thoroughly to make them align with the topic of the book; *searching for traces of the Infantile in psychoanalytic therapy with adults*.

I end this preface by thanking all the patients who have given me their informed consent to appear as clinical examples in the book. All names have been changed, and all details enabling their identities to be disclosed have been changed or deleted. My respect for their suffering and willingness to struggle with it in therapy is as great as is my gratitude for their generosity and understanding that it may help other therapists develop skills with their patients.

Beginning my thanks with deceased colleagues who were a great inspiration, I mention Eric Brenman, Irma Brenman Pick, James Grotstein, Jean Laplanche, Donald Meltzer, Johan Norman, Per-Anders Rydelius, and Andrzej Werbart. Among present-day clinicians who have inspired me, I want first to mention Florence Guignard, who coined the concept of the Infantile in a manner that is similar though not identical with how I am using it. Another influence has been her welcoming me to the SEPEA (Societé Européenne pour la Psychanalyse de l'Enfant et de l'Adolescent). Un très grand merci! Among other influential colleagues, I wish to thank Joseph Aguayo, Keren Amiran, Jacques Angelergues, Christine Anzieu-Premmereur, Evrinomy Avdi, Tessa Baradon, Anders Berge, Alexandra Billinghurst, Heribert Blass, Stefano Bolognini, Larry Brown, Susan Donner, Bernard Golse, Michael Feldman, Peter Fonagy, Francis Grier, Talia Hatzor, Susanne Hauser, Susanne Hommel, Angela Joyce, Hugo Lagercrantz, Françoise Moggio, Daniela Montelatici Prawitz, Sylvain Missonnier, Donna Roth Smith, Rolf Sandell, Dominique Scarfone, Clara Schejtman, Michelle Sleed, John Steiner, and Elizabeth Tuters. My thanks also to the colleagues in my international supervision seminars, and to Idit Dori, Anne Rilliet Howald, and Fabienne Wälli Phaneuf who inspired me to launch them. Among presidents of WAIMH, World Association of Infant Mental Health, I thank Miri

Keren, Tuula Tamminen, Antoine Guedeney, Kai von Klitzing, Campbell Paul, and Astrid Berg.

My sincere thanks also go to the Bertil Wennborg Foundation for supporting my research and writings over the years, and to the Mary S. Sigourney Award Trust for making me a recipient of their award 2024. Last but not least, my warm thanks go to my wife, colleague, and co-author of Chapter 6 in this book, Majlis Winberg Salomonsson. Without her support, patience and interest, this book would never have been written. Also, a big hug to the youngest members of our extended family; Noah and Leo, Hugo and Axel, Olivia, Oliver and Ruben, and little Love.

Stockholm, Midsummer Day, 2025
Björn Salomonsson

Chapter 1

Introduction to a kiss and to a concept

We will now move from the unfathomable Universe to the banal habits of everyday life. Whenever we human beings set up a meeting, big or small, at home or at work, we arrange for something to eat and drink. When we go to bed, we follow our personal routines with pillows, setting the right temperature, pulling down the curtain, placing a glass of water at bedside, and so on. When we wish to show our love to a child, a relative, or a lover, we kiss them, though in different ways. In our closet, our favourite cardigan and slippers have been there for ages. These habits are so ingrained that if we skip them, we get distressed and annoyed. And they are so rooted in us that we forget to ask ourselves whence these quirks came and why we stick to them so fervently.

These habits revolve around simple wishes and needs of food, sleep, body temperature, human closeness. I conceive of them as residues from our infancy. In those days, we protested when we were tucked in a new bed, did not receive the breast at once or felt it smelled differently, heard an unusual sound, or did not get the same spoon as yesterday. I guess this parallel will meet with little protest, and we need not invoke psychoanalytic concepts to explain such remnants from our personal history. In brief, we know we have them but do not need to talk much about them. In analytic terms, they are *ego-syntonic* patterns. Consequently, they can hardly have anything to do with a book called "Traces of the Infantile in psychoanalytic therapy with adults". The title carries us to the clinical domain where, obviously, what I call *the Infantile* seems to cause our patients trouble of some sort.

The Infantile – what then does that term cover? Something to do with babies, evidently, but what more? Let us move to the territory of psychoanalysis and how the term is used there. In 2021, the International Psychoanalytic Association (IPA) held its biennial congress. The main theme was "The infantile". Note that I use the capital letter in the book, whereas "the infantile", as in the congress, is also an accepted way of writing. We will return to this important detail in Chapters 2 and 12. The congress should be an excellent source for establishing the meaning of the term in the psychoanalytic sense.

DOI: 10.4324/9781003640363-1

But, as the titles of the three keynote papers indicate, such a mission was fraught with problems: "The infantile: Which meaning?" (Canestri, 2021), "The infantile: Its multiple dimensions" (Tanis, 2021), and "Constructing the infantile" (Litowitz, 2021). The titles indicated that the term seems vague, complex, and far from standing on solid ground.

To avoid the term's ambiguity, we might take recourse to the person hidden inside the term, the infant or the baby. In a congress devoted to "the infantile", we would expect to also find seminars on how real babies appear under normal and stressful circumstances and how they and their parents can be helped in therapy. But such events took place only to a limited extent. Does this mean that "the infantile" has nothing to do with babies? Or is there another and specifically psychoanalytic perspective on those mental events that deserve the epithet infantile – even if they occur in people who have left infancy? But why then call them infantile?

One answer is that the *psychoanalytic* meaning of "infantile" differs from the traditional *medical* one. If a paediatrician speaks of "infantile colic", he refers exclusively to a little baby's condition. In contrast, think of a psychoanalyst who notices that a patient avoids his/her[1] eyes recurrently after the weekend breaks in therapy. He might well conceive of this pattern as the patient's "infantile manifestation" of emotions that emerged during the recess. His argument would be that separation anxieties typically emerge and peak in infancy, and that the patient's present anxiety and helplessness resemble that of a baby, alternatively that it is even causally linked to it. In this psychoanalytic usage, the term infantile thus does not refer to a well-defined age or series of events. Rather, it subsumes sensations, emotions, behaviours, and psychosomatic phenomena resembling a baby's emotions, mentation, or behaviour. We will soon compare this term with "the Infantile" – a term used in this book's title – to see if the two are identical or not.

One speaker at the congress, Jorge Canestri (2021, 563), stated that "when 'the infantile' speaks, the speaker [the patient] does not know it... he needs a 'narrator', i.e. a psychoanalyst in the transference situation". It is thus *the analyst's* personal experiences, unconscious prejudices, impressions in the session, and theoretical studies that make him interpret a clinical situation as being coloured by "the infantile" of the patient. He may thus be facing a patient who behaves, speaks, looks, and sounds in ways that remind *the analyst* of an unhappy baby. If so, he may choose to bring this up with the patient. Alternatively, he may choose another interpretation that addresses more "developed" or "adult" levels of the patient's personality.

Now, what one analyst regards as an infantile manifestation may not be regarded as such by another one. This brings in the well-known critique of psychoanalysis that it is based on the analyst's guesswork rather than on "objective" findings. In the preface, I argued why psychoanalysts can never make epistemological claims similar to those of astronomers or other natural scientists. As André Green once said in a debate, psychoanalysis is not a science in the ordinary sense but a "disciplined conjecture", a position omni-present in his writings. But I would not be an analyst if I were awestricken or paralysed by this inevitable subjective element of my findings and conclu-sions. On the contrary, psychoanalytic training inspires us to include a *meas-ured* and *well-reflected subjectivity* when being with, and trying to understand, our patients. Here comes the first one.

Colin: a first-time father

Many years ago, long before I started working with psychoanalytic parent-infant psychotherapy (PIP), I came across a young man who elicited my inter-est in what I today would call *the Infantile and its traces*. My contact with *"Colin"* took place in a psychiatric outpatient service. I have no notes from our work, so any quotes to follow are merely my ways of portraying more vividly his suffering. As I recall Colin, he seemed intelligent and affectionate when he spoke about his son, who at that time was around one year of age. When the son was much younger, Colin's dedication had been interfered with by an infatuation with a woman other than the boy's mother and his wife. The reason he sought help was his anxiety about it and why it had happened. He wanted to do this before he and his family were to leave Sweden for their home country. From the onset, it was thus clear that this was going to be a brief contact.

My first dialogue with this academic in his thirties showed that the birth of his son had not been an entirely happy event. I got the impression that he now sought help to relieve himself of the guilt, sadness, and disappointment with himself that he felt as a first-time father. The focus of our brief contact was this turmoil, which had shaken him deeply since he had always looked forward to becoming a father. He thought it had to do with his strict and distant father. Although he liked his father and learnt much from him, they didn't have a warm and confident contact. Now that he had become a father himself, he wanted to be kinder and more present than him. When the first son, whom I call *Eric*, was born, Colin felt joy, pride, closeness, and a desire to protect him and his mother. The fact that father and son looked alike had created a special bond between the two.

Some days after Eric's birth, Colin suddenly lost his appetite. Normally a gourmand, he was stunned at this shift. He seemed psychologically minded, so I ventured an interpretation that I would reconstruct as follows: "Perhaps you were jealous when seeing your son breastfeeding. Losing your appetite might have been a cry for help from a boy who felt abandoned. No food or comfort left for you, as it were." I recall that he turned thoughtful, sad, and ashamed of being envious of his son.

Colin now moved on to a more embarrassing topic. When Eric was four months old, he fell in love with a colleague at his office. Or rather, he felt that she "dragged him" into desiring her. They never had a sexual relationship, but kissing was a bliss. He felt ashamed, helpless, and guilty towards his wife. After some months, his infatuation abated. This was the time when he started thinking about contacting a psychiatrist. Now, he told me, he had found a calmer way of collaborating with the colleague. Colin still did not grasp why it started, but he knew he had to end it.

Colin did not understand why he became enthralled by a woman whom he liked as a colleague but was never really in love with. He felt passive, surrendering to a force he didn't understand – except for one thing; she admired him, which boosted his ego. Later and unexpectedly, he mentioned that when he himself was four months old, he had been hospitalised at length due to severe eczema. He knew that breastfeeding was terminated abruptly. When he asked his mother about it later in life, she was still horrified thinking of visiting her son in the hospital.

His mother had also told him that when he returned home, he developed a voracious appetite for butter. When speaking about this, Colin was taken by an association to his fascination with his beloved's lips. He spoke of their gloss and smell of butter. Thus, it became even clearer to him that his infatuation was not really about sexual intercourse but more like fusing with her. This reminded him of kissing his first girlfriend in his teens. Colin also mentioned an elder sister, whom he was deeply attached to. However, she moved abroad in his adolescence, and their connection was slowly weakened. He suddenly recalled that the first time the colleague and he were kissing was on his sister's birthday. He was intrigued and bewildered by this coincidence.

In our brief work, he became more tolerant of himself as a father. He had always longed to be a father, but when it happened, he felt that forces stronger than himself overpowered him and pushed him in directions he had never foreseen. Less burdened by shame and intolerance with himself, Colin dared talk with his wife about the deeper roots to his behaviour. She showed understanding, which decreased his guilt and liberated more commitment with Eric.

As for Colin's life before fatherhood, he led an ordinary family life. His professional achievements were excellent, and he had close male friends. But with girls it had been more difficult when he was a teenager. He spoke of himself as inhibited and too close to his protective mother. Becoming a father toppled this construction. When Eric was born, Colin briefly turned into a man with some traits of a starving and depressed baby. His infatuation with the colleague some months later could be seen as a desperate reaching out to an idealised version of the mother, whose continuous presence had been interrupted in his first year of life. During his second year, his sister was born, which probably made him feel disconnected from his mother a second time.

Some years after Colin had terminated our brief contact, he wrote a letter that their second child *Nolan* was born a year ago. Like Eric's delivery, Nolan's birth went well. He conveyed his love of Nolan and that he saw him, in comparison with Eric, more like a separate individual. When he resumed work, he was overwhelmed a few times by longing for little Nolan. He went home, cried for a while, was comforted by his wife, and returned to his job. His letter indicated that, today, he could handle better his baby-self-identification and focus on fathering his two children in a more mature way. He added that Nolan had developed a skin rash when he was around five months old. The mother, still breastfeeding, changed her diet and the eczema healed rapidly.

Later, when I had become a psychoanalyst and reflected on Colin's eczema, I wondered if it was a psychosomatic expression of a conflict between container and contained (Bion, 1962) – that is, if it might have articulated a deep scar in the earliest mother – infant relationship. As argued, his stormy reactions after Eric's birth suggested that he was overwhelmed by a hitherto concealed wound of his psyche. Did this even mean that his eczema was actually a psychosomatic reaction to a disturbed mother – infant relationship? If so, did such a relational disturbance contribute to destabilising him after Eric's birth and making fatherhood a double task: to care for both Eric and the distressed baby within himself? At this point, I am cautious of suggesting that Colin's infantile eczema emerged in the wake of a primeval relational disturbance. His son Nolan's food allergy suggested a biological factor in Colin's eczema as well, and the relationship with his mother had been close but did not contain mistrust, hostility, or detachment – at least as I remember it.

Traces of the infantile in Colin

Colin was a reasonably well-functioning man with a personality structure most therapists would call neurotic. He was inhibited, somewhat anxious with women, and low-keyed at times but not clinically depressed. His ego strength had sufficed to steer him away from any breakdown or serious psychiatric symptoms. He said that when his son Eric was born, he took part in the delivery with pride and joy, but then a symptom emerged; he just didn't feel like eating. Let us assume I was stretching my imagination when I interpreted his appetite loss as an unconscious identification with an abandoned baby. Indeed, you do not need to accept my idea, but it would be more difficult to deny that when Colin fell – or plummeted – in love, he regressed towards a more infantile functioning. The sudden and witless sinking in the arms of a woman because she admired him – and not because he was in love with her – points in this direction. Other indications are the bliss when kissing her and his fascination with her lips' butter scent which, after all, is a somewhat oblique way for a man to appreciate a woman.

The psychoanalytic concept I use to account for Colin's upheaval when he became a father is *regression*. In Freudian terms (S. Freud, 1900), it was both temporal and formal. Temporal, because Colin had been "harking back to older psychical structures" (548) when Eric was born. Formal, because he used "primitive methods of expression and representation [that] take the place of the usual ones" (548). The appetite loss was an embodied, implicit, and unclear way of expressing his emotional turmoil. We may call it a trace of his feelings and experiences around feeding.

In other words, while Colin in many other aspects functioned on an adult level with preserved cognitive, intellectual, and ethical standards, there was a parallel track in him: *the traces of the Infantile* kept twinkling ominously as if coming from a distant galaxy. He did not perceive the signals and precisely therefore they could exert a powerful influence. To reformulate the astronomy metaphor in psychoanalytic concepts, the reason that the traces were so powerful was that they were *unconscious*. Colin did not feel any jealousy towards Eric, he just wasn't hungry. And he discerned nothing about the connection between his infantile trauma and the infatuation with his colleague. At the time, he felt "it just happened". Could we say that his devastation and jealousy were *split off*? If so, the term "split" cannot refer to the fact that he could not recall his baby hospitalisation. After all, suggesting that every infantile amnesia represents a split in the personality is to stretch the concept way beyond its psychoanalytic meaning. Alternatively, the split might cover the lack of emotional contact between being a proud father and feeling depressed and "just not hungry". I will soon return to the term splitting and my second reservation about it in this case.

Why were Colin's experiences of the original trauma unconscious? Because he felt guilty or ashamed about them? No, this was not a repression in the traditional sense, as if he had unconsciously pushed aside something embarrassing, forbidden, or reprehensive. Two factors prevented "classical repressions" or "repression proper" (see Chapter 12) from dealing with his experiences. First, their affects were different from the ones that we normally handle by repression; they were overwhelming, horrendous, and linked with helplessness and abandonment. Second, as a baby, Colin had only been able to signify them in a most primitive way. Therefore, and instead of repression proper, they expressed "a first phase of repression, which consists in the psychical (ideational) representative of the instinct being denied entrance into the conscious. With this a fixation is established" (S. Freud, 1915a, 148). This was Freud's way of establishing the concept of *primal repression*. He referred to impulses that had never been conscious (S. Freud, 1915b, 181) and were also barred entrance to the Conscious.

Freud's model has been questioned (Balestriere, 2003; Maze & Henry, 1996) on logical grounds: one cannot repress something one never knew anything about. To solve this problem, I have suggested (Salomonsson, 2014a) we apply a semiotic perspective on the concept of primal repression. Such a perspective is not at all new to modern psychoanalytic theory, and I will develop it in Chapters 2 and 12. In my formulation, primal repression refers to impulses that indeed were *registered* from the very beginning but *signified in an archaic mode*. Such primitive signs might then be mentally elaborated – albeit in a primitive mode – as a flush of affect, a shiver, a transpiration, a current of unpleasure, a motion in the body, a grimace, an affront or delight at a certain odour or sound, a dream fragment, and so on. In Colin's case, we could fantasise such ways of signifying as "stretched out in panic", "butter smell is marvellous", "lips heal every pain", "itch is help-lessness", and so on.

When such experiences were frightening, incomprehensible, and over-whelming, they were retained as a *living fossil* (Salomonsson, 2014a, 121). The term expresses a contradiction: "fossil" refers to an archaic, vague, and rigid representation of a dead object, whereas "living" indicates that it is still active. Kissing his colleague is a neat illustration. It may have looked like two adults kissing and relishing it – like lovers do. But in Colin's experience, there was idealisation, devotion, sinking in her arms plus the taste of butter. They all pointed back to his infancy, not in any direct and explicit way but as a shadow, a trace, or a fossil that yet was alive.

Now we will return to my reservations about the term splitting in this case. Freud (1940) used it to describe how some of us manage to simultane-ously maintain two attitudes towards reality: full acceptance and total rejec-tion of it. He used the term to comprehend the inner world of patients with perversion. Later analysts like Klein and Kernberg applied it to children and to personality disorders in adults. But Colin was neither a child, a pervert, nor a borderline person. He was more like a depressive man who became overpowered by the reminiscences of his infancy that until now had been living in a "fossilized" form, as a facet of his Infantile.

Interestingly, Laplanche and Pontalis (1973) speak of splitting not as a mechanism but as a "phenomenon" that "has a descriptive value but no intrinsic explanatory one" (428). If we analyse a child, a psychotic, or a fet-ishist thoroughly, the patient might arrive at speaking about, and struggling with, two wholly contrasting positions in the mind. It is different with the "living fossils" that inhabit the Infantile. To illustrate, an analysand might get in contact with totally opposite feelings towards the analyst, such as grat-itude and resentment. When such a split becomes evident to my patient, he faces a choice: to forgive, or continue a hopeless war with me and himself, too. In contrast, had I been able to analyse Colin, he might reach contact with his helplessness and panic in the transference relation. I would be satis-fied if he became empathic with himself and wary of his destructive behav-iour when he felt abandoned. But I would not expect him to explicitly link his affects with the dramatic events in infancy. Those episodes were primally repressed – that is, registered on vague, global, and nonverbal levels – but they were not split off.

Let us continue imagining Colin in an analysis where he had realised that his lover resembled his mother in certain aspects. Perhaps, he would also discover that as a boy he had loved his mum who was "so beautiful". To explain why he had not understood deeper the parallel between his boyhood adulation and his present romance, we could invoke the traditional usage of the term repression. When "regression proper" is at work, present and past urges can be re-translated in psychoanalytic treatment. Colin could then have worked on this insight and feel ashamed, guilty, romantic, or relaxed about it. In brief, he could work on his personal version of the Oedipus conflict.

Things are different with primally repressed impulses; they are about accents, odours, faces, and other impressions that are preserved as still life paintings. Slowly, they sink to the depths of our mind where they sometimes contribute to secure attachments, sound-object relations, and a stable self-esteem. However, when trauma occurs, this process is interrupted, and primal repressions take another and more threatening route. If trauma becomes overwhelming, as I think happened when Colin was hospitalised, the psychic apparatus is overcharged by affects that cannot be represented as thoughts and then later be translated into words. Instead, a *trace of the Infantile* is created; a chip, a dent, in an otherwise smooth surface. I refer to further discussions in Chapter 12.

Doctors have a special term, *locus minoris resistentiae*, meaning the place of least resistance. This refers to a place in your body where you, for example, once suffered a fracture or contusion. When that part suffers some little injury later in life, the old trauma flares up, and healing becomes more painful and protracted than if there had been no previous damage. Colin's personality was "smooth" in the sense that he did well at school and work, had friends and hobbies, and was a likable guy. But when his life course passed across the dent – or the locus – the trace of the Infantile was activated. Perhaps he had tried to prevent this from happening when, as a teenager, he did not dare approach girls he was fond of. But when his first son was born, there was no way out. He could not stop himself from tumbling right into the fissure of the dent.

Although our contact was brief, Colin also came to grasp why his mother used to call him "an eczema child". Colin was puzzled about this label since he had no further skin problems in life. Only in our work did he understand that his mother had not got over what had happened. The last time we met, he told me about an event in preschool when it was time for the oldest children to start school. There was a girl whom he was fond of. When he saw her leaving preschool for the very last time, he felt an intense pain which he could recall even today. He thought it was because she was sweet and gentle – and that he would never see her again. He added that today, when his wife was about to travel overnight, he would feel a painful pang. In our dialogue, he associated this to the preschool drama. We talked about this story as also relating to the fact that our contact was about to end, and I represented the girl whom he would never meet again. Today, I think the tragic notion extended even further backwards. I surmise that preschooler Colin's suffering at the girl's departure was linked to his lengthy separation in infancy. In that sense, his reaction in preschool was a screen memory and a trace of the Infantile. The girl's adieu was engraved in his memory because it latched on to another, earlier and much severer, experience in his infancy. The common tragic twinge of the two events could be described as "I will never see Mummy again".

Psychoanalytic formulations of Colin's state of mind, then and now

My brief contact with Colin enabled him reasonably well to defuse his guilt and agony about the events around Eric's birth and thereafter. Evidently, his suffering was connected to the theme of infancy by the simple fact that it started when his son was born. We also uncovered its roots with what happened in his own infancy. But owing to my lack of experience, his wish to move on in life, and the family's upcoming departure from Sweden, a deeper penetration was not possible. Today, I would suspect that his personality structure implied a greater risk than he and I realised at the time. I support this suspicion with the stark contrast between this man's achievements, his deep wish of becoming a father, and then his falling headlong after Eric's birth. Had he remained in Sweden, I would surely have recommended that Colin embark on psychoanalysis.

Today and decades later, two phenomena stand out that help me discern deeper the unconscious roots and the psychodynamics of Colin's suffering. I conceive of them as two juxtaposed identifications: one with his father and one with his "baby self". The relationship with his father was ambivalent, a mix of love, pride, anger, loneliness, and mourning. When he became a father himself, he was overjoyed and proud but did not grasp that he was standing on shaky ground. This was not only due to his distanced relationship with his father, which he seemed reasonably aware of. More importantly, an unconscious identification with a baby seemed to interfere with his paternal identity. I did not feel this identification sprang from seeing himself and his son as copies, as if Eric were a narcissistic prolongation of himself. Colin could speak of the boy with love and as a little person with unique characteristics. But beneath this, he could but glimpse another baby, namely his own baby self. When he lost his appetite after Eric's birth, I conceive of it as based on an unconscious identification with a baby who cannot reach the mother. Such a drama occurred when he was hospitalised. Probably, the separation from her was too abrupt and fraught with anxiety to enable him to conceive of the vanished breast and realise that it was out there somewhere and would return later.

How might a baby be affected by such a skin rash plus a sudden termination of breastfeeding and separation from the mother? With panic, longing, confusion, sadness, helplessness, somatic collapse? Probably, although such terms may seem too advanced for a four-month-old child. Yet it seems too restrictive if we refuse to conjecture anything at all about his mental state at the time. We can guess that Colin suffered from an infantile depression (Keren & Tyano, 2006; Ornstein, 1998; Spitz, 1965). To this was added the difficulties for him to develop a capacity "of tolerating a no-thing" (Bion, 1965, 106), namely to view the mother as a container to help him tolerate her absence, retain her as an internal object although she had left him and his skin was itching, and make use of this object to bear the panic of abandonment. In other words, I assume he could not use *thoughts* to tackle his anxiety and depression. This overwhelmed him and necessitated that he build up solid primal repressions, a term that I will discuss in Chapters 2 and 12.

Colin could not create a thought, or an implicit sense of security and a *primal representation* (Salomonsson, 2014a) such as "Mum's gone but she'll be back". Instead, he perhaps experienced a scary hole inside that must be displaced far from consciousness. Note that when we met, he had no explicit memories of the hospitalisation. Linking his loss of appetite and the infatuation with the hospitalisation was a joint reconstruction. An important tributary was what today I would call my countertransference. I was moved hearing about the little chap in the hospital bed. I was also shaken by the contrast between his composed personality and the havoc and helplessness around his helpless infatuation. Knowledge and emotions around an early separation in my own life were probably also stirred up as I listened to him. However, in those days, understanding such aspects of countertransference was less available to me. There was another tributary that I could not make us of then since I was unaware of its existence. I refer to the vast amount of findings from infant research. Today, we know that babies react vehemently to sudden changes in the emotional environment and communication (Adamson & Frick, 2003; Mesman, van IJzendoorn, & Bakermans-Kranenburg, 2009; Tronick, Als, Adamson, Wise, & Brazelton, 1978). An abrupt termination of breastfeeding and daily interactions with his mother, plus a transfer to a hospital in another city, would definitely count as such changes.

Simone, a woman girl

Although I cautioned earlier that Colin's personality structure implied a greater risk than we realised at the time, he managed to stabilise – as far as I know – his relationships with his son, his wife, and himself. With other couples and individuals in similar circumstances, things may run another course, with locked positions and bitter resentment. This may be due to the specific nature of the trauma, the participants' flexibility and commitment to each other, and their willingness and courage to grapple with heartbreaking feelings.

I will now introduce another patient who shows similarities and differences with Colin. *Simone* is a married professional woman with children. She seeks advice in a harrowing moment in life. She is in love, head over heels, with a man she met in the neighbourhood. Now and then, they meet in a nearby coffee house. She wants two things: to hear him say that he is attracted to her and to her solely – and to kiss him. For her, it is his lips – not his male body – that captivate her the most. Their chats are filled with mutual assertions that the other is perfect, beautiful, and irresistibly alluring. In these respects, Simone resembles Colin. We recognise the enthrallment of the lips, the idealisation of the partner, and the desire to be viewed as someone beyond compare, which enhances one's self-esteem.

Apart from the many differences between the two, my methods of treating them have also differed. I have already described my lack of experience when meeting Colin. With Simone, I am an experienced analyst with lengthy experiences of treating adults, including mothers with their babies. She starts therapy twice a week. If I compare my ways of working long ago with Colin and today with Simone, I am now better prepared to listen to her when she speaks of the primal relationship with her mother.

Simone: "My mother is emotionally far away when we meet. She says the right things to me, but she doesn't absorb what I or the children tell her. Last week, we had set up to meet at a coffee house. She didn't show up! I phoned and she had totally forgotten about our date. She gave me a whitewashing explanation but didn't seem to care, actually. I know she cares for me, but I don't know how. There is a kind of screen between us."

For Simone, it is even worse to realise that the relationship with her daughters is like the one with her mother but in reverse. When they snuggle up to cuddle her, she feels a shameful resentment and even disgust. She's a very conscientious mother but must force herself to relish the girls. She knows they long for a closer contact, but she is as helpless in satisfying their wishes as when trying to evoke her own mother's love. Her father was never very present in her childhood, which has caused her much resentment, but she finds it much easier to be with him and never doubts his affection. They chit-chat and laugh together. "He takes life on an easy note, he's not the most profound guy in town", she says.

The first year in therapy is filled with stories of *Martin*, her lover. Or that word is a bit inflated, because she only wants to kiss him. They talk as well, but slowly she realises that their dialogue consists mostly of mutual adulations. One day, she speaks with him about her political views, which are quite divergent from his. She gets afraid that she risks toppling their relationship if they enter deeper in the discussion, so she stops. The next session, she is back to an enthused account of their recent rendezvous. They have sex only rarely, and she speaks very little about it. We learn that their foreplay thrills her much more than the complete sexual union.

More and more, Simone discovers that she and Martin are like two sailors clinging to each other while the tempest is raging, and their vessel is about to be shipwrecked. When they're alone together, there is only bliss, and nothing evil will befall them. Afterwards, there is guilt and anxiety that she is destroying her life. We compare her situation to that of a drug addict. With some grim humour, the two tell each other that they need to be filled up with each other, as when a heroin addict panics to fill the syringe, inject the drug, and get high. At this point, I assemble Simone's account of her affair with Martin with how she conceives of her mother.

Analyst: "You cling to Martin's lips and devotion. It reminds me of a baby who searches her mother's eyes and breast and cannot come to rest until the two are united again. Why this despair when Martin and you are apart? Why is it only the kisses you long for? You never speak of his male body."

Simone: "I see what you mean, but I can't do anything about it. I feel guilty, not only towards my husband but also towards Martin, since I don't know what I want with our affair – except that I can't be without him!"

Analyst: "You and Martin cling to each other, but is it pleasant and joyful? Perhaps, but there is a lot of unspoken uncertainty and anxiety as well. Could this be related in any way to how you've described your mother's restrained way of relating to you? You did tell me that she was depressed when you were a child. Did that make you bewildered and uncertain in your relationship with her? And today, is this why you need to constantly 'refill' with Martin's lips?"

I interpret that Simone's affair with Martin is a kind of remedy for a traumatic relationship between her as a baby and her mother. This line of thought is based on her account that when she was a child, her mother was treated for depressions for years. The parents divorced later, and the mother was left with the main responsibility of the children. But Simone's response to such interventions is rather bleak. She does confirm her shallow and disappointing relationship with her mother. She also recognises, though with hesitation and some unease, my comparison of a baby's lips reaching for mother's breast with her yearning to kiss Martin. But she feels no emotional resonance when I connect her adult present with her infantile past.

Simone is caught up in a cocoon with Martin. Life outside has little attraction to her. This is becoming a technical problem in her therapy: "I know this can't go on, but the thought of breaking up fills me up with such panic that I rush back to him". Thus, my interpreting Simone's infatuation as a trace of her Infantile leads us nowhere. I think this is because she fears that if she were to realise how her Infantile impacts on their relationship, it would end her desire and lead to loneliness and catastrophe. Yet, when we talk about the affair's long-term futility and how it affects her and Martin's families, she is an interested though guilt-ridden participant.

I realise that, similarly to a drug addict in the concrete sense, Simone brings into therapy an enticing but malevolent competitor with our work: her obsession with, or addiction to, Martin. It opposes my efforts at helping her and her pronounced strivings to exit her blissful maelstrom. When swirling around in it, she listens to alluring promises of bliss, calm, and a pain-free existence, like the kicks an addict gets from the drug. When we speak about her infatuation, her insight is rationally and emotionally well anchored. But when leaving my office, she gets excited again about an upcoming meeting with Martin. In a similar vein, when I suggest that her infatuation, which started before therapy began, could be seen as her effort at avoiding similar feelings for me, she shrugs her shoulder in disbelief. "You're too old", she says.

Yet some factors make the equation crumble. Neither she nor Martin is eager to start a new life together. There is thus a blissful standstill in their relationship and no dialogues about the future. Simone discovers that she is like a child awaiting an upcoming birthday party. Hanging out with Martin is fun, being at work or at home is boring. Taking care of taxes and bank credits is dreary like a cloudy summer's day. In such dialogues, and when she speaks of kissing Martin, she gives me the impression of being a teenage girl. The only time worth being in is *now*, and the only object worthwhile is Martin's lips. Simone says she and her husband *Guy* once loved each other passionately and recalls years of warm and satisfying sex with him. But over the years, feelings dried up, and today, the relationship is polite and factual with no physical or emotional intimacy. One day, when she is in agony and remorse about her secret relationship, I tell her:

Analyst:	"Why don't you talk to Guy about your affair with Martin?"
Simone:	"He'd throw me out of our home on the spot!"
Analyst:	"Are you sure?"
Simone:	"He has his principles. He's a straightforward and honest man, actually."
Analyst:	"Then maybe he would at least listen to you."
Simone (crying):	"I can't do it. He'd stay in our home, and I'd lose contact with the kids."

I will not go into detail about what happened next, but in brief, Simone overcame her resistance to talking to her husband. To her surprise, he did not kick her out of the house. He behaved in a dry but correct manner, leaving it to her to decide if she wished to continue with Martin and divorce or to stay with her present family. This was, of course, a relief but also forced Simone to compare the two relationships. She began thinking that it was more important to try to repair her relationship with Guy – or decide to end it – than to continue with her affair with Martin. This, of course, implied a long and painful journey involving Guy, their children, and Martin.

Beneficial effects of an erroneous idea?

We will leave Simone here, at a time that for her and the others involved is still precarious, worrying, and woeful. A reader might ask why I have included Simone's case. After all, likening her blissful yet desperate relationship with Martin to a construction of her as a baby and her depressed mother was *my* hunch and not hers. Furthermore, she didn't buy it. One might also object that change in therapy emerged only when I queried why she did not talk with her husband about her turmoil – not when I interpreted the resemblance of today's She & Martin and the prehistoric She & Mother. Even though Simone was lukewarm when I linked her infatuation with an aspect of her Infantile, I contend their relationship had an infantile quality: her hungry rapture when they kissed, uninterest in a more mature erotic relationship, indifference in seeing him as an individual person, and her craving for him to vow that she is the world's only beautiful woman. Lately, she has revealed a profound and acute anxiety and rage if Martin tends to briefly pay attention to someone else. No matter how much of the "drug" she consumes, her basic security remains brittle. All in all, Simone begins to grasp that she is ensnared in a dreamworld that prevents her from becoming a mature woman.

My reason for including Simone's case is to show that though a therapist's assumption may simply be wrong – or wrong at the moment – this is not a waterproof argument for remaining silent about it with the patient. First, she did not dismiss my suggestion that her infatuation with Martin might serve to "heal" the wounds of the infantile relationship with her depressed mother. Her response was more like, "I don't know, I have no memories from those early days". But interestingly, she has recently told me that she and her mother never look into each other's eyes. Physical contact with her mother is also unsettling, as when sitting next to her in the sofa to watch television. They thus avoid two essential modes of emotional interchange: touching and looking at each other. She discovers that her real problem is that the intimacy she yearns for with men, her children, or mother instantly elicits embarrassment and even disgust.

The period in life when such communications and yearnings are most salient is, of course, infancy. As for gaze avoidance, I have observed it many times in work with infants and depressed mothers. When a baby cannot capture the attention and devotion of the mother, especially if she is postnatally depressed, the maternal internal object can turn into an impenetrable and scary presence. As a result, the baby may avoid mother concretely. More exactly, she shuns the external representative of the scary internal object by looking away from Mum's face, notably her eyes. This is not an infrequent finding in parent-infant therapies, with much pain for the mother – and for the baby (Cowsill, 2000; Fraiberg, 1982; Kernutt, 2007; Salomonsson, 2015b, 2021). All in all, when Simone claims she has "no memories from those early days", she is, of course, right. But as I see it, certain traits in her interactions with her mother point to a "dent" or a "hole" in their primal relationship.

Another facet that I think relates to Simone's problem with emotional intimacy is that she has staunchly avoided coming to me or to her job without makeup. Lately, she gained courage and arrived without foundation on her face. I then perceived her skin as greyish and a bit lifeless. The experience combined an objective observation with my countertransference reaction to a disappointing object. I can swear neither that her skin was greyish nor that any such colour indicated some breach in emotional contact with her mother in infancy. But I do regard the event as reflecting my countertransference that mirrored an interaction of a depressed baby and her disengaged depressive mother. This would reflect an important point, which I will also illustrate with the case of Bess in Chapter 2 and others in the book: the Infantile emerges not as a specimen to an observer-analyst but in a *relationship* with intense and mutual involvements of patient and analyst.

My conjecture is thus still that the intimacy of Simone and her mother was mangled and that the infatuation with Martin was consequent upon it. Though she remained doubtful to my suggestion, it brought about gradual and important changes in some other positions of hers. When she started therapy, she suffered from a boring marriage that she did not dare repair or break up. She spoke of a complete happiness with Martin but did not know what to do with it. As our work progressed, she realised that they had neither a full-bodied erotic passion nor a deepening relationship.

Why was she infatuated with Martin and why couldn't she leave him? In sessions, she often asked herself these questions. To further develop my conjecture, I think her present affair illustrated Freud's famous explanation of "why a child sucking at his mother's breast has become the prototype of every relation of love. *The finding of an object is in fact a refinding of it*" (S. Freud, 1905b, 222, italics added). Simone's dilemma was that she tried desperately to find and repair an object that, however, was damaged. I refer to the challenge that she, like many babies of depressed mothers, must tackle. When refinding the original maternal object and looking into its eyes seems impossible, the baby can invent an "as-if-refound" object. She must have a pacifier for years or becomes restless or depressed. Adult Simone tried to find such a substitute object in Martin, whose pacifying lips she *must* have – and *now*. This explains why the construction was brittle and why she did not dare to get to know him as a present-day man. There were sessions when she did not dismiss my parallel between present and past relations. Then she looked sombre and said, "this thing about me as a baby and my mother, it feels like a hole, I don't dare approach it".

Simone's spontaneous use of the word "hole" brings to mind reflections by analysts describing psychological catastrophes in adults (Baranger, Baranger, & Mom, 1988; Cohen, 1985; Green, 1998; Grotstein, 1990; Tustin, 1986). Eshel (1998) refers to "individuals whose interpersonal and intersubjective psychic space is dominated by a central object that is experienced essentially as a 'black hole'" (1116). They feel gripped by its pull, or they become petrified in their relationships to avoid being pulled over the edge into the "hole". Many authors agree that such phenomena also appear in persons with a neurotic personality structure. So far, Simone's and my work has centred mainly on disarming the crisis in her relationships with Martin and Guy. But she does intuit a scary domain in herself. She also grasps that her love of Martin is peculiar in that it fills up a void inside her. So far, she is standing on the brink of the hole but has not dared to look steadfastly into it.

When I suggest that Simone needs to have her "hole" filled up, I am relying not on Tustin's (1986) concept of the hole in autistic disorders but on my work with infants and children. A two-year-old girl in therapy with her depressed mother spoke unequivocally of her fear of "them holes" and later made drawings expressing her terror (Salomonsson, 2013a). This model links with the one of Grotstein (1990). He suggests that a failure of maternal reverie, insufficient holding, and an uncontaining environment can lead to a "black hole" in the child's psyche.

In my hypothesis, Simone's project of "refinding" the lost maternal object in Martin aimed to replace her infantile powerlessness and suffering with the bliss in kissing him. It helped close her eyes to the insight that every love relationship has limits. She wanted to stay with him forever – but the concept of time meant little to her. When she pulled back a little, she saw that he was not really intriguing as a man – if one considers that word in its entirety. For example, she dared not open up to him about her frailties, inconsistencies, or "bad and silly thoughts". And true, Martin could not change the course of time. She was terrified of getting older and could not imagine that a woman of fifty can lead a content and passionate life. Consequently, she was horrified that Martin would lose interest in her.

My parallel between Simone's relationships in infancy and today was, to be true, my construction. Some facts supported it: her mother had been treated for depression for years, but I did not know much more. And there were other signs of disharmony in her family of origin. With Martin, kisses were only rarely followed up by intercourse. But this all sounds like a meagre support for a rather elaborated construction! Yet I claim it was of great help to Simone. True, she could have used it to feel sorry for herself and accuse her unpropitious fate, mother, or husband. Yet she did not use my idea for such purposes. This was because I showed empathy with her predicament – and I addressed her as an adult woman wanting to take responsibility and agency of her life.

I thus think it was the combination of approaching her infantile and adult aspects – her kissing and adulating self as well as her responsible and caretaking mature self – that enabled her to launch a momentous and difficult shift in her life: to move on from being a girl of 40 to being a woman *d'un certain age*. This work implied not only investigating her "addiction" to Martin but also taking responsibility for what to do about her marriage.

Summing up so far how I use the Infantile concept, I view it as part of our personality that may reside in the background without necessarily causing much trouble. However, sometimes like in the case of Colin – and, in my view, of Simone as well – it gushes forth unexpectedly and inexplicably. When this causes suffering we must, of course, bring out the heartache and talk about it. This being said, I am very far from claiming that the Infantile is the cause of all emotional suffering and that we must bring it up in every situation or case. The Infantile, as we will see throughout the book, is also a font of creativity, spontaneity, intimacy, and *joie de vivre*. But sometimes a therapist intuits that "the ghosts in the nursery" (Fraiberg, Adelson, & Shapiro, 1975) are present, active, and threatening – but deeply unconscious to the individual who is haunted by them. Talking with Colin how he might have been affected by the eczema, the abrupt weaning, and the hospitalisation helped him understand in retrospect his infatuation with his colleague. As for Simone, my referring to her Infantile did not create a groundbreaking "aha-experience". But combining it with interventions of how she avoided handling her present marital conflict gave her empathy with herself and a resolve to do something about it. As for her feared "hole", a terrifying experience that I think today's infatuation seeks to remedy, it still awaits further analysis.

Finally, as we learn from Colin's and Simone's cases, we can live a life whose beginning was marred by painful experiences which, however, have not harassed us for ages. They are successfully fossilised, as I call it. Then one day, a crisis develops in a love relationship, at work, in our health, and so on. The fossil comes to life again, aspects of the Infantile hit us like a bolt, and we fall to the ground. We get infatuated, enraged, ill, depressed, and helpless. Throughout the chapter, I have used some imageries to describe such phenomena, but I have also applied the Infantile as a metapsychological term. The time has come to discuss it deeper.

Note

1 Of course, a psychoanalyst or a patient may be a woman or a man. Therefore, I wrote "his/her" here. However, I think such double words are cumbersome, and I find it even more inconvenient to use the modern "they" as a gender-neutral but singular pronoun. I will henceforth speak of the analyst as "him", simply because I am a man and do not wish to conceal that aspect of my subjectivity.

Chapter 2

The Infantile
Evolution of a concept

This chapter will discuss more thoroughly the concept of *the Infantile*. We will focus on its metapsychological anchorage and on the phenomena covered by it, namely how they surface in everyday life and in psychoanalytically inspired therapies. True, phenomena that can be attributed to the Infantile can emerge anywhere and anytime, but only in the analytic consulting room can we study them with our method and help patients suffering from them. As we shall see, it is also through this method that we can link the Infantile with the corpus of psychoanalytic theory.

One might think that the Infantile refers to a specific age: approximately the first year of our lives when we were "in-fans", a word that refers to someone who is unable to speak. But this is not the whole story. As a psychoanalytic term, the Infantile does not even – in isolation, that is – refer to the little babies we see at home or in our consulting rooms. Rather, it covers certain phenomena that may occur in persons of any age whom we encounter in everyday life and in psychotherapy. Recall Colin with his appetite loss and infatuation or Simone with her compulsion to kiss her lover.

Why do I refer to Colin and Simone as illustrating the Infantile? Could we use other terms, for example, that they behaved, felt, and thought in primitive or immature ways? Yet such adjectives cover the same psychological phenomena as the ones I claim pertain to the Infantile, at least sometimes. They refer to manifestations that occur early in a person's life and are simple and unsophisticated in affects, representations, worldviews, and communication modes. One day, they may recur in the adult as "traces of the Infantile" echoing past behaviours and experiences. Someone applying another perspective on my two patients could describe them as weak, hypersensitive, irresponsible, or overly demanding. But that would not make us understand more of what is going on inside them.

A second alternative is to use another psychological theoretical system. Yet I won't go into them. This is because the book addresses clinical events that were understood through a psychoanalytic mode of investigation, technique, and theorisation. True, other theories have much to say about how human behaviour reflects humankind's prehistory, as in evolutionary

DOI: 10.4324/9781003640363-2

psychology. Or they develop models of our cognition, as in theories underlying cognitive behavioural therapy. Yet I argue that no psychological theory system comprises as much as the psychoanalytic regarding human behaviour and representation, cognitions and affects, the individual in solitude and in interactions with others, being influenced by past and present events, and developing from infancy to adulthood.

Consequently, this book applies a psychoanalytic perspective to the term under study: the Infantile. Or should it be written infantile? Does it matter if we view it as an adjective or a noun? As an adjective, Freud used it frequently, most famously in his work on infantile sexuality (S. Freud, 1905b). He also wrote about infantile anxiety (1925–1926), helplessness (1927), neurosis (1918), and so on. Unfortunately, he oscillated between using the prefix "infantile" for babies or *Säuglingen* – whom we today regard as being up to one year of age – and for older children. In *Three Essays on Sexuality* (S. Freud, 1905b), he insisted that "infantile sexuality" occurs in newborns. But he could also claim that five-year-old Little Hans suffered from "an infantile phobia of animals" (1909, 101). At other times, he was more specific about when a symptom manifested, as when he suggested that "the earliest anxiety of all – the 'primal anxiety' of birth – is brought about on the occasion of a separation from the mother" (1925–1926). Only rarely did he illustrate such helplessness in detail. An exception is the "Fort-Da" vignette (1920, 14). Freud's personal involvement in observing the boy has been discussed in depth (Shapiro, 1996; Whitebook, 2017). Here, I only point out that his detailed and vivid rendition of the little boy's game with the wooden reel was about his grandchild mastering the pain of abandonment from his mother, Freud's beloved daughter. I suggest that this personal involvement enabled Freud to open up to his own Infantile and thus identify with how the boy handled his emotional pain.

The first time I encountered "the infantile" as a concept was in an issue of *Revue française de psychanalyse* (2015/79/5). The theme was "The sexual infantile and its destinies". In this vast collection, senior French analysts discussed the concept, mostly from theoretical perspectives. Their take was mainly to link it with Freud's (1905b) concept of infantile sexuality. It surprised me that they (Chervet, 2015; Golse, 2015; Ody, 2015 and others) did not extend the concept to incorporate real babies as seen in everyday life or in psychoanalytic infant observations. This is all the more remarkable since parent-infant psychotherapy (PIP) was being practiced since long in Paris. My experience was similar to that of the International Psychoanalytical Association (IPA) congress 2021: much talk about the infantile but very little about real infants.

The Infantile according to Florence Guignard

What about the history of the concept of the Infantile, namely the word used as a noun? As far as I have been able to research, the credit goes to Florence

Guignard, an analyst of Swiss origin and active in Paris. Incidentally, the issue of *la Revue* mentioned above contains no publication by her, though she had published papers on the topic years earlier (2021, 2022). Perhaps, this was because the issue of *la Revue* used the term infantile in Freud's sense, as cited above. Guignard's reason for using the capital letter is, as expressed in an interview (Guignard, Levy, & Ungar, 2021), that she refers to a *structure* that is "soft but complex". Traditionally, psychoanalytic structures and sub-structures are written with an initial majuscule. One example is Freud's (1923) terms the Ego (*das Ich*), the Id (*das Es*), and the Superego (*das Über-Ich*) in his structural model. These nouns refer to structures as the mind's gross building blocks that have a direct bearing on our personalities. They are relatively stable though they develop over the years and may oscillate and even deterio-rate when we become physically or mentally ill. Guignard does not, however, place the Infantile on the same conceptual level as Freud's three classic struc-tures. She rather uses the majuscule in the Infantile to place it in line with other concepts that have a certain "noun-like" character (Guignard, 2021), such as the True and False Self (Winnicott, 1960), the Self (Kohut, 1971), and the Third (Benjamin, 2009; Britton, 1989; Ogden, 1994).

Here is Guignard's definition of the Infantile. It is...

a strange historical/ahistorical conglomerate, the crucible of primal fanta-sies and sensorimotor experiences that can be stored as memory traces, the Infantile may be regarded as the psychic locus of the first unrepresentable emergences of the drives. All that we can ever know of this "advanced action" is its representable derivatives, in the form of infantile sexual the-ories on the one hand and memory traces on the other. The Infantile is a basic structure on the fringes of our animal nature, the depository and container of our drives, be they libidinal or hateful on the one hand or epistemophilic on the other. It is that combination of drive-related and flexible structural elements that makes a person who he is and not some-one else. Irreducible, unique and hence universal, the Infantile is therefore the entity that will usher in our mental life, through all the developments of its psychic bisexuality as organized by the Oedipus complex. A psychic place of primary and unrepresentable drive emergences on the boundary of the Ucs. and Pcs., the Infantile is the culminating point of our affects, the locus of hope and of cruelty, of courage and unconcern; it operates throughout life, in a twin spiral of process and assignment of meaning, and can even be discerned in the most severe pathologies, provided that these are not confused with its normal mode of organization. And if the Infantile in us continues until our dying day to operate simultaneously at the level of secondary Oedipal processes and of primitive mechanisms, this is because it partakes of the astonishing force of the drives, the fantastic unfolding of which can be observed in the rhythm of psychic development at the very beginning of human life.

(Guignard, 2022, 5)

Guignard's condensed and poetic writing can help us chisel out the concept of the Infantile. *First*, it refers to *temporality*. The Infantile, she says, "ushers in our life" and is "the crucible of primal fantasies". It also evokes "the rhythm of psychic development at the very beginning of human life". We know that Freud (1915b, 187) mentioned the blunt disrespect of temporality in the processes of Unconscious, as when our fantasies mingle events that occurred in the past, now, or in the future. Thus, a little girl may dream of marrying Dad tomorrow, and an old man can fantasise of jumping around on the moon. The Unconscious couldn't care less that such ideas affront the constraints of time, distance, age, natural laws, logic, and other trivialities.

Freud's concept of the Unconscious is thus rooted in infancy, but it is not limited to that period of life, which Guignard seems to do with her concept of the Infantile. Yet a paradox can be observed as she speaks of the Infantile as a "historical/ahistorical conglomerate". If it is "the psychic locus of the first unrepresentable emergences of the drives", the word "first" must refer to a time period, that of infancy. In contrast, "ahistorical" must relate to something timeless or eternal. I interpret her position as follows: the Infantile refers to a specific and historic time of life, namely infancy – but it also transcends that period and continues to "our dying day". I hope the book, especially its final chapter, will clarify further the question if the Infantile is a "structure, developmental period, cluster of experiences, or what?", as one caption there expresses it.

Second, Guignard (2022) speaks at length about how the Infantile is represented in us – for example, as nonverbal emotions and "hallucinatory and protosymbolic retinue of preforms that are constantly in all our mental activities" (5). The quote shows the interest among many French analysts in how we humans signify our emotional experiences. Some other authors are Anzieu (1989), Rosolato (1978, 1985), Green (1999), and, of course, Lacan (1975). We also note similarities with writers from other cultures (Bion, 1962; Bruner, 1990; Gaddini, 1992; Litowitz, 2011; Mancia, 2004; Van Buren, 1993; Winnicott, 1962). Their semiotic terminologies did not exist in Freud's era. We could say that Guignard, more clearly than Freud, links what we perceive in real-life babies with what we as analysts deduce goes on in our older patients. My additions to Guignard's view of the Infantile are twofold: (1) to illustrate how an analyst's immersion in psychoanalytic therapies with babies and parents (PIP) enables him to get "under the skin" of experiences in the baby-mother interaction and the countertransference and (2) to show how the analyst can transport such clinical experiences to make him more sensitive to related phenomena in adult therapies and more adroit in linking those patients' present and pristine experiences. When I bring out PIP therapies as inspirational sources, point (1) refers to the historical aspect of the Infantile, whereas (2) refers more to its ahistorical aspect, to use Guignard's expressions.

Third, Guignard's Infantile concept has very much to do with emotions. It is the "culminating point of our affects, the locus of hope and of cruelty, of courage and unconcern", and it contains both libidinal and hateful drives.

It is not a heavenly and stagnant abode but a place of passion, in that word's double sense of bliss and suffering, delight and tribulation, war and peace. The English version of Guignard's book translates the French *creuset* into "crucible" with its more haunting connotation, as in Arthur Miller's play of that name. To speak with Klein (1975, 54), it is a place where "the life and death instincts and therefore love and hatred, are at bottom in the closest interaction, negative and positive transference are basically inter-linked".

To Guignard, the Infantile represents the constant pulse of instinctual drive forces and exists on the frontier between the unconscious and the pre-conscious system. Maybe Freud would have argued that this pulse was what he meant by the Id (1923). To object, we could remind him about his claim that such unconscious/preconscious pulses also exist in the Ego and the Superego. Indeed, all three Freudian structures contain primeval, untamed, and unconscious parts, the Id more so than the others. We will have to wait until Chapter 12 to see why I regard the Infantile as having another meaning and another specific position in psychoanalytic metapsychology than the Id or the Unconscious.

Guignard's rendition of the Infantile strikes many chords in analysts and therapists who want to enlarge their scope of what goes on in the transference and the countertransference. In the preface, I played with a metaphor of astronomy and suggested that the analytic instrument is our "telescope". Now, the word *scope* comes from the Greek verb *skopein* (σκοπεῖν) meaning *to look* and the prefix *tele* (τῆλε) meaning *distant*. Thus, tele- is apt for the objects that astronomer watch. But since I, in line with Guignard, regard the countertransference as totally essential for discerning the patient's Infantile, we should perhaps invent another word for our analytic instrument, such as the "endoscope", where *endo* (ἔνδο) means *into*. True, the term is already annexed by the medical sciences, but we can suggest here that *endo*- means that an analyst needs to look both into his patient and into himself.

Guignard's writing is firmly anchored in the Freudian conceptual apparatus. She follows a French psychoanalytic tradition, which demands that a new idea, concept, or enterprise be anchored in these terms. Concepts like the drive, the Unconscious, and psychological economy are salient in their texts, which makes them cohere with classical analytic theories. The emphasis on drives and their roots in the Unconscious is also fruitful, since it clarifies what psychoanalysis is about: to disrobe the Unconscious and show how it affects our habits, dreams, fears, passions, and behaviour in the analytic consulting room.

Challenges

Yet there are also challenges when I seek to integrate Guignard's concept with my clinical practice. I come from a tradition in psychoanalysis and research that is anchored in an empiricism demanding that new ideas be supported by clinical material. In contrast, Guignard and many of her French colleagues rarely illustrate their texts with case histories and detailed patient – therapist dialogues. This makes it hard for me to put clinical "flesh on the bones" of their theorisations.

So, how do I suggest what a situation typical of the Infantile might look like in a baby or in an adult? This is not easy to answer, partly because we cannot *establish* what goes on in a baby's mind. Neither can we settle beyond any doubt that a phenomenon in an adult patient reflects her primordial life experiences. Just like astronomers, we must content ourselves with looking for traces. What this means and how it is done in clinical contexts, mostly with adult patients but also with some children, are the book's overarching themes to which we will return repeatedly.

When I just suggested that the term "analytic endoscope" implies to look into oneself and into the patient, it shows that an analyst does not observe the Infantile as an unequivocal event, experience, or behaviour in the patient. This is why Canestri (2021) says that "the 'in-fans', the one who cannot speak, needs a narrator – a psychoanalyst in the transference – to be able to hear again the 'silent' language" (560). He clearly refers to analysing adult patients. He and Guignard seem to agree that the Infantile is something that the analyst intuits and constructs by making use of what the patient communicates. Guignard says that for this to come about, the analyst must listen carefully to the countertransference and to his Infantile. This may result in an affect, hunch, metaphor, or an explicitly formulated intervention. Such affects may be subtle or overwhelming, clear or hazy, pleasant or stressful, vivid or dull. Hunches and metaphors often emerge as an imagery in the analyst in response to the countertransference, as we will see in Chapter 11. Other interventions that resulted from my listening to the countertransference can be found in most chapters of the book. They show how central I regard, as does Guignard, the role of countertransference in detecting and containing the Infantile of the patient – and of myself – in the session.

The idea with the term "endoscope" is that the psychoanalytic instrument looks in two directions at the same time. The sceptic may ask if this means that patient and analyst concoct a story that links the patient's past with her present suffering. In a way, this is so, although the word concoct is way too harsh and dismissive. When Guignard (2022) discusses the Infantile, she shifts her emphasis "from the subjective towards the intersubjective and… from the analyst to the analytic relationship" (4). This shift reflects an ongoing and giant change that started a century ago in psychoanalytic therapy, the "intersubjective turn". It implies that we focus on the patient's, as well as our own, external and internal object relations as well as their interplay. Today, psychoanalysis is thus seen more as a collaborative effort between clinician and patient. I won't go into this big and contentious issue in modern theory and practice, except for submitting references for the interested reader (Bohleber, 2010; Benjamin, 2009; Levenson, 2005/1983; Renik & Spillius, 2004; Mills, 2005; Stern, 2004).

The intersubjective or relational turn has also contributed to a greater focus on the countertransference, which no longer is seen as an obstacle that the analyst must "overcome" (S. Freud, 1910, 144). We rather see it, as already Heimann (1950) suggested, as referring to "the emotions roused in the analyst [which] will be of value to his patient, if used as one more source of insight into the patient's unconscious conflicts and defences" (83). In brief, the analyst is no more viewed as an outsider cognising about the patient but an insider in emotional connection with her. He uses both vantage points to understand the patient and convey alternative perspectives to her. The main test is not whether our – or the patient's – ideas are veracious but if they are meaningful to the patient and will lead the therapy process forwards. The book contains many vignettes for the reader to assess if and how my patients were helped by my perspectives – or if addressing the clinical material on another level or from another viewpoint would have been more apt and helpful.

If the analyst must use his personal Infantile to construe that of the patient, this puts an extra weight on the clinician's mental balance, says Guignard (2022). Like in every human being, the analyst's Infantile is ticking in the background, influencing his personal sufferings and, as we soon shall see, his joy and creativity. We hope that owing to his training analysis, he shall have a reasonably unhindered access to his Infantile. Yet, inevitably, some aspects will "remain unanalysed in his own analysis" (8) and seek to find expression in various ways. Another caveat is that if the analyst wants to help a patient become more acquainted and fearless of her Infantile, he needs to have an Infantile that is "cathected particularly strongly and permanently" (9). That is, the analyst must halt the normal process of repression in himself. This entails a "constant risk of collusion between the Infantile-in-the-patient with the Infantile-in-the-analyst" (10).

The analyst thus pays a price by staying close to his Infantile – otherwise, he will be deaf to it. He feels – and should feel – the disarray and loss in his own Infantile when similar feelings emerge in the patient. To protect himself from such pain, the clinician may develop narcissistic defences and collusions with the patient. This could result in a blind spot, causing the analyst to react with "stopper interpretations" or "pseudoassociations" (Guignard et al., 2021, 14). The analyst is always, in one way or another, pressured by the analysand's Infantile, as in her or his wish of being cured, salvaged, or vindicated. Guignard cautions the analyst to remain in the anguish of uncertainty. She sorts out three traps, into which the analyst may fall in a clinical standstill. He may blame the patient, rely extensively on analytic theory, or refer to the analysand's personal history, "especially if it includes one or more apparently severe traumas" (12).

Since I suggested in Colin's and Simone's cases that events and experiences in their infancy played an important role in their present suffering, I wonder if I am committing the error that Guignard (2022, 12) is warning of: making "repeated references to an event in the analysand's history deemed significant by the analyst". If so, this would exemplify what she calls a "blind spot denoting the meeting place of the Infantiles of the analysand and the analyst" (21). This might lead to a mutual cecity and deafness – in short, a collusion to avoid "the full – i.e. transferential – analysis of the psychic trauma" (12). It would push the patient into a Cyclops-like view of her internal world: "My analyst tells me who I was and who I am. Like a passive baby, I must swallow his wisdom." Such unconscious oppression by the analyst may lead to a False Self developing in the analysand – and in the analyst as well.

Another way of expressing this dilemma is that when the Infantile of patient and analyst get out of phase, the same thing happens as when the impact of two waves delete each other. This is the blind spot, where the analyst feels helpless or stupid and does not capture the message from the patient's Infantile. These moments appear as a notch in the ongoing rhythm between the participants. The analyst becomes tempted to establish "law and order" in the analytic field and thence his stopper interpretation, *interpretation bouchon*, to speak with Guignard. But if the analyst acknowledges what is going in the interchange of transference and countertransference, he can discern aspects of the patient's Infantile that she still cannot verbalise and confront. He can thus avoid that *his* Infantile will set up a "protective shield against stimuli and container for the infantile elements in the transference/countertransference relationship" (Guignard, 2022, 11). Note her position that if the analyst can localise the blind spots, this may allow the analytic process to be resumed with the patient.

One such moment, when I referred to a patient's personal history, was when I suggested that Simone's infatuation with Martin was linked with interactions in infancy with a depressed mother. Was this a stopper interpretation expressing a collusion between Simone's and my Infantile? I will bring in factors speaking for and against this critical question. She was not taken by my idea. Had I kept repeating it, this would have pointed to such an unconscious plot. Yet she provided many details which, as I argue, support my suggested link to her Infantile: the gaze avoidance between Simone and the mother, the revulsion of intimacy with her and others, and the obsession with her lover's lips. Maybe, she will one day understand more of her fear of tumbling down into emotions that she subsumes under the term "the hole". She and I agree that it probably refers to experiences early in life – though we do not know what they were like. Bringing together these considerations and reservations and turning my "endoscope" inwards to the countertransference as well, I find it hard to discern in this particular case the *bouchon* (cork or stopper) implied in Guignard's term.

Both Guignard and I claim that the analyst needs to be in contact with his or her Infantile and that this also puts a weight on our analytic functioning. Do I then mean that the analyst needs to be childish? In a sense, yes. He needs to be playful and flexible, with a fluid access to more primitive levels of his mind, namely to his Infantile. Of course, he also needs to be in contact with the more mature personality levels in himself – and know how to differentiate his Infantile from that of his patient. Such demands, ranging from being like a playful child to more of a dispassionate captain, may sound overbearing and incompatible. On the other hand, analytic work is often interesting, breathtaking, and full of surprises and joy in seeing relationships moving forwards, not the least when troublesome and anguishing journeys have been traversed ensemble. The analyst's Infantile, far from being bad and harmful, is also a rich font of creative insights that may substantially help the patient.

Guignard thus emphasises the vitalising and creative aspect of the Infantile. They reflect moments when the mother played with her joyous child and contained her distress. Just like a play can be initiated by mother and/or baby, this also occurs in psychoanalysis. We will soon get to know Bess, a woman patient, where the "play" was initiated via two images that popped up in me and which I conveyed to her. This led to the history of her infancy that we now could link with a present crisis in a love relationship. I hope the reader will discern other similar moments in the book.

Before moving on to my patient Bess, I must take up a wrestling match with myself. In 2007, I published a paper, "Semiotic transformations in psychoanalysis with infants and adults" (Salomonsson, 2007a). I struggled with a question; my analysand Monica, also mentioned briefly in Chapter 3, suffered from severe anxiety. She expressed it in words but also through jerks, sighs, and moans on the couch. She did not speak about infants or her infancy, but her movements made "a strong impact on me of an inconsolable baby" (1205). Reflecting on her bodily communication, I wondered if it was perhaps a direct continuation from her infancy. Alternately, my baby connotations might be mere imaginations without any explanatory value. Finally, I wrote that maybe they represented a "transformation" (1207). But if so, I could not decide *what* had been transformed.

In that paper, I wanted to avoid any essentialist conception to the term transformation, as if some unknown dingus had remained in her throughout life but was now expressed in a different form. When I suggested that Monica's present anxiety represented a transformation of infant distress, I merely referred to a *semiotic* transformation or a shift of signs. Over the years, her distress had been transformed into another mode of signification, from a primordial experience to her present jerks. Then what was this primordial experience? Could we ever reach it to get an answer? I argued that the answer was no.

I return to this question here because some circumstances have helped me come a bit closer to this "primordial experience" though – mind you – I still claim that we will never arrive at its pristine origin. One factor is my accumulated experience with patients like Colin, Simone, and others to follow. They revealed palpable or plausible early childhood traumas. In parallel, the more babies I have met in PIP or consultations, the more solid is the ground I am standing on when I suggest that, for example, "this woman's jerks look like the motions of a distressed infant. Maybe there's a link?"

Before continuing my wrestling match, I will briefly return to the comparison of astronomers and analysts. To me, it is hard to discern any elemental difference between stating that Monica's jerks resemble an infant's motions and an astronomer's remark, "The patches on this photo look like the ones we investigated earlier and proved were galaxies. Consequently, the patches here probably also represent another galaxy". As said earlier, astronomers actually study emissions from celestial bodies very far away. They can provide solid arguments that the stars are still out there, but they would agree that their conclusions are based not only on certain observations but also on probabilities.

Yet the astronomer could provide another support for his or her conclusions: the natural laws of the Universe. At this point, we analysts stand speechless. No law states that all jerking babies become jerking adults or that all jerking adults were once jerking already as babies. Analysts' support comes from another direction: our subjectivity when we capture observations and allow them to grow into *Erlebnis* or emotional experience in dialogues with the patient. Anyone is free to dispute it, of course. But I can always retort with, "You don't acknowledge any resemblance between babies in general and my patient Monica. OK, give me another hypothesis and let's see if it helps us understand her suffering better". All in all, I hope this passage can give us more assurance as to the value of construing symptoms and emotions in our patients as "traces of their Infantile".

Returning to Monica's jerks, when I applied the transformation concept to them, I used a concept from Bion (1965). Now, a new problem emerged. Bion had suggested that when A is transformed to B, an *invariant* of A may remain. But already when Bion exemplified with a painting of poppies, we run into problems. We can hardly say that its invariant is "poppy" or "poppiness". I argued in the paper that Bion's problem was that his invariant concept relied cursorily on Kant's "thing-in-itself" which, as Kant said, is always unknowable. What both analysts and astronomers study are transformations of signs, whose essence, *das Ding an sich*, cannot be verified. When they interpret observations, both rely on theory and experience. The astronomer's telescope is directed towards the stars. The analyst's "telescope" – or two-way "endoscope" – is turned to the patient and to his own self. This is the background when we say that the Infantile is emerging in a clinical situation. As Guignard emphasises, our interpretation rests on how we experience the *analytic relationship*.

My wrestling match ends with avowing that I have changed position since the 2007 paper. Then, I was more cautious in attributing any causal links between experiences in infancy and adulthood. My digression to semiotics and the critique of Bion reflected such prudence. Today, I argue that my experiences of therapies with babies and mothers have provided me with more support in "thinking along the paths of the Infantile". Thus, when a patient and I reconstruct events or experiences during infancy, and if we do it thoroughly, at length, and correcting it under way, it has a greater heuristic value nowadays compared with how I conceived of it two decades ago.

We will now follow another patient to see how I made use of my Infantile to help a woman overcome her obsession to boss and control her partners, which had made her destroy previous love relationships and toppled her into a depression. We will follow as my Infantile came up with a metaphorical imagery. When I mentioned it to her, she suddenly spoke of what her mother had told her a long time ago about events in her infancy. In this way, the Infantile of the patient and myself collaborated in a fruitful and helpful way.

Bess

Bess is approaching 40. She seeks therapy fearing that her dreams of starting a family and becoming a mother will never materialise. All her love relationships have failed because she, after some time, realises that she has allowed herself to be treated nonchalantly by her partner. Or she has found some minor fault with him, leaving him on the spot and feeling firm and proud of herself. But therapy has revealed deep fears of being rejected. They have emerged in dreams where friends ignore and reject her. In the transference, similar fears have emerged when I have taken a week's leave. When returning to sessions, she has complained about traffic jams, poor weather, and so on. I felt they represented accusations that I had abandoned her and wasn't there when she needed me.

Bess started twice-weekly psychotherapy a few months ago. She begins a session by speaking of an event yesterday. She and Fred, her partner, went to the gym. Afterwards, they were to buy food, have dinner at home, and take a walk in the summer evening. After the gym, Fred got an idea: "Let's go right home, get a blanket, and relax in the park for a while". She got upset, "We said we'd go home for dinner at first! Why this change of plans?" Fred withdrew from his idea, but she started feeling she had been rude to him and unable to "think outside the box".

In therapy, Bess's reliance on plans and vexation when they are changed have been addressed. Love relationships have capsized because her boyfriends could not accept it. She sighs, "I'm such a control freak". This epithet has helped us understand how she has sabotaged her love relationships. But this time, I feel it does not adequately cover what happened between Bess and Fred. I envisage their dialogue on my inner scene and feel silently, "What a sad ending of an event that could have been so nice for the two lovers!" There is something more to the scene than stating that one lover is controlling the other. In resonance with Bess's expression "control freak", I get a second image of a toddler who, if she doesn't have it her way, gets furious. I convey this image and she hums in vague confirmation but also as something she already knew about. Her meek response makes me doubt that the toddler imagery really captured why she got angry at Fred. She is not obsessive or rigid, and her reaction to his suggestion seems to convey something beyond a wish to control him.

She now provides a detail from yesterday's squabble:

> First, I thought Fred's idea was nice, to sit on the blanket in the evening sun. But then I got hungry and yelled at him, 'But what are we going to eat, we haven't gone shopping yet!?' He said we'd bring some potato chips from home. At that moment, I exploded. 'We've agreed we shouldn't eat chips more than twice a week!'

Again, her statement about chips reveals a need to exert control. But this time she also gets sad about how threatening it is for her to accept the unexpected – especially when it is nice and alluring, and maybe even more so when it touches on hunger and food.

Bess: "I know my chips comment sounds crazy. In fact, it might have been nice in the park with Fred. I rejected his ideas that were actually warm and welcoming!"

Her discontented realisation that she disposes of good things yields my third image, which is also nourished by her reference to the chips. I think of them as a treat that children indulge in but that their parents think is unhealthy. Maybe there is both a gorging child and a forbidding parent inside of Bess? Then how is the interaction working between the two?

Analyst: "I'm thinking of a baby fretting at Mum's breast, the first place where we negotiate our needs and wishes. Mum offers the baby her breast but must also consider her own needs. The baby is hungry but also takes Mum's reactions into account. Such negotiations take time to develop. Your dialogue with Fred makes me think of you as that baby. First you felt content about the plans for the evening. Then Fred disturbed your safety with his idea, and you got upset that it was 'bad food'."

She adds details about her love relationships. She has not been able to show, outside of home, that the two are in a relationship. Kissing outdoors has been impossible, "because everybody sees we're together. Why do I hide the good thing that we're in love!? Fred's idea was actually cute!"

I suggest: "You're like a little girl who feels safe only when her daily routines are followed exactly and she just gets 'good food'. When Fred disturbed your state of mind, you got annoyed and started to wail. Now you realise that his idea was sweet. One wonders why you saw it as threatening at first."

In tears, she interrupts me. I have seen her crying many times when we touched a painful issue, but now it is different. Her face becomes soft and mellow, like that of a child.

Bess: "Maybe I didn't tell you, but I was born prematurely. Only two weeks. At first, they put me to Mum's breast, but then they took me to an incubator at the neonatal care department where I spent about a day. Mum often talks about how hard it was for her. She was young, newly arrived in our country, and upset that I had a severe disease."

Our dialogue now takes two directions. One links my imagery of a mother and a baby to her quarrel with Fred, the other goes to her relationship with mother today:

Analyst: "I was talking about the 'negotiations' between mother and baby. The two need to get to know each other, understand their wishes and adjust as good as it gets. It takes time and contains both bliss and stress."

Bess: "When you say bliss, I think of Fred's idea. It would really have been nice, and we didn't need to go to the supermarket! But I got so mad at him! Such events have ruined many relations. I can't stand having schemes interrupted! But this time, I rethought the event and realised I'd overreacted. I apologized, and things felt better."

Analyst: "You said that after delivery, you and Mum were separated. We don't know how you reacted, but Mum evidently was fraught with fears and still keeps returning to it. Could we envisage a scene early in your life, where those 'negotiations' between you two floundered? That your feeling of security was not established smoothly, and you replaced it with becoming a control freak who must have schemes to feel safe?"

Bess: "Of course I don't recall how I felt when I was born. But I do grasp better why I destroy relationships when they get deeper. I start trusting the guy – but then I conjure up scenarios where he abandons me, and I break up before he does it. So many relationships destroyed... I get sad. Mum often talks about the events after birth. We've a good relationship, but I haven't grasped how deeply they affected her. I feel sorry for her."

The next session, Bess tells me of her mother's birthday party some days ago.

Bess: "Mum's is so eager to take care of me, asking what kind of food I prefer and that I don't need to give her any gifts. It's as if I occupy a special place in her mind, that I'm brittle in some way, though I don't know why."

Bess has no memories of her life postpartum, but her mother does. To speculate, they have left a "psychological scar" in her relationship with her
daughter.

Bess: "I don't usually think about these things. After all, when leaving
           the neonatal ward and returning to Mum, I was OK."
Analyst: "You were in good health, but I guess your mother was fear-
           stricken, which prevented her from viewing you as a healthy girl."
Bess: "Well, I was hospitalized a little later because I didn't gain weight.
           It lasted some time, and we had to return for regular checkups. I
           don't know why I didn't gain weight."
Analyst: "We don't know, but your mother seems to have lost some confi-
           dence that everything would be OK with you."

One month later, Fred's apartment is renovated, and he moves temporarily to
Bess's flat. They are a bit scared because things happened quickly in their
relationship. They've become seriously fond of each other, and they have fun.
But one day, Bess tells me they had a big fight. He was with his pals and came
home a bit later than agreed. She became cold and dismissive. The episode
was preceded by some days of increasing coldness between them. Now that
Fred got home after being with his friends, he called her Bessie. She retorted
furiously, "My name's Bess!" This escalated into a quarrel filled with
wounded feelings.

Bess: "At that moment, I really hated him and wanted to get rid of him."
Analyst: "Any other feelings?"
Bess: "I was dead scared he was going to leave me."
Analyst: "So it was both 'go to hell and don't come back' and 'for heaven's
           sake, don't ever leave me'!" Perhaps a bit like the baby and mother
           we've been talking about. All negotiations capsized. Go away!
           Stay! No, to hell with you!
Bess: "I noted one thing. Not only were my thoughts as categorical as
           you say. I couldn't even bare looking at Fred."
Analyst: "Some babies avoid mother's eyes when they seem to have a shaky
           relationship with her."
Bess: "My mother told me that I didn't look at her for quite a few years,
           also when I was no longer a baby."

Psychodynamic formulations and therapeutic technique

As a consultant at a Child Health Centre, I have met many mothers calling
themselves "control freaks" because they constantly check the baby's sleep,
diaper, motor patterns, and so on. Any worry about the baby's appearance or
behaviour grows into intense anxiety, which can be stilled only by a renewed

scan of the baby. They live in a spin of panicky thoughts and checkups of the baby. When analytic therapy was possible, we discovered that mother's control contained unconscious anxieties of abandonment or guilt and shame because she felt that the baby – or herself – was far from perfect. This made her unable to relish the baby and pushed her to act as his inspector.

Bess is not a mother but a "control freak", she says. Her self-diagnosis has not helped her relax. When she used that word in our dialogue, I felt frustrated in that we already knew about it but not *why* she is that way. My resentment was also reflected in my first internal imagery of the lovers in the park, as if I identified with being snubbed of a delightful stroll in the greenery. At this point, the two images, first of a defiant toddler and then of a distressed mother-infant dyad, popped up in me. Let us now look at this passage along Guignard's (2022) thoughts about how the Infantile of patient and analyst meet and interact in a session. At first, there was my disturbed reaction to her rejection of Fred's idea. To this was added Bess's facile explanation of her being a control freak.

On the spur of the moment, Bess had reacted to Fred's idea as if it were a threat. Talking with him elicited her shame of being controlling, but she had no contact with longing for a picnic with him. Or rather, his invitation ignited both her preconscious desire to cosy up with him and her age-old unconscious conviction that such a situation would become messy, painful, and filled with mutual misunderstandings. Her only way out was to quarrel with Fred, be ashamed, and, finally, admonish herself by sighing, "I'm such a control freak!"

Let us now envisage that, instead, I had responded to her self-critique by suggesting we investigate her control freak pattern further. I might have conceived of Bess's need of control as issuing from an anal character (Abraham, 1923) with its "conscientiousness in carrying out small duties and trustworthiness" (S. Freud, 1908, 169). Yet Bess has very little of typical anal traits like being overly cleanly, parsimonious, or obstinate. She is a good-natured, relaxed, and warm person – until she encounters a gentle proposal from somebody she is attached to – like Fred. I concluded that if I delved into her control-freak identity, this would have exemplified Guignard's "stopper interpretation". It would have prevented Bess from realising that her toughest challenge was not to abstain from controlling Fred. It was rather to accept his idea *precisely because it was lovely*. His proposal of a stroll in the park had touched her Infantile, which went into a spin of affects, hopes, longing for the loved object, and snubbing it.

The session interchange helped Bess grasp her habit of breaking up with men when she has become emotionally involved with them. Her problem was not, as she previously believed, that she had met the wrong guy or couldn't stand his "annoying behaviour". Instead, her problem emerged *because* she was about to fall in love. The verb "to fall" depicts vividly Bess's fear of falling into dependence, longing, opening up for concealed desires, and, of course, the fright that such emotions would end up with her being abandoned by Fred. When these desires from her Infantile now became evident and accessible for further processing, she dared being more resolute and openhearted in her conflicts with Fred instead of throwing him out of the door. She realised that beneath her stern and controlling behaviour, she was dead scared that he would scram.

My imagery of the wailing baby, and her apropos comment about the premature birth and separation, enabled her to link her love problems with the events in her infancy. True, she did not explicitly remember them, but we built a model that helped her become *less incomprehensible to herself* which, after all, is a worthy goal of a psychotherapy. She also became aware of some incongruencies in her relationship with her mother, such as mother's exaggerated concerns about her daughter and Bess's avoiding mother's gaze in her childhood.

I have submitted the vignette to show that the therapist needs to be open to signals from his own Infantile. This happened when I identified with being cheated out of the stroll in the park. The imagery of an interaction of a whining baby and a helpless mother was created in a similar way. This identification was also ushered in by her reference to the chips, so tasty or unhealthy, depending on whether you adopt the parent's or the child's perspective. In the imagery, I "was" a yearning baby who didn't get what I wanted. As I then communicated such identifications – in the form of images – it yielded surprising results: Bess's ensuing story of her birth and her insight that the good things about love scared her. The vignette thus shows that *the discovery of an aspect of a patient's Infantile frequently goes via the therapist's contact with his own Infantile.*

In this dialogue, my metaphoric images played an important role. In Chapter 11, I will suggest that they appear especially when the countertransference contains frustration. One may see it as a *mise en acte* or *enaction* (Lebovici, Barriguete, & Salinas, 2002, 181) of my grievance. This term does not refer to a clinician projecting distress into the patient to feel better himself. Rather, it may help him understand what he, for now, cannot capture as an ordinary verbal interpretation. It is a *screen-thought in the form of an imagery* that is preliminary and needs further investigation. When we suggest it to the patient, we also hope it is more palatable to her and easier to process further. *Such metaphors are a vital and fruitful aspect of containment.* If anyone thinks this technique is exclusive or idiosyncratic, I would object in line with Ogden (1997) that "a very large part of the way in which patients speak to their analysts, and analysts to their patients, takes the shape of introducing and elaborating upon one's own and the other's metaphors" (724).

Lebovici suggests the therapist to be "taken over by the situation" (182) in a "hysterical identification" with the patient. He speaks of PIP work but also argues for it in adult work. "Hysterical" denotes the analyst's ability to enter in rapid and fleeting identifications with a patient. This does not imply an over-identification where the therapist exclaims how terrible it is for the patient. As shown in Bess's case, the therapist's Infantile is involved as well, as when I identified with being barred from the outing. But importantly, I processed her story and my reactions to it, and then the metaphor popped up which I communicated to her. This "screen-thought" was fortunate in that she responded with her premature birth and separation. The ball was rolling; we could connect her negative response to Fred with the early relationship with her mother. This is very different from being hysterical in the sense of dramatising and claiming that one totally understands the patient's feelings, the danger that Guignard warns of when speaking of stopper interpretations (2022, 12).

My thoughts about metaphorising interventions will continue in Chapters 3 and 11. Here, I just want to add that a metaphor is strong and useful when it is evocative, simple, dreamlike, condensed, and captivating. I would dub my baby imagery such a metaphor in that it condensed blissful longing and painful rejection as well as human relationships and food. A metaphor is weak when it feels inexact or senseless or its import is evident only to its creator, here the therapist. The patient may respond with "Yeah, so what?", implying they will have to search in other directions. Such development is also described in Chapter 11.

If I speak of Bess reacting like a baby, I should also bring her mother into the story since "whenever one finds an infant one finds maternal care, and without maternal care there would be no infant" (Winnicott, 1975, XXXVII). Bess told me later that family members fled to Sweden because of political persecution in their home country. Her mother arrived in her late teens with relatives remaining over there. A lonely young woman, she married a compatriot who had been living for some time in Sweden and was probably more settled here than she was. Shortly thereafter, Bess was born. Therapy has ignited Bess's interest in the family atmosphere. Most of her relatives now live in Sweden. "We have fun and like each other, but nobody EVER talks about the persecution in our home country." There is a silent family agreement to let bygones be bygones and adapt to a secure life in Sweden. She wonders if this has prevented her mother from talking about her first months in life. "I don't know if such a dialogue would have made my love life easier, but at least I'd have understood myself better."

As for Bess's relationship with her father, it is good and friendly but not intimate. I sometimes wonder if he, as a result of Bess's projections onto him, bears some of the brunt that originally pertained to the mother – daughter relationship. Or, alternatively, that he did not grasp to what extent his wife suffered in the beginning of Bess's life and thus could not help defusing sufficiently the panic in the mother-daughter dyad. In my experience, it is sometimes difficult for men to understand the depth and complexity of the emotions flooding a first-time mother. Needless to add, this challenge also applies to grasping their own emotions, as, for example, in Colin's case.

I will summarise this chapter by returning to the Andromeda metaphor. Bess's "Andromeda" was her premature birth and brief hospitalisation, experiences that were real and undisputable. Over the years, they were subjected to diffractions, elaborations, and primal repressions. The session was about a banal yet frightening quarrel with her partner. My imageries were created in my analytic "endoscope", as fantasies engendered in the countertransference and rooted in my Infantile. Then Bess provided a memory – though not of the original "Andromeda", namely of an explicit memory of her first days of life. Instead, she became aware of memories stored in her Preconscious of what mother had told her about events after delivery. This put her in contact with emotions anchored in her Infantile: longing, despair, fear, and so forth. She understood that similar feelings had been roaming about when Fred suggested the outing and she reacted aversively and incomprehensibly. This insight paved the way for Bess to handle such future situations more gently and constructively and, last but not least, to do so in a continuous dialogue with her partner.

Chapter 3

Parent – infant psychotherapy as source of knowledge of the Infantile

There is an inherent contradiction in the book concerning *observation* and *conjecture*. I have repeated that I could not *observe* the Infantile of Colin, Sabine, and Bess. I needed to circumscribe the argument into saying that I was intuiting when I said their behaviours, attitudes, and sufferings reflected things, feelings, events, and interactions from their first years of life. In this way, the word "infant" concealed in our term "the Infantile" needs clarification. In the following chapters, I will argue that an important source for this investigation is my experiences of psychoanalytic Parent-Infant Psychotherapy (PIP). Mind you, however, that not even a baby's Infantile is within my or anyone else's direct reach. We must deduce it by searching for its traces by looking and listening to body movements, odours, miens, and more. Yet this embodied communication takes place in the here and now of the PIP session and thus is also observable. But in work with adult patients, it is different. Colin's kissing the colleague had occurred *recently*, but his hospitalisation was *then*. When I claim that his infatuation reflected his Infantile, I presuppose that it had a link, it was a trace, of what happened in his childhood. In Guignard's terms, it was historical/ahistorical.

Let us get back to the astronomer. If it were possible for him or her to reside in a galaxy today and be in instant contact with a colleague on earth, the two could check when and how an event in the star corresponded with a specific phenomenon in our night sky. Similarly, had I been able to sit by Colin's hospital bed and talk with him about his love affair, we could have understood more of their links. Of course, this idea contains many logical errors. Whereas astronomers would assume that the light from the star is not affected much by its long journey to earth, things are different with human beings. Colin's journey in life was subjected to various influences, just like in any other individual. When he was kissing the lover, he was a man with decades of experiences. The same goes for Bess in the previous chapter; she made a forty-year-long journey from her neonatal care to rejecting her partner's alluring idea. Colin and Bess as babies and as adults were thus very, but not totally, different. I argue that, today, they retained some *similarities* with

DOI: 10.4324/9781003640363-3

their baby selves, and we might discern them as *traces* involved in their afflictions as adults.

I seem to be trapped between two contradictory positions: empiricism and inductionism, or between observation and conjecture. Strict empiricism holds that only the observable is true. In this view, since I had not observed Colin's life as an infant, linking the love affair with his hospitalisation was unfounded. Inductionism implies that my hunch about the links between his life now and then was legitimate – though only as credible as anyone else's hunch – and that it needed to be verified or at least supported through deductions and abductions. This touches on an eternal debate on truth and verification in psychoanalysis. My own discussions (Salomonsson, 2014a, 2020) were inspired by PIP, not the least because that method pushes us even further to apply inductive reasoning; since the baby doesn't talk, we must induce very much of what he feels. Still, the baby is there in front of me as therapist, enabling me to observe him or her with all my senses – thus to support my empirical stance.

Reverting to my adult patients, can't I then assume anything about their infancy experiences because I was not there when they occurred? And had I been there, through some fantastic time machine, couldn't I have said anything about the infant's experiences because he didn't talk to me about his tribulations? Am I stumbling about in an epistemological fog? I think this is not the case, actually. I will now claim that the two positions merely seem incompatible. In fact, they constitute a paradox, namely a *seeming* contradiction.

A sheer empiricist way of learning about the world is a mirage since our observations are always influenced by our existing theories, beliefs, and expectations. Thus, they cannot be purely objective, neutral, or "theory-free". Among important philosophers criticising such a monistic empirical doctrine are Kant, Hegel, Husserl, Wittgenstein, and many others. On the other hand, the problem with a sheer inductive epistemological stance can be illustrated as follows: if I heard a patient complaining or being ecstatic about kissing his lover and I then would claim that he had an infantile trauma, this could certainly be prejudiced nonsense. What we humans do from infancy onwards is to make summarising guesses about inner and outer reality. The man sighs, "kissing her wasn't nice at all. It's always the same with women." He and I need to rely on abductions and deductions to establish what makes him translate yesterday's kiss into a disenchanting and irrefutable truth.

To summarise, we have transformed what seemed like an epistemological trap into a paradox. A paradox cannot be resolved, but once we acknowledge this fact, it can become an intriguing object for further investigations. Here, I am influenced by the philosopher C.S. Peirce's (Kloesel & Houser, 1992, 1998; Misak, 2018) suggestion of combining induction, deduction, and abduction to extend one's understanding. His idea is that such a combinatory method enables us not to reach the irrefutable Truth but rather to come a bit closer to it. This is one of the hallmarks of his pragmaticist position. By heeding and applying it, we will find that the paradox becomes easier to sustain and capable of yielding new insights and research.

In my view, PIP is a new empirical field in which babies, a new group of patients, are studied and treated with their parent(s). It also expands the field of the therapist's inductions, not the least by taking countertransference even more seriously as an instrument for understanding the plight of the patient. My interest in the links between present pathology in adult patients and what they told me about their infancy was further ignited when I heard Johan Norman (2001, 2004) presenting his parent-infant work. This led to training in psychoanalytic PIP, which was initiated by Norman and formalised by the Swedish Psychoanalytic Institute. It is time to recount more of what PIP is all about. We will investigate if PIP can function as an empirical instrument that brings us a bit closer to the Infantile. Let us therefore learn more about this method.

A brief exposé of PIP

Once, I was asked by some young students about PIP. They were neither parents nor did they have any psychotherapeutic training. I decided to describe PIP without any professional terms. I told them about a mother who had arrived with her baby at my office. She seemed unhappy, sad, and tense. Her feelings about motherhood were painful. Tense and ashamed, she said, "I don't know if I love my baby". I observed that the baby was flailing and grunting and that there was a frown on his forehead. Sometimes, he avoided looking into his mother's eyes.

The students protested.

> Of course, there were two suffering human beings here – but not two patients! A patient speaks with a therapist in a dialogue, but babies can't speak. The mother came to you because she was unhappy with her baby, but that didn't make him a patient!

They got surprised when I claimed that I do address both mother and baby, "because I don't want to talk with the mother about the baby but also to the baby". Many were incredulous of my stance.

To sharpen my argument, I told them:

> If a mother tells me she doubts if she loves her baby, I will, of course, pay attention to her pain and shame. But I will also address *him* in plain and simple words, for example, 'Peter, your Mum is not sure if she loves you. That's painful to her. She doesn't want you to see that she's in pain, but perhaps you note that something changes in her when she is in trouble. Maybe there are two tense people here, you and Mum. I'm interested in

helping us find out why Mum, maybe you too, are not as happy as the two of you wish'. After a while, the boy's flailing movements may abate, and for a second or two he is looking steadily into the mother's eyes.

Another student demurred,

> This mother is depressed and needs help! Addressing the baby seems far-fetched and even cruel. How do you know the boy discerns her depression or understands your speculative interpretation! And how do you help the mother when she hears you're talking to the boy about connections between his and her distress?

The critique covered major questions about the character, aims, techniques, and results of the PIP method. I will approach them here and in other chapters in the book.

As for my argument that infants of depressed mothers may react aversively to the mother's emotional state, it has been supported in a host of studies (Blandon, Calkins, Keane, & O'Brien, 2008; R. Feldman et al., 2009; Field, 2010; Tronick, 2007b). Similarly, the Still-Face experiment demonstrates such sensitivity in the baby (Adamson & Frick, 2003; Conradt & Ablow, 2010; DiCorcia, Snidman, Sravish, & Tronick, 2016; Mesman et al., 2009; Tronick et al., 1978). All in all, babies respond quickly and with emphasis to their mothers' emotional state whether it is happy, anxious, angry, or depressed.

The students' remaining objections were more clinically oriented and required therapy material about verbal interchanges, other communicative modes like movements, eye contact, tone of voice, cries, bodily tension, and sweat and, not to forget, my often intense and oscillating countertransference reactions. Many languages, such as German, have a special term, *Gesprächstherapie* or "conversation therapy". This term may be sufficient to describe adult therapy but not PIP. When the students contended that Peter was not a patient and my address to him not psychotherapy, they overlooked that we were not doing mere *Gespräch*. We also exchanged miens, gestures, tone inflections, looks, and so on. That they affected him was suggested by his reactions to my address: he calmed down and his jolting movements decreased. Simultaneously and intertwined, these effects also emerged as the mother felt relieved by my baby address.

Thus, to me, the shibboleth of whether a baby is seen as a patient or not depends on whether we *regard and relate to him as taking an active part in the session* – or not. There is a consensus among PIP psychotherapists, though with some variations, as to how much they emphasise this therapist-baby dialogue (Anzieu-Premmereur, 2017; Baradon, Biseo, Broughton, James, & Joyce, 2016; Emanuel, 2011; Fraiberg, 1980; Keren, 2011; Lieberman & Van Horn, 2008; Norman, 2001; Paul & Thomson Salo, 2014; Salomonsson, 2014a, 2018; Tuters, Doulis, & Yabsley, 2011). A brief canon of the theory and psychotherapeutic technique could be formulated as follows. PIP thera-pists observe and communicate with mother and child. They acknowledge that the baby does not understand the lexical levels of language – and they also acknowledge his ability to pick up and react to emotional communica-tions in the session. They capitalise on such capacities by addressing the baby about what they surmise are his dilemmas, feelings, behaviours, and so on. Thus, therapists transmit to baby and mother a readiness to contain their distress. They presuppose that the baby pays attention because he or she senses their willingness to be a *Nebenmensch* or "a fellow human being" (S. Freud, 1895/1950). Until now, the environment, not the least the parents, has met the baby's distress by caring, comforting, or feeding him. Now he meets someone interested in understanding the anxieties in baby and mother and bringing about positive changes in them.

Can we speak about the Infantile in an infant?

The students posed important critical questions. Another one that was not on the agenda on this occasion, but which is an overarching topic of this book, is how the Infantile of the adult corresponds with that of the baby. Such questions will be easier to approach once we have clinical material from PIP treatments. But first, we need to talk about the "Infantile in an infant". Wouldn't that be a tautology? No. As I emphasised earlier, the terms are not interchangeable. The adjective "infantile" refers to a child who is 0 to 12 months old or, alternatively, a child who has not yet learnt to speak, whereas the noun "the Infantile" designates some sort of psychological *structure*. To cite Guignard (2022) again, the Infantile is a "crucible of primal fantasies and sensorimotor experiences that can be stored as memory traces" (5). But we can't just say that they are stored in the Infantile in an original form. It is not a question of ordinary repression, as when a child "forgets" what Mum said and hogs the cookie.

   In contrast, the Infantile harbours the first *unrepresentable* emergences of the drives, says Guignard. When using the term "memory traces", she relies on a long psychoanalytic tradition of searching for suitable concepts that give us an impression of how a baby might signify his perceptions. Freud called them "*Wahrnehmungszeichen*" (S. Freud, 1950 [1892–1899], 234) – "signs of perception". He had in mind primal and loosely arranged registrations. Though they are "non-repressable, foreclosed, non-fantasizable", they act "upon everyone's psychic and/or somatic life" (Balestriere, 2003, 63). To describe what kind of traces the Infantile is made of, I use terms like "sig-nifications in archaic modes", "living fossil", or "primal representations". I thus object that drives in the Infantile would be unrepresentable or even unrepresented. In my view, the Infantile consists of traces such as wishes, fears, and riddles that indeed are signified – but in such enigmatic, diffuse, and incomprehensible ways that we cannot access them directly. It's like when you try to focus on a tiny object with the blind spot, namely the little spot on the retina where the optic nerve exits. Then you can't see the object! You have to encircle it and perceive it sideways using other parts of the retina. Similarly, this is how we can access our Infantile.

If you accept my way of thinking, you might nevertheless claim that it cannot be applied to infants. You might argue something like, "Everything is open and unfiltered to infants. They have not developed psychological tools to help them sort out stimuli into psychological elaboration." Well, I disagree. I consider infants, and quite young at that, to possess such mechanisms. I have elaborated this notion and suggested that, in infants whom I met in PIP, it was at times possible to discern signs of transference, defence, language receptivity, primal repression, trauma, sexuality, and, last but not least, a capacity of very early signification of the baby's experiences (Salomonsson, 2007b 2013a, 2013b, 2014a, 2015b, 2017, 2025). We will soon meet Nicholas, a baby who already at two weeks of age seemed to have divergent registrations of feeding at the right and left breast. I will also hypothesise why this had happened.

I would not be surprised if you protest that I am attributing too much of advanced mental functioning in a baby. But wait a second! We know that babies only a few days old react specifically to the "smellscape" (Porter & Winberg, 1999) of the mother's breast, and they can differentiate between the odour of their mother and of other mothers. You might claim that "it's just a reflex". True, but what makes it difficult to accept that a baby creates some sort of primitive mental representations of the two women (e.g., "she is familiar" or "she is alien"), although the explicit meaning of these words is way beyond the baby's toolbox? And what would prevent us from thinking that such a baby might add some emotional tint to the representations, such as "nice" or "not nice" or simply "+" and "–"?

Theresa and her son Nicholas, two weeks old

The PIP case that contributed to my focus on the Infantile in adult therapy – although at that time I didn't know of the term "Infantile" as used in this book – was actually my very first one. I still recall when I first met Theresa with her son Nicholas, two weeks of age (Salomonsson, 2007a). She had got a wound on the right-hand nipple. It soon healed, but her nurse recommended that she contact me. Her ambivalence was evident when she told me on the spot, "Motherhood isn't my thing!" She seemed trapped, angry, and desperate, constantly worrying about Nic. When sucking the breast, he jerked and tossed his head as if shunning the nipple – or sucking it as if trying to swallow it. This made smooth nursing impossible. To see Theresa's anguished face while Nic fussed was poignant and alarming. Something must be done quickly unless their relation would get stuck in mutual resentment. Here is an excerpt from the first session:

Theresa:	"When he doesn't clutch the nipple or he bites it without sucking, I panic. Where's the design for all this? I tell him to stop crying and start sucking!"
Analyst to Nic:	"I wonder why you are so troubled at the breast. Maybe you remember that it hurt Mom when you sucked her. You didn't understand why she pulled her breast back. Perhaps it filled you with something bad inside. You didn't like Mom's breast then. Is this why you don't dare to suck it?"

It soon became evident that Nic was cautiously paying some attention to me. I turned to him now and again, to explain the pain of his hunger and that he was caught in a memory trap:

> You sense the wonderful milk. Then you recall Mom's 'Ouch' when it hurt her breast. You didn't like that. Now you turn away from the breast and throw your head back. Then you get hungry and want it anyway. And Mom gets stressed.

In connection with this book's focus on the Infantile in adult psychotherapy, the following insight emerges now, two decades after I worked with this dyad. At that time (Salomonsson, 2007a), I had published the article that aimed to integrate experiences of adult therapy and PIP – but I did not use the term "the Infantile". I had started, not so long ago, to work in PIP and did not fully realise its value for understanding the Infantile in my adult patients as well. The 2007 paper combined the case of Nic with that of Monica, a patient mentioned in Chapter 2. She was a reserved, intellectualising, and tense analysand. She was often ironic and disparaging, and I got vexed and frustrated at times. Her anxiety emerged on the couch in stressful ways of swaying and sighing. Sometime after her analysis started, I met Nic and Theresa. This PIP work offered me a new look at Monica. Working with the mother-baby dyad made me observe that Nic's jerks, twitches, and groans were quite similar to Monica's body language. This perception made me more empathic with her, and after much work, she became softer and dared dedicate herself to a man she fell in love with. In brief, PIP treatment inspired a more solid and confident contact with what I today would call Monica's Infantile.

Another person who helped me in my work with Monica was Theresa, Nic's mother. She and I saw that Nic's fretting was confined to the right-sided and previously injured breast. My first idea was that her breastfeeding pain had frightened him and made nursing complicated, notably much more on the right-hand side. So much for Nic. Gradually, facets in Theresa's personality emerged that we metaphorically referred to as her right- and left-sided parts. In her "left-sided" part, she thought of Nic as sweet and lovely and of herself as capable and devoted. Often, however, she felt unworthy as a mother. Such resentment of herself and of Nic was then plain to see. A brief squabble at the breast fired this "right-side" aspect and threw her into depressive self-hatred.

After a few months, Nic's breastfeeding issues had disappeared completely. I conceived this occurred because he had made peace with his mother or had integrated what we might call his "right-sided" and "left-sided" – in Kleinian terms, his bad and good – internal mother objects. I felt it was time to end PIP, but Theresa insisted on continuing on her own to better understand why she still felt like a bad mother. She continued in individual therapy with me for three years. Some issues made traces of her Infantile emerge more clearly. One was the strained relationship with her mother, an orderly, matter-of-fact, brisk woman. She was devoted to her daughter and grandson, but their dialogues were factual and without a deep connection. I thought Theresa had not found in her own mother someone to latch on to, as it were. This contributed to her panic when Nic fussed at her breast. I conceived of her as having an unhappy baby representation in her Infantile. My guess was supported when she revealed two shameful secrets. One was her long-lasting teenage anorexia. The other was a masochistic bent, which had made her abide with a rather self-centred partner. It also contained some sexual preferences where she desired to be treated in a rude way.

Theresa's personal therapy showed how a mother's Infantile can affect and be affected by her baby's distress. True, she had many constructive, responsible, and caretaking psychological assets. Let us call them her "Adult". But beneath it lay a dormant Infantile of a fretting baby who was longing for – but not reaching – a calm and containing maternal presence. She did well at work, and until now, she had been satisfied with her family and intimate life. Before Nic's birth, her Infantile and the Adult had lived in peace. Their conflictual potential was unleashed a few days after delivery. In the ward, she felt "like a queen". But on her way home, she panicked about what she had set going. It was as if her Infantile screamed, "stop the cab, I wanna go home, I didn't ask for this intrusion in my life, I'll never make it". Those images clashed completely with her expectations, responsibility, and wish to take care of her baby. "I was appalled and paralysed", as she told me.

The PIP therapy provided two teachers, Nic and Theresa, for my learning more about the Infantile in the adult. When Nic shunned the nipple that he had charged with bad memories, it exemplified a memory function of storing bad experiences and his avoidance of them. His way of "thinking", or whatever we should call that very primitive mentation, could be formulated as, "if I avoid that pink protruding thing on this side of her, I might escape this aching thing inside of me". To exemplify with an adult patient, something similar may have been going on in Simone in Chapter 1. The bad experience she wanted to avert was something that she called an eerie "hole inside" and which I conjectured was in some way linked with her mother of infancy. Kissing her lover was a way of filling up that hole, like a balm that could heal everything gnawing at her mind.

This chapter's caption suggests that PIP can help us understand the Infantile in adult individuals. One could object that most of what I learned about Theresa's Infantile emerged in her individual therapy, after Nic had left the scene. However, I contend that I grasped much about her Infantile already in the very first PIP sessions. Her helpless and callow tone of voice was moving when she said, "The best time is when Nic's asleep. When he wakes up, I don't know how to play with him!" Nic was only a few weeks old, but Theresa already felt her duty and impotence. She prayed he would become independent quickly. But she also feared that he would become a teenager and suffer conflicts like the ones she had with her mother. The bottom line was that she felt unable to provide the love, devotion, and care that her child needed – because she herself felt like an unhappy child.

I have presented this case to show how the Infantile of mother and baby emerged and interacted and, at least initially in PIP treatment, did so in anguished and non-productive ways. Yet Nic was only two weeks old, which makes it seem far-fetched to already divide his personality into the Infantile and "the Adult". I will therefore bring in another case of an older baby (Salomonsson, 2007b), where such divisions were feasible.

A mother and Karen, eight months old

Karen is eight months old, demands nursing continuously, and cannot fall asleep unless mother yields to her insistent demands for the breast. She cries easily and her mother is exhausted and helpless – but she has a light tone of voice when telling me this and dismisses my comment that it must be hard for her. I feel she fears her unvarnished affects about Karen, such as that she is annoyed with her. This makes it hard for her to contain the girl's affects. Perhaps, Karen's whining for the breast is related to her mother's way of handling this affective situation? I reflect on my countertransference feelings of our artificial and shallow contact. Meanwhile, Karen whines and starts crawling. She tumbles at a little stool in my room and starts to cry.

Mother to Karen: "Oh dear! You fell and hurt your head."
Analyst to Karen: "Well, actually you look angry when you're looking at me. You might wonder what kind of man you have come to, with my stupid stool … Yes? … But it wasn't that dangerous."

Mother seems to sugarcoat her daughter's reactions, whereas I suggest Karen actually got angry with me and my stool. This illustrates my conviction that what a baby needs most of all is, to paraphrase Freud's "*J'appelle un chat un chat*" (S. Freud, 1905a, 48), for us adults to call affects by their real names. Thus, I tell Karen she looks angry and thinks my stool is stupid. She calms down but whimpers still, while mother describes how Karen wakes up in the night and only the breast will soothe her.

Mother to Karen: "When we wake up in the night, the only thing that helps is the breast at once, otherwise you become So Sad."

Analyst to Karen: "One could ask: do you get sad because you don't get the breast? Or, do you get Angry?!" Karen roars and I comment, "Well, that does sound quite angry!"

Karen stops crying. Up till now, she has been governed by an Infantile that cajoles her that the breast is her only solace and that, if she does not get it, she has every reason to be "So Sad". If the breast but yielded to her demands, everything would be fine! But from the vantage point of more "adult" or mature parts in her personality, this is untrue. She will not benefit from her mother's disingenuity or feeble surrender to her claims. Only honesty and containment from adults will help her develop what I would call a healthy Infantile and show her that she needs to allot it a "nursery". In this psychic space, her Infantile can inspire her to dream, fantasise, and become creative. Guignard (2022) also stresses that the Infantile has creative aspects. To illustrate with Karen, I will refer to a vignette towards the end of therapy. The mother is now more able to differentiate when Karen is angry or sad. She has also developed a wish to find out why Karen has this or that feeling. Karen arrives at a session newly awakened and a bit hungry. She looks at me earnestly and I wait. Unexpectedly, she crawls to a cabinet with illuminated little figurines that capture her attention. She reaches for its doorknob. She knocks at it and moves her hand to her mouth, as if swallowing something. She gives a laugh, which mother meets. Mother says to Karen, "You're having a drink at the milk-bar, aren't you!"

Karen's little theatre shows her integrating my interpretations of her anger with Mom's breast and her fears about it. The punchline of this "Play of the Infantile" is

OK, I've got it. Sometimes when I feel hungry, I'm actually annoyed about something else. Or, I am truly hungry, but then I've got to do my share and scream at the breast to make it come to me. But in my theatre piece, I just knock at the pitcher and get what I want.

Mother's "milk-bar" pun shows a similar playfulness; she has grasped Karen's demands without being ensnared by them.

It is time to sum up what Nic and Karen and their mothers taught me about the Infantile. First, I refer to the intensity, vivacity, and consistency in the babies' positions vis-à-vis their mothers. In Nic's case, I would express it as

> Mum, once you fussed when I sucked the breast on that side. This proved to me that it was no good, so every time you put me there, I had good reasons to fuss. I also suspected you've got a two-sided relationship with me, one that I didn't grasp.

In later years, and now I'm speculating, this might have been transformed into a trace of his Infantile, such as a pessimistic attitude of "when I desire someone, some fuss may always intervene". Second, the mother's ways with her baby were influenced by unresolved issues from her Infantile. To exemplify, Theresa's personality contained a frustrated baby aspect that was discontent with not having all the attention. I sensed it emerged in how she handled Nic – and he reacted to it.

How many Infantiles take part in a PIP therapy? At least three, I would say: that of the baby, the mother, and the therapist. The last of these participants takes us to the question of countertransference in PIP. In Chapter 2, we learnt that Guignard emphasised how the analyst detects traces of the Infantile by listening to the countertransference. She referred to work with adult patients, which I have illustrated with Colin, Simone, and Bess. At times, I felt frustrated and confused with them, but they also evoked my concern and sympathy. Their helpless suffering created an echo, a resonance with similar feelings in me, which made me better comprehend their quandaries. The book's upcoming vignettes with adult patients contain more vignettes with references to my countertransference.

PIP as a teaching template for adult psychotherapy

Let us return to Colin in Chapter 1. When I met this young man, I had no experience of PIP. If I had such knowledge then, would I have behaved, thought, and focused differently? Indeed, I think so. Many PIP colleagues have confirmed that their ways of working with adult patients have been affected by their PIP experiences. Unfortunately, they have not written much about this interesting phenomenon. I will now address some specific points about PIP as a "teacher" in adult psychotherapy. In brief, such work has changed my view and practice of adult therapy regarding

- Embodied communication
- Countertransference and empathy
- Reconstruction of infantile experiences
- Attention to verbal and nonverbal communication – in patient and analyst
- Analytic technique

Embodied communication

PIP sessions illustrate that babies are very sensitive to the emotional states of their attachment figures. They may become distressed, fussy, or sad or avoid mother's eyes when she is depressed, worried, hostile, blaming herself, and so on. Also, they can become upset when a mother is chatting insensitively or covering up a painful issue. In reverse, they also react with joy and relief when mother breaks through such spurious communication and starts to speak sincerely or "*parler vrai*" (Dolto, 1994b). I will address this in Chapter 8. As for studies of mother – baby – therapist interactions on multiple communicative levels, I refer to Chapter 9. I emphasise already here that babies are also sensitive to the therapist's nonverbal cues. This can affect PIP therapists and make us more observant of, and able to speak about, an adult patient's sigh, tone or tremor of voice, body tension, odour, evasive eye glances, strokes at a specific body part, hand gestures, and so on. Such embodied communications are, I contend, easier to recognise for a therapist who also has worked with PIP.

How might PIP experiences have affected my stance with Colin? I guess I would have been more observant of his body language, look, tone of voice, and posture. I would also have been more aware of how such components in me; that is, my body language would have affected him at the spur of the moment. My thoughts would thus have revolved around our interaction – in both the verbal and nonverbal sense. Had I done this, I would have acted in accordance with Merleau-Ponty's (1962) tradition that we can "never experience independent of our bodily existence in the world" (Frie, 2007). In brief, PIP work makes it clearer that we are all "body-subjects".

Countertransference and empathy

Another example of an increased sensitivity due to the therapist's PIP experiences concerns the countertransference. When Colin told me about what had happened to him after his own and his son's births, and we guessed how they might be linked, I was moved – but did I really let it find its way into me? Was I able to enter what Racker (1968) called a *concordant identification*? Note that "concordant" literally means "with one's heart". Was my heart in tune with Colin's in these sessions? To what extent was I active in imaginative thinking, which "always involves a dynamic object relationship in which the self is absorbed creatively with its object" (Grier, 2021, 457). Such relationships may also resonate with one's own life experiences. I gather that the ways I absorbed Colin were also rooted in my personal history of an early separation, as noted in Chapter 2.

Another take on this question is possible. Despite my empathy with Colin, I may unconsciously have expressed some dislike of what he had done to his wife. Obviously, his behaviour had immature and self-centred components, and my reproach might have found its way through a frown, a tone of voice, or a turning away that he could interpret as rejections. The more an analyst is aware of the countertransference, the more adept he becomes in understanding the patient and helping him or her to understand himself/herself and become "the master in his own house", to paraphrase one of Freud's lectures (S. Freud, 1916–1917, 285).

Reconstruction of infantile experiences

Another fruit reaped in PIP is that it gives the therapist a more solid ground to reconstruct, with the patient, links between present and past. This idea will be expanded in Chapter 7. Returning to Colin, he came to me with self-reproaches and bewilderment about his infatuation. He knew about his hospital stay in infancy but did not link it with his passion. He needed my help to link the two and understand that, although he wished to be a responsible father and a role model for his son, his Infantile took over screaming, "I'm forsaken and helpless, I'm stuck and deserted in an alien place. Mummy, come here and bring me home!" The reconstruction did not imply that he unearthed the external events when he was hospitalised. This he knew already. Rather, it consisted in detecting its link with his relations to women and to his colleague in particular, as if pleading to her, "Lips, bring me home!"

How can I claim that PIP experiences have inspired me to do more reconstructive work? The answer is quite simple. Psychoanalysis as a discipline started with adult patients talking about their present suffering and then turning to their childhood experiences. Only one generation later did children enter a few analytic consulting rooms, and it took two more generations to allow babies there. Yet all the years before PIP arrived, analysts talked about and conceived of the infantile mind and its repercussions in the adult patient. What distinguished the PIP therapists was that they met baby and mother in concrete interactions. Evidently, all such screams, sighs, laughter, contact, and lack of contact have lent more concreteness and substance to the Infantile than the speculations in analytic "pre-PIP" writings because one "leg" was missing then: the empirics of PIP. This footing gives PIP therapists an increased propensity to reconstruct, together with their older patients, traumatic influences from infancy that may impact on their present distress.

Attention to verbal and nonverbal communication – in patient and analyst

In PIP, the borders between nonverbal and verbal communication are particularly blurred. Additionally, nonverbal communication is even more in focus in PIP than in adult therapy. Nowhere is the expression – that psychotherapy is but a "talking cure" (S. Freud, 1893–1895) – as questionable as in PIP work. Here, verbal and nonverbal communication go together like the warp and the woof in a weave. If we do not consider nonverbal communications as equally informative and influential, therapy risks becoming meaningless or false in Winnicott's sense (1960). In PIP, this confluence is plain to see: a baby's smile, cry, odour, grin, a raised eyebrow or a mother's pained face or grey hue, the analyst's startle or concerned mien; these nonverbal cues plus the parallel verbal communications form the entirety of PIP practice and will also raise the therapist's awareness of such complex communications in his adult patients.

Therapeutic technique

In PIP, things happen at split-second speed (Miltz, Pennicott-Banks, Avdi & Baradon, 2023) between the participants. One can note, as in videorecorded PIP sessions, that a therapist's expression of consternation is almost instantly followed by the mother's anxiety and the baby's closing down. We can conceive of such interchanges as occurring between container and contained – impersonated by therapist and baby or by baby and mother. The therapist thus becomes a keener observer, which he can transfer to sessions with adult patients.

Furthermore, these up-tempo interactions seem to foster more improvisation and volatility in therapeutic technique. When the PIP therapist is speaking to the baby, the mother, of course, hears and reflects on it. And when he speaks to the mother, the baby listens, looks, and reacts more often than we think. There are many "balls" in motion, some slow and others speedy, some almost imperceptible and others overly clear. The PIP therapist thus becomes trained in agility, nimbleness, speed, and improvisation. These assets are actually similar to the capacities that many parents with infants develop quite quickly, especially the ones whom PIP therapists do *not* meet: those who are harmonious, happy, and content with their babies.

I am still eager to show how I approach the Infantile in my adult patients. I also wish to elaborate how PIP experiences can hone a therapist's capacities of perceiving the Infantile and make use of them to help the patient. In the next chapter, I will present a case where I have preserved extensive notes from our contact. Bianca was in psychoanalysis with me 30 years ago. Some five years after termination, she contacted me again. She was grateful for the analysis because her life was much better. But she was also critical that I had not understood how hard it had been for her to speak out in the analysis about her embarrassing thoughts and feelings. Instead, we had tumbled into disputes of dominance and surrender. True, she recognised such interactions from her love relationships, which she could handle better today. But she still regretted that we had not reached the depth of understanding that might have made her become more on speaking terms with her Infantile, as I would express it today.

Chapter 4

Bianca

A swaddled woman

Bianca was 30 years old when she contacted me. After one crashed marriage, two abortions, and several failed relationships with men, she was at the end of the road. A friend who had been in psychotherapy recommended her to contact me. She seemed a capable and independent woman, the eldest of three siblings in an immigrant family. Bianca had arrived in Sweden at the age of five and, as it later emerged, some years after her parents. She spoke with me of her sense of loneliness that increased notably when her father died and she, an 18-year-old and recently married young woman, felt devastated.

It did not take long for us to decide to start an analysis. It would last six years, with a frequency of mainly four times a week. Bianca appeared genuinely interested in reflecting on herself. To exemplify, she told me that the days before her first interview, she felt "like before an exam". She thought of contacting Enzo, one of her boyfriends, to get his support. She described him as "a sleazy twerp", but she needed him because she was nervous about coming to me. Then she asked herself, "what do I want by phoning Enzo, actually?" She realised that it would end up in a sham comfort, so she did not contact him after all. At the end of one of our first encounters, she became sad. She had just talked about her family's return to their country and then about her father's death a decade ago. She stood up crying, and I suggested to her that these situations resembled each other: her family leaving her, her father dying, and now she was about to leave me. She nodded in agreement. The scene was moving, and I said goodbye to her with the sense of an intriguing and moving analytic journey ahead of us. As we shall see, it was to become much bumpier and more unsettling than I had envisaged.

My life as a "pre-PIP" psychoanalyst

I met Bianca long before I had any experiences of working with babies or children in a psychoanalytic setting. A decade earlier, I had started my analytic training with *The Interpretation of Dreams* (S. Freud, 1900), where he analysed his dreams in terms of professional ambitions, victories, failures, and his struggles with incestuous wishes. His analyses were creative, smart,

DOI: 10.4324/9781003640363-4

and relying extensively on his verbal associations. Reading them, I felt a bit like solving a crossword. But Freud's personal struggles also found many echoes in myself.

Then came a chapter, "The psychology of the dream processes" (S. Freud, 1900, 509), where he delineated the origin and purpose of dream formation. In the midst of this dense and complicated chapter he spoke at length about babies! This was surprising to me. His idea was that a baby swings between states of contentment/pleasure and their counterpart, panic/unpleasure. What often ignites unpleasure is a budding hunger or some other distress, which the baby tries to subdue by hallucinating the bountiful and appeasing breast. This is the prototype of a dream: a primitive "mental movie" about something which, once we have analysed the dreamer's associations, we can interpret as depicting a wish of being satisfied. For the baby, this solution cannot work for more than a short while. For the dreamer, it lasts as long as the dream goes on and until one wakes up to reality. There are many differences, of course, between babies and dreamers. The baby's worldview is restricted, for example, in that the breast is felt to be the only conceivable source of satisfaction. In contrast, the dreamer has acquired many more and varied "dreams" and passions throughout his life, many of which are doomed to remain unfulfilled.

The interpretations of the dreams in Freud's book veer towards conflicts – not the least the Oedipus complex – that afflict people older than babies. Yet his theory of the origin and function of dreams refers much to infants. But was Freud then speaking of babies he was interacting with, or was the baby a theoretical construct? This was unclear. I was surprised at and curious about the prominence of babies in Freud's writing, but two matters were unclearly described: the "feel" of the baby's alarm and how it appears in his contact with the mother.

The "relational turn" in psychoanalysis emerged as future generations of analysts came up with a deeper understanding of a baby's distress and how it can be handled – with or without success – by the parent. In this sentence, we only need to replace the word "baby" with "patient" and "parent" with "therapist" to grasp the enormous consequences that these findings and insights post Freud have had for psychoanalytic practice. For example, "countertransference" is viewed and utilised differently today than in Freud's days. To him, it was a "result of the patient's influence on [the analyst's] unconscious feelings, and we are almost inclined to insist that he shall recognize this counter-transference in himself and overcome it" (S. Freud, 1910, 144). It took a generation or two for analysts to realise that Freud was certainly right that the analyst needs to continuously be aware of and grapple with the countertransference – but to insist that he should "overcome" it is futile and may lead to a one-eyed and even authoritarian analytic technique.

The case of Bianca shows a young analyst at work. I was eager to understand the strong and often painful affects that emerged in me. I was aware of the intensity of our interactions in sessions. Also, I sometimes discerned in her quarrels, accusations, and dependence on me a desperate baby trying to survive in a world where grownups fail to handle her emotional needs. Still, I had a lot to learn about such a baby and how to handle her in sessions. In this education, Bianca was an essential teacher. But there was a long way to go before we could reasonably resolve our transference-countertransference conflict or – to put it more robustly – our battle at the couch.

The story of Bianca's and my joint analytic work contains an overarching plea for an approach, which is as important for an analyst working with a patient as it is for a mother caring for her baby: to combine a clear view of the violence, self-centredness, and exacting demands of a baby or, as here, of Bianca with empathy with a poor baby or patient who feels she has nobody to turn to for help – or is ashamed of doing it. This will lead to some conclusions at the end of the chapter.

The analysis

My notes of Bianca's analysis cover one hundred pages. The second entry is quite different from the first. She has left her reflective position and is now into a "heavy resistance", as I formulated it then. I realise she does this because of strong affects, which she fears will flood her. She knows she is supposed to say whatever comes to her mind but cannot do it, "because you'll think I'm talking nonsense!" Psychoanalysis is thus a humiliation, from which she tries to escape by literally jumping up from the couch. Her inferiority feelings are matched by an arrogant and ferocious attitude. Already in childhood, she was called "Little Franco". Pacing around in the consulting room, she can be snappy and arrogant, but after a while, she fiddles with a plant or a blanket, calms down, and returns to the couch. "It is impossible to speak with you about my thoughts. I'd become totally ashamed!"

Bianca reports dreams, often violent with blood and murder. In other dreams, she and I play together, she asks if I've got children, and I answer yes. In one such dream, she is naked and abashed, feeling even more so when my next woman patient interrupts our play. I interpret the dream as her longing for the affection of a man/father, her efforts at seducing me, and her shame when our intimacy is interrupted by the woman/mother. I interpret it as an Oedipal scenery. Bianca has the reputation of a flirty seductress, but I am more taken by her panic and shame on the couch. Such feelings prevent her from even finishing a sentence like "I had a dream last night…", followed by a lengthy silence. This sets in motion impotent feelings in me, and she reports similar emotions in herself. I ponder, "Get yourself together and speak out!" She says, "It is not true that I can't tell you what I had in mind, I know I wouldn't die if I did it. I do the same game with men".

Bianca is a teaser – and some men get turned on by it. As for me, I feel there is something childish and helpless about her rather than a sexy *femme fatale*.

Two more details support this track: she is a kleptomaniac and obsessed with her weight. She steals trifles or drab and colourless clothes, which she then rarely uses. Abraham (1927) is reported as saying: "Cleptomania refers to the fact that a child feels injured or neglected in respect to proofs of love, which [she has] equated with gifts, or in some way disturbed in the gratification of [her] libido" (Allen, 1965, 573). In my words, Bianca's stealing reflects conflicts about longing for emotional nourishment from a mother whose warmth and generosity she does not trust. It's as if she must snatch pieces of the breast and then accuse it of providing mere trash. As for her relation to food, she has never had anorexia or bulimia, but she checks her weight constantly and is eager to appear like a thin, sexy, and gorgeous woman. Thus, Bianca's stealing and weight fixation indicate that her identity as a "man-eater" conceals another aspect of her personality that is in harsh conflict with her nourishing but stingy mother.

Bianca's swinging in the transference is seen in the following incident. She starts a session by saying she is afraid of becoming pregnant again. She then says she went to a swimming pool and thought of me. Tonight, she will babysit for a friend. She blurts out, "I know you're thinking that I want to become pregnant with you, all analysts think that way!" In fact, that was far from the top of my mind. I was taken by her longing for me in the pool, as if she were floating in an amniotic fluid. Also, I know that pregnancy is an inflamed theme, in view of her abortions and failed love relationships. Once again, she wards off serious questions and fragile feelings by quarrelling.

Sessions with Bianca thus swing between moments that are dramatic and heated and others that are tranquil and reflective. True, she can be fussy and rowdy, but when such storms have waned, she can get in contact with very painful feelings. After a year in analysis, she has a dream:

Bianca: "You were of my nationality. You were the father of another Bianca, actually I have a cousin of that name. She was in therapy with you. That was not appropriate, so she must switch therapist to Natalia instead [the friend of my patient who once recommended her to start treatment with me]. Then there was a murder, somebody was chasing a little child, you lifted it up and held it in your arms, it was cute."

Bianca associates the child to a TV programme about children from Colombia who were adopted to other countries. She recalls their screams when they were abandoned by their mothers. Now, Bianca starts a new quarrel, I don't recall about what. I suggest that often she starts fussing with me when feelings about longing and sadness appear – and that they are to do with abandonment. This idea is also supported by the previous session, when she had talked about her country of origin and its ethnic conflicts and her "ridiculous" given name. Making me her compatriot in the dream is a comfort that gets smashed by the fact that my daughter is in therapy with me. This proves that I am not to be trusted, and that the contact between me and my daughter must be terminated.

Bianca interrupts, this time not with a storm of attacks but with a sad and calm tale of her childhood. The family was poor, and both her parents emigrated to Sweden to get work while she was taken care of by her paternal grandmother. She lost contact with her father from three to four years of age and with her mother from 3½ to 5½ years. When she was four years, Bianca's father travelled back to their country of origin to bring her to Sweden. But the paternal grandmother refused to give Bianca to him, so he returned to his wife without their daughter. Not until she was 5½ years old did the entire family settle in Sweden, where two sisters were born. It is plain to see that the crying Colombian children aroused deep identifications with abandoned, exposed, and powerless children.

My acting out

Sometime after the "Colombian session", I felt we were more in sync. True, she often continued to swing between two poles. One was a hardboiled, sexy broad who lured "disgusting weirdos" to bed. Another was a weeping, sobbing girl with feelings so overwhelming that she couldn't handle them. She did realise that the only possible way of reaching some inner calm and harmony would be to accept my commitment and concern. She acknowledged her problem with the two equations of Love = Humiliation and Dependence = Slavery. Sensing that I cared for her made her feel disgusting, ashamed, and ridiculed. Feeling that she needed me was equal to ending up in a creepy submission to me, her narcissistic and excited exploiter. But the fact that Bianca could talk about herself in this quite sophisticated way supported my feeling in sync with her. In other words, I sensed we had a tenable working alliance.

Maybe, I naïvely expected that she would make use of her insights faster or more thoroughly than she appeared to do. Today, I would argue that she was on the road of tracing an essential aspect of her Infantile, "the Colombian child". But she often digressed by starting quarrels with me or her partners. I made notes about "her conflicts around gender identity. The longing girl is perhaps a girl without penis and self-confidence. Is the aggressive and fussing broad equipped with a fantasized phallos?" Today, I would emphasise more *my own fear* of "being in the crib" with Bianca, namely sharing her emotions of an abandoned and inconsolable child. When she donned the role of a *femme fatale*, I now regret that I did not respond by a more composed, waiting, and less active position. I showed her that I was seeing through her invitation and did not want to tango with her. But had I been "in the crib" with her, it might have brought us closer to an exposed, vulnerable, and thin-skinned aspect of her Infantile. As we will soon learn, it is no coincidence that I use a word referring to the skin when depicting this frail and reactive aspect of her personality.

Was I belligerent, cocky, brash? Did I feel like her male partners, getting simultaneously excited and furious? To me, these explanations do not fit. My challenge was rather that Bianca had a weapon that I found so hard to avert: *her silence*. Not silence in a sad, withdrawn, or contemplative way. No, a silence which she sensed was provoking me. At first, she could awaken my commitment by declaring that she had something to say – and then a blank silence. One Monday hour, she said: "I had a dream..." Then followed an almost total silence till the end of the hour. I sensed both her pressure and pleasure. When a few minutes remained, I said: "Either you tell me the dream, or we finish the analysis".

I am still ashamed about this episode thirty years ago. Did I really want her to quit? Definitely not. Did I really think she would leave? No, I did not. Was it an empty threat? No, neither that. Today, I come to think of a situation that I've seen many times with mother – baby dyads: a depressed mother, at the end of her tether with her baby, calls out, "If you go on screaming like this, I'll go crazy" or "I'm never gonna have another child. My God, you're just TOO MUCH!" But this connection between a mother and a baby, or me and her, was not accessible to me at the time.

My ultimatum was an acting out of my frustration, disappointment, humiliation, and rage against the ways Bianca was treating me. Had I restricted myself to "tasting" my feelings and reflected on them, this could have been helpful to her. But I did something beyond this by threatening to end her therapy. Our contact was such that I did not really envisage her terminating treatment, but I was indeed surprised by her ensuing immediate comment:

Bianca: "You're right. I needed this. In the dream, I was with Enzo. Very arousing. He fiddled in my anus with some kind of pill that he had divided in two. He pushed it into my anus, it was disgusting and exciting. Then a man with a machine gun shot into a crowd."

There was no time left for talking about the dream or what had happened between the two of us. The next day, we talked about the dream, and I interpreted it in terms of the transference relationship. I suggested she wanted to get me worked up to the point when I "stick it up in her behind" in the form of coarse comments and threats, like my ultimatum yesterday. At first, she responded with "that's the most stupid thing I've ever heard" but then she turned sad, telling me of her previous marriage with Oscaro. He was only capable of anal intercourse or masturbation in solitude. "I accepted that life with him! How could I?"

The following sessions, Bianca complained of her menstrual cramps. And she just had her wisdom tooth extracted. My notes indicate that I was thinking,

It's as if when you show me your front side, I'll see a bleeding, defective woman whom I despise. If you show me your backside I'll get worked up, and then we're into a violent and horny intercourse, but our emotional contact is turned off.

Thus, Bianca could envisage neither that a man would want to see her beautiful and loveable body and mind nor that he would want her to see him in the same way. Their eyes, the windows of the soul, should not meet in mutual recognition, curiosity, warmth, and respect. As I shared this notion with her, she responded, "Yes, I want to be a man, I was always looking at the boys' dicks. But then I thought they were laughable. My own sex was ridiculous, too, that's why I let men do what they want with me." She agrees when I suggest that she hates me because I am a man – and because I'm a man, she loves me. I tell her, "This is very difficult for you", and she nods in silence.

As always in psychoanalysis, things are complicated, the more so when we think of them in retrospect. My ultimatum was a threat, and as such, it was unquestionably my error and responsibility. But what followed laid bare her conflicts about being a woman and how to relate to men in ways that were not degrading and contemptuous. The session climate now changed, and there emerged more of tolerance and less of belligerence in her. Was she right when she responded that my ultimatum was right and that she needed it? From what followed immediately in sessions, my answer would be yes. We needed to work through her excited anal game with me. But in a larger perspective, I would say no. Not only was it imprudent, but it also slowed down our search for traces of the Infantile awaiting to be revealed and worked through.

One example is when she spoke of a newspaper article about Socrates and Plato with the famous story about the cave. After much sweating and hesitation, she brought the article to a session. Bianca was far from experienced in philosophy, and she was embarrassed about her initiative. But the text fascinated her, though not because of the philosophical allegory per se. No, she thought of her analysis as a cave with the two of us inside and then coming out in the unpleasant and glaring light. She also spoke of my ceiling lamp as the cave's opening. Analysis would be like the two of us entering her interior, understanding her thoughts. Following this she burst out, "Gosh, my thoughts are so utterly ridiculous!"

Themes followed about babies and children, both her longing for them and her dread when she read about child abuse. For example, she needed to go to an antenatal clinic to check if she had a venereal disease. Seeing pregnant women in the waiting room, she got devastated – but she could approach it:

> Sometimes when I leave the session, I touch your coat in the waiting room, thinking how much I like you. Sunday, I was at an afternoon party, there was a baby, I played with her. But WHY doesn't Jane, my boss, give me the free hours I'm entitled to? Damn her!

These passages indicated Bianca's turn – from a phallic girl heating up the man to penetrate her anus to a "woman in progress". She began fantasising of being a mother in a love relationship. This inevitably led to a new challenge:

the relationship with her own mother. This was seen when she jumped from her comment about the baby to her anger with the female boss. Accusing the boss, Bianca failed to discern that she needed not more free hours but a freer access to an introject that could offer love, trust, touch, and calm eye contact. The fact that her accusation emerged after having told me about playing with the baby indicates that this was a maternal introject. We will now follow how this brittle and torn introject evolved in the analysis.

The baby slips into sessions

One and a half year into her analysis, Bianca is in her quarrelsome mood again.

Bianca: "There's no relationship between us! As soon as I don't talk about you, you don't like it. I could've cancelled this session since I've an important seminar this very moment."

Analyst: "You didn't cancel…"

Bianca: "It was impossible, I couldn't phone you that late. Bah, all this is nonsense, I know, I'm just making it up."

Analyst: "You know you're making it up and that you long to come to me, and then you say we don't have any relationship. Yet, you know that's a lie."

Bianca: "I'm not lying! Well, I do, but when I tell you that I brush you off, it really FEELS like that to me."

Analyst: "So this seems to be the only alternative left to handle your feelings for me. One could say that for you, the truth is unbearable and the lie is tolerable."

Bianca: "That's true!"

Why can't Bianca admit that she abstained from cancelling the session because she eagerly wants to see me? Why does she contend that I am so self-centred? Why claim that we have no relationship? One could object that it is because of the ultimatum. But I retort that, no, I like working with Bianca, I do want to help her, and I believe I am capable of it. I also feel she senses all this. Posed with this cobweb of contradictions, I suggest to her, after the just-cited interchange:

Analyst: "All your passions, you think I am so beleaguered and sick of them, as if I just can't stand your feelings for me. To me, your passions also seem like those of a tiny child."

Bianca: "I'm thinking of my Mum, hehe (laughing mockingly at herself), sure, she didn't love me, hehe (turning serious): My Mum. I — know — she — didn't — love me. Bah, I wanna cry. No! What time is it. Eww, 12 minutes left. I get cold now. I thought about it, sometimes when you look warm, I turn cold.

Analyst: "What do you think about it?"

Bianca: "I don't want to think about it! Away with it all!"

After we have talked about this theme some more, I add:

Analyst: "You've tried to convince yourself and me that you must annoy me, and then I won't stand it and I would do away with you. Is this because you fear that I cannot stand when you long for me, think of me, and want to be with me, all because you're repugnant to me?"

When leaving this session, Bianca is thoughtful and calm. The next day, she starts another power quarrel, though in a milder, subdued, and playful way. Suddenly:

Bianca: "I read a newspaper article about newborn triplets. They were so sweet!... There's a photo in the family album, I was swaddled as a baby... Now I'm thinking of my marriage, so pervert, how could I stand it!?"

When Bianca gets in contact with her yearning for me, she has often switched to pestering and attacking me. As we have learnt, she is now beginning to bear with her yearning and speak about how it scares her. She gets cold and wants to cry or run away – and she mentions babies. Now she adds something new and essential: she was *swaddled at length as a baby*. This disclosure emerged after 1½ years of analysis. Even today, I recall the chill and empathy that I felt when I heard, however briefly, her mentioning the swaddling.

The next entry about the swaddling appears only two years later in my records. I find this utterly strange. Did we not talk about it when she mentioned it? We certainly did, but the question is *how*. What about her descriptions of psychosomatic phenomena, such as her coldness when she speaks of me as a warm person? And her sweating, jumping up from the couch, snapping her fingers, cracking her finger joints, and more? I noted them, but it was hard to broach the topic because of her shame and my unfamiliarity with talking about such embodied communication.

In my notes, I discern several reasons for the "swaddle pause", the time from her mentioning it till we began talking at length about it. She often returned to accusing me of being cruel and indifferent, that analysis was a humiliating power struggle she was bound to lose. She added accusations against her father of being a selfish man who idealised his daughter but then beat her up when he was drunk. She challenged lying on the couch and began sitting in the armchair – and she got surprised that I did not coerce her back to the couch. In retrospect, I wonder why she was silent about being swaddled or transmitted it like a gleeful and factual aside comment. I guess this factor plus my irritation with Bianca made me impervious to the full impact of what today I would call a maltreatment of a baby girl lying swaddled in her cot while her parents were working in the fields.

The swaddle was thus in the background, and the excited anal game continued, with me and her partners. She would make men horny, wanting to be penetrated anally, feeling disgraced, and wanting to leave but being unable to do so. True, themes of children reappeared more frequently, but not as the cute baby she had just read about. Instead, her dreams, associations, and daydreams involved aborted foetuses; starving, maltreated, and murdered babies; and girls who underwent genital mutilation or were prostituted. My notes exude hopelessness during the two years after Bianca had mentioned the swaddling for the first time.

> She's like a baby, filled with toxic feelings that need to be expelled through projective identifications, where I assume the role of a diabolic non-understanding man. She has no vision of a relationship where the other person contains her pain. In a normal relationship, the child becomes more skilled in signalling what it wants, and the parents more skilled in reading and containing them. But not so with Bianca, who seems to be in a constant colicky state throughout her life, including the years since she started analysis.

Today, I think this note overlooks another perspective, namely that the "toxic feelings" might have to do with her trauma of being swaddled. It seems to have left her with a stunted capacity of containing strong feelings, whether they concern hostility and humiliation or warmth and tenderness. Bianca addresses this difficulty: "I can't go on like this, I can't walk around town and start crying when I think of you, I've got a job to do! I will end up in an asylum!" Other stories show that Bianca has often experienced how her pleas for help have been misconstrued by her family and neighbours. True, she seems to have voiced her complaints only rarely, but one must also consider that adults around her have responded in a blunt and clueless way. Once in her teens, she yearned for her sisters and grandmother who had returned to their native country. A neighbour in Stockholm noticed she seemed gloomy and asked her about it in a friendly way. Bianca replied she had a toothache. In response, the lady sent her to a dentist for a tooth extraction. Bianca then phoned her mother for comfort, but she thought her daughter was drunk. In brief, this is a story of blunt and concrete treatment by the adult world of a teenager who is in acute emotional distress.

Such ways of feeling contained by her kin are visible in how she treats herself. This period in analysis is replete with promiscuous enactments, where she acts like a "Rambo-like" sexy woman. Having sex with married men adds to her excitement. She has a dream:

Bianca: "I dreamt that a married man and I hugged each other. His wife saw it. Then there was a farm with green apples that I really wanted. Another man was deep-frying them. I was enraged with him. Then, the first man and his wife came out of their house, they were nice to me. And the man who was deep-frying gave me a gift, an exclusive lipstick."

"Then I had another dream about a baby I couldn't handle. They hadn't changed diapers for a long time. The baby smelled of poo. I asked how I should handle the baby but got no response... You know, my grandmother told me that when we were little, they swaddled us so tight that the diapers were fuming when they took them off. You could hold the baby like a package!"

In the dream, she tries to conquer the Oedipal rival, the man's wife. But the couple supports her in becoming an adult woman who has to find her own husband. The second man's gift of the lipstick can be interpreted as an affirmation of her femininity. As for the apples, she tells me that the ones hanging low in the tree were yellow, but she wanted only the green ones from the treetop. This makes her think of when as a girl she was offered the best piece of the chicken, after her father but before her mother and sisters. Little Franco claimed her privileges and got them. But then the second dream's stinking baby portrays her impotent suffering. She now seems ready to face the truth: neither seizing another man's wife or the best chicken piece, nor triumphing that I don't like her, is of any help. *She must get to know the stinking baby.*

I was shaken by her associations to the swaddling and wrote in my notes, "I have never witnessed so concretely the link between an infantile trauma and an emotional disorder in an adult". Was the swaddling a trauma per se? Of course, being swathed for nine months must be an unimaginable experience. Maybe there are moments when the swaddle feels comforting or supporting, but as soon as the baby wants to move or when sweat begins to trickle, feelings of panic, imprisonment, impotence, and a psychosomatic overflow must occur. Beyond the swaddling per se, another factor contributed to the genesis of trauma, namely what I would call an underdeveloped culture of containment in the family. Bianca could not force out empathy and containment from her kin. In this hopeless situation, she began experiencing the swaddle no longer as a sweaty and stinking bandage but as a hard but also libidinised shell which she used to exclude both concrete and psychic reality. It protected her from painful external stimuli and from internal disintegration.

The swaddle, plus the uncomprehending containment she encountered, prevented her from developing a Skin-Ego, *une moi-peau* (Anzieu, 1995).

Her skin was healthy and covered her body adequately, but she had dermal symptoms like blushing, sweating, and swaying between feeling hot and cold. In brief, I conceive of Bianca as a thin-skinned person protecting herself with a tough armour. The skin phenomena and her behaviour in sessions indicated that the swaddling and the childhood milieu had prevented her from building up a healthy psychological skin that would allow her to experience and handle her feelings and thoughts. Readers familiar with the work of Esther Bick (1968/2011) will recognise in Bianca "the development of a 'second-skin' formation through which dependence on the object is replaced by a pseudo-independence" (135).

Bianca's problems with her Skin-Ego or second skin explain, in my view, what often happened when she listened to me and felt understood. In a second, our interchange became dangerous because she felt as if being without skin. One saw this concretely when she shuddered and turned cold and warm in touching dialogues. We also saw it in roundabout ways when she got explosive, derogatory, and deriding with me – not because, as she said, I wanted to humiliate her but because *she felt exposed in her humiliation and excoriation*. This also explained why, after I had suggested these ideas to her and a session approached the end, she needed to collect herself at length. It was as if she must get dressed again, albeit with a second skin or with a ragged Skin-Ego.

Donald Meltzer (1967, 1992) and Meltzer and Harris-Williams (1988), the American-British psychoanalyst, was an important source of inspiration to me over the years. In a supervision session, I presented this hour to him. He emphasised that

> The important point for your patient is when the swaddle is removed. She experiences it as an exposure of her as a shitty, peeing and steaming baby – not as a situation where one cleanses her and takes good care of her. In her fantasy, she has been swaddled because of her violence, which must be controlled in a concrete and absolute way. Swaddling creates a sharp split between calm and violence, there exists nothing between swaddling and exposure as a pee-baby.

I concurred with Meltzer that for Bianca to enter my office was like having the swaddle ripped off.

> Yes, and your problem as analyst is that when you think about her instead of ripping off her swaddle, she feels exposed. This leads to violent comments and attacks on you. Even if the swaddle might make the baby feel safe against her own violence, it only increases her exasperation. Entering your office, which she unconsciously experiences as removing the swaddle, exposes all her accumulated violence. Then the war between the two of you starts and escalates.

Meltzer also linked the swaddling to Oedipal sceneries. In Bianca's imagination, the parental couple swaddled her to get away from their baby and be alone in lustful enjoyment. In the two latest dreams, she tries to become part of this couple by seducing a married man. But neither he nor his wife wants to play along, and in the second dream, Bianca must face the painful truth about her as a swaddled baby. But this proximity to her pain is brittle. In a second, she can transform her concordant identification (Racker, 1968) with the poor swaddle-baby into a complementary one, in which she craves to be penetrated and despises her shit-identity.

In this situation, the analyst's main challenge is to transform these models into elements she can use for thinking about her present life. For example, how can she feel that my suggestions are not excited and sadistic intrusions into her anus but *ideas* for her to consider? Many of our interactions have turned into fights, where she sees me as cruel, dismissive, or contemptuous. Then, thinking is out of the question, and she has no way out but to fight back. But as we also have seen, the golden possibility of encouraging her thinking is when she gets moved, speaks of someone or me being gentle to her, and then reacts aversively. If I manage to remain calm and reflecting and find a way of formulating her dilemma, and if I do this in the brief moment of opportunity between her emotive and angry states, then she may experience my comment as helpful and interesting.

A year before termination, I made notes that her exposed self was like a skin that was much more sensitive to love than to hatred and insults. She called it her "love allergy". What if it overwhelmed her and she couldn't go on working? What if she exposed her passions to me and I would think she's disgusting and sweaty, like that baby she fears so much? Also, exposing herself by taking off "the swaddle", namely removing her hard shell and talking earnestly about her passionate self, would lead to an emotional flooding and to death. Or at least this was what she feared.

I think today that I was not fully aware of the *concreteness* of her fears. True, we had reached a climate where she trusted my empathy when I spoke of the swaddling as detrimental to her. But in retrospect, I don't think we talked about the concreteness, even the lethal danger, of "feeling her feelings". The three words evoke W. R. Bion's (1962) concepts of the alpha- and beta-function and the contact barrier. They help us understand a clinical problem: Bianca's tendency to experience my interpretations as attacks or denigrations concealed another difficulty: *thinking* about her emotions was impossible and was replaced by experiencing them as material and nasty objects. When Bion writes that "both good and bad breasts are felt as possessing the same degree of concreteness and reality as milk" (34), "breasts" refer to emotional experiences that the infant can construe as things inside and outside of her. Bianca was sometimes in the throes of such psychic functioning. In Bion's terms, she was overwhelmed by beta-elements which, as we know, can be "remarkable for their concreteness" (55). Sweating, shivering, and jumping from the couch indicated that she felt inundated by such elements and must physically protect herself from them.

In retrospect, I think I was too preoccupied with conceiving of our communication as a traffic of projective identifications. As said, Bianca could meet interventions with "I know you're thinking that I want to become pregnant with you, all analysts think that way!" or "You think I'm talking nonsense!" Such words revealed her to be in the realm of projections ("you think...") and showed that she felt I was there as well. She took my interventions as proofs that I was discharging my malaise by projecting beta-elements onto her, and she retorted likewise. We could think of her swaddle as a deficient contact barrier that sometimes was working like a machine gun. It fired at any contact efforts from me or others. When this occurred, the contact barrier, a concept close to the Skin-Ego and the second skin, could not allow impressions to be transformed from beta-elements to alpha-elements. "Out with it" was her philosophy. And then she cried at her destruction and solitude.

The end of the analysis

Bianca's analysis lasted six years. The end was heralded by some remarkable changes in her life. She fell in love with a man, *George*, and they began a relationship where they talked seriously and empathically with each other about wishes, fears, and hopes for the future. This included sharing dreams of having children together. He was not prone to play anal games with her, neither in sex nor in other interchanges. Some dreams revealed her struggle of yielding to temptations of such games, but also a counterforce to them. This was one such dream:

Bianca: "I dreamt I was an officer, it was unclear if I was a man or a woman. I ordered my soldiers to rape children. Some refused because it was wrong to act like that. Then I dreamt that I pushed an oblong wooden piece into my anus. Ashamed, I did it on the sly, but George woke up. We talked and I remember he used the word 'vagina'".

There was thus a temptation of anal excitation with its components of domination, perversion, and cruelty. I think the officer and the soldiers who were prepared to obey his orders were partners in Bianca's anal world. But now she had another kind of partners, too: the soldiers who refused to rape children. She also partnered with George, who noticed her "tricks" and talked with her about them. He also showed that he coveted her vagina and not her anus. He represented a kind of man she had recently discovered: a man who wants children with a woman he loves, or a male colleague who compliments her work achievements without a secret plan of penetrating her behind. This gentle, concerned, and solicitous view of men was still developing.

She showed this in her recent decision to volunteer in a charity, which would have been way beyond her horizon some years earlier.

At the time of these dreams, termination was looming in the air. She felt content with what we had achieved in the analysis, and she had learnt to better understand the warning signals from the perverse corners of her mind and not to act them out on the spot. George got a new job in another part of the country, and they decided to move there and settle as a family. Some years later, I received a letter with a photo of her firstborn, a sweet girl. Bianca's love of her was translucent.

Bianca's critique

Some years later, Bianca asked to see me. The family's move had worked well, they had two children, and she was content with her new life and her relationship with George. She attributed these improvements to her analysis and was grateful for it. She recalled vividly her former lifestyle and how we talked about it in analysis. Our inflamed interchanges were well remembered and embarrassing to her, now that we talked about them. She remembered her accusations that I didn't care, that I despised her, laughed at her, and so on. But Bianca also wanted to criticise me for one particular thing.

Bianca: "I know that you did care for me in the analysis, otherwise I wouldn't have come here today. But there is one thing I feel you didn't understand… that I really COULDN'T talk to you sometimes, when I lay on the couch, thought of something, was sweating, jumping up and down. It was totally IMPOSSIBLE!"

Analyst: "You sound very serious, and I recognize the situations you are referring to. How do you think I responded to you then, in those impossible situations"?

Bianca: "You seemed to think that I COULD talk if I only stopped fussing. I know I was fussing, but I also told you, at least sometimes, that it was impossible to act otherwise. Then and there, I don't think you believed me but rather, 'pull yourself together, girl'."

Analyst: "I recall such moments, and how we talked about our divisions of roles. I was supposed to be excited and enraged, and then you could leave me because I was so cruel. Or the obverse, as when I said 'Either you talk, or you quit the analysis'. I guess you recall my menace and that I apologised for it. You have all reasons to be angry with me for my remark. But you seem to have come to talk about something else."

Bianca: "Sure I remember, and I know I was part of it by being provocative with you. But I'd say there was too much emphasis on this pattern and too little on the fact that I just COULDN'T talk to you."

Bianca was deeply earnest in trying to make me understand her critique. She was neither attacking me nor coercing an apology from me. Our few meetings ended with my thanking her for her sincerity and courage to voice her criticism and my resolve to think about it further. I felt she had an important point but could not verbalise it beyond her own formulations. What did she mean, that it was totally impossible to say what she had in mind? When fussy, she could indeed talk about my office, mien, clothes, voice, and so on. In other moments, it was impossible for her to speak at all.

How can we understand this paradox? To answer, let us move the emphasis one word to the right to discern another meaning. Instead of writing "I just COULDN'T talk to you", I will write "I just couldn't TALK to you!" In other words, "I couldn't talk to you, but I could communicate in many other modes". The shift highlights the disparity between verbal and nonverbal communication and the grey zone in between. Especially, experiences with PIP have familiarised me with reading embodied language in babies who are kicking, wringing, fidgeting, sighing, crying, and screaming. This occurred in therapies when parents had contacted me because they were desperate, despondent, and ashamed of their "failure as parents". Their complaints, too, often contained much nonverbal communication, such as changes in the tone of voice, facial expressions, tears, gestures, and eye contact.

These therapy situations of being subjected to communications that oscillate between the verbal and nonverbal – while I feel impotent, confused, and helpless – create a specific pressure in the countertransference. Though I may feel competent and experienced, at the same time I can feel stupid, ignorant, overwhelmed, and scared. To paraphrase Bianca, many times I have felt "I CAN'T understand what's going on!", which can be exasperating. Such countertransference pressure can reveal how a parent or baby is feeling, especially if I refer to our knowledge of how projective identifications work. With Bianca I used such knowledge, as when I discerned how I identified with internal objects that she projected on me, and thus I was supposed to assume the role of an excited and punishing anal intruder. Recognising such patterns enabled me to get into more of a concordant countertransference (Racker, 1968), which helped me exit such jams with Bianca. She conveyed that she had noted my persistence in investigating our respective parts in this "game", and she was grateful for it.

But Bianca insisted there was something I had *not* understood, and I now gather that she referred to her being overpowered by the "mute theatre" on and beyond the couch. I allude to her tapping on the wall, cracking her finger knuckles, sighing, sweating, being cold, being warm, sitting up, nipping my pot flowers, stroking my coat in the waiting room, sighing, giggling, and so on. This theatre has many similarities to PIP work with a distressed baby and her frustrated mother. The interchange between Bianca and me also contained much embodied communication on her behalf, whereas my own signals were more subdued – or I was less aware of them? I think Bianca's slap-bang changes may have dislodged my resonating analytic instrument (Balter, Lothane, & Spencer, 1980; Brown, 2009; Norman, 1994). This prevented me from disregarding, at least for the moment, her words and just looking at and "inhaling" her body language – and sensing the concomitant and resonant body movements in myself. In another mindset, I might have grasped that Bianca couldn't *talk* – but that she did express herself in other faculties. My notes are replete with observations of her nonverbal communications. Today, I would be more committed to addressing them with her, yet knowing that she might feel shamed by me and tempted to start a sadomasochistic squabble.

As I read my notes after more than 30 years, I am taken by Bianca's repetitive quarrels with her boyfriends and with me. I am also startled that after her first account of being swaddled, it took a long time before we set out to talk about it thoroughly. My notes are, of course, incomplete, but I still feel we both tended to avoid the swaddle theme via our sadomasochistic bickering. She had all reasons to avoid it since it evoked such agony. I would not state that I wanted to avoid it as well. The problem was rather that I had too little clinical experience with real babies and mothers. Or was the problem that I had too little contact with my "internal baby" or my Infantile? Was I afraid of it?

I would be foolish to answer, "I'm not at all afraid of my Infantile". Babies may be cute, but their minds harbour everything from bliss and joy to woe and grief. Remnants of these feelings and vague reminiscences rest in all of us and in me as well. My answer will follow another track, which will lead me to echo one of my major arguments for encouraging and inspiring analysts to include PIP in their practice. When we work with an adult patient, we meet several decades after the building blocks of his or her Infantile were laid down. We are really working *après-coup*. Though the patient may be immersed in today's qualms and crises, we know that the linchpin was driven into the patient's personality very long ago. Conversely, working with a baby and a mother is quite different even though we, so to say, tackle the same building. We confront their despair and helplessness here and now. Their drama is unravelled before our eyes while we are under pressure and forage for an idea, a comment, or a stance that might be of help.

I believe many therapists are attentive to their Infantile and also have come to understand it better through their training analyses, where the future analytic candidate can surrender his or her Infantile in the hands of the analyst. Starting a modern training in psychotherapy or psychoanalysis, the students will do infant observations that will bring out such layers in them, too, and make them even more acquainted with their Infantile. Yet infant observation does not entail the dare and responsibility of *treating* a baby and mother in therapy. In my view, there is a difference between doing training analysis and educational infant observations compared with parent – infant psychotherapy.

In PIP, one is confronted with a derailed mother – infant interaction and an urge to do something about it. Now! I argue that direct contact with babies – as a clinician in a position of responsibility – can be an essential asset for therapists or analysts, regardless of the age of their other patients. Such clinical contact with babies and parents goes way deeper than observing infants, reading about them as theorised in the psychoanalytic literature, or learning about the Infantile in one's personal analysis.

To sum up, *the study and practice of PIP treatments lead us to the earliest stages of life – especially situations of dyadic distress in various forms and backgrounds. Such experiences can influence therapies with adults in decisive ways.* This is a major reason for me to write this book.

Some late conclusions after the pre-PIP period

If we want to find traces of the Infantile in the patient, we cannot investigate it like a pathologist looking for a derailed cellular development in a sample. No, the "sample" is here, in front of us, with us, at times even like inside of us. In other words, we can find traces of the Infantile in a patient only if we can find similar, though not identical, traces in ourselves. The Infantiles of the two participants need to resonate to become visible and manageable. As Guignard (2022) puts it, when we are working with the Infantile, we need to shift our emphasis *"from the analyst to the analytic relationship*, and from the child to the Infantile" (4, italics added). This is no easy task since every analyst has blind spots, and his repressions "will draw into its wake not only the aspects of the Infantile in himself that did not find expression or remained unanalysed in his own analysis, but also what I shall call the basic components of his *Weltanschauung*" (8). Thus, the analyst needs to move from a hierarchical to a democratic view of therapy, from a clairvoyant to a probing vision of our task, and from seeing himself as a theatre director to a fellow actor on stage with the patient.

I have come to reevaluate my readings of post-Kleinian authors addressing pathological organisations (Rosenfeld, 1971), psychological retreats (Steiner, 1993), and the risk of reassurance (M. Feldman, 1993). I have learnt enormously from their writings and supervisions, not the least their sober eyes on the destructive relationships that can develop between analyst and analysand and turn into negative therapeutic reactions. The same goes for their insights of the load on the analyst who strives to become aware of his own contributions to the destruction. Here, Betty Joseph's (1989) contributions are groundbreaking as well.

My experiences of PIP and, as we have seen, adult patients like Bianca have demonstrated the baby's despair and extreme dependency on the caretaker – whether mother or analyst – to mitigate the distress. PIP babies have shown under my skin that their hopeless, terrible, and backbreaking behaviour, fantasies, and demands point to their helplessness and total desertion. My colleague Joseph Aguayo and I (Aguayo & Salomonsson, 2017) argue that Melanie Klein "downplayed the mother's impact and provided no model of how it works in interaction with the baby" (398). Perhaps, she did not have "a terminology to cover the interactions among external objects and how they impact on the participants' internal worlds" (399). It may be that her influence, so important to the cited authors and to me, has subdued the notion that treating babies could be valuable for more deeply understanding those interactions that they have described so persuasively.

It is all the more interesting that some publications by the authors just mentioned show an empathic interest in the "real baby's" suffering, namely in infantile trauma. I refer to articles on the Oedipus drama (Brenman, 1980; Steiner, 2018). Eric Brenman, with whom I was in group supervision in the nineties, shows great empathy with Oedipus's prehistory when his father left him to die in the wilderness as an infant. "It is difficult to imagine that any analyst would believe that he was furnished with a good enough environment or objects to deal with his problems at the start of life" (57). Steiner digs into the trauma when baby Oedipus had his ankles pierced and was left to die on Mount Cithaeron: "We no longer believe, as we used to do, that babies feel nothing and remember nothing. I think that we are obliged to assume that such trauma would have left a significant scar, both physical and psychological" (555).

Steiner finds it "remarkable that the trauma has not featured prominently in discussion of the Oedipus Myth" (555). This, of course, goes back to Freud, who used the myth to denote the child's desire for one parent and fear of the other's ire, something that in his view happens later than in infancy. In my terms, Freud overlooked the traumatised Infantile of Oedipus, whereas Brenman and Steiner acknowledge it and discusses its various repercussions in adult Oedipus. It will be interesting to one day investigate whether the "London post-Kleinians" were inspired by infant observation and observational research. In Chapter 10, I argue that this happened to an analyst of another tradition, Jean Laplanche, when he elaborated his notions of infantile sexuality and enigmatic messages.

The other side of the coin is to adopt a shallow, concrete, and mere empiricist view on infant development and interactions, a view that I am cautious about. We can, of course, observe what babies or patients are doing. But when it comes to understanding what goes on inside of them, we must go beyond sheer observation and also rely on guesswork, intuition, and, why not, the observer's countertransference. Especially the last of these factors is not consistently addressed by infant researchers such as Tronick, Stern, Trevarthen, and Feldman. My critique also concerns the absence of psychoanalytic concepts to formulate what may lie beneath the baby's overt behaviour in their observations. I miss concepts like a baby's conflict, defences, and sexuality.

To exemplify, Stern (1985) criticises Klein's postulates of "the infant's basic subjective experiences as consisting of paranoid, schizoid, and depressive positions. These assumed infantile experiences operate outside of ongoing reality perceptions. Here, too, the units of a genetic theory are fantasy-based" (254). To me, his critique is redundant: a theory of the baby's mind must rest on observations *and* on the fantasies of us adults who observe the child. If not, we are left with a dull vision of the infantile mind. Having seen so many babies, smiling and babbling happily or crying helplessly, I cannot doubt that in the first scenario, the baby had some notion of a good object, experience, worldview, World of Feelings, Mindscapes (Stern, 1990), or whatever we call it – whereas in the second he felt everything was "just bad". This pleasure/unpleasure dichotomy is a central pillar in psychoanalytic theory and, I argue, it is also observable in babies. To conclude, when I say I miss psychoanalytic concepts, my critique is not a mere question of terminology. I argue that to form viable imageries of what might go on in a baby's mind, we need a psychological theory that builds on the individual's emotional experiences. In my opinion, psychoanalytic theory meets these criteria, though, which goes without saying, it needs to develop further, not the least in the domain of the Infantile.

Bianca today

As I am preparing this book, Bianca contacts me, many years after the analysis. She says she leads a good and meaningful life, but she wants to talk to me about her concerns regarding one of her children. I bring in an observation here that refers to our discussion of containment and the swaddle. In the beginning of a consultation nowadays, she can suddenly become flooded with an emotional stir, often of warmth and contentment of seeing me. When speaking about her child, she can become worried or upset. She may also blush with tearful eyes. But I no longer see any reactive hostility or unbearable humiliation when something that I suggest to her yields a positive or negative emotion. In other words, her object relations, with me and others, have become much more stable and rewarding. True, she still has intense feelings, and one can see her efforts at subduing them with "psychological swaddling" as she gets in contact with her rage or tears. But it is as if a more healthy "psychological skin" quickly comes to her help and calms her down. This calm also implies that she can mentalise how she and the other are feeling and thinking.

Chapter 5

Parent – toddler therapy
Indications of the Infantile

If there is an Infantile in every one of us, this must apply to toddlers as well. An interesting topic of study would then be to what extent a toddler's mind is influenced by his surrounding and by his Infantile. If we compare the two groups of toddlers and babies regarding language, motor, and conceptual abilities, there are, of course, vast differences. But there are also similarities concerning their dependence on the parent's presence and support. When the latter fails, both baby and toddler can be distressed, though in disparate ways. As I met such toddlers in my consultant work at the Child Health Centre, I decided to transfer the parent – infant psychotherapy (PIP) method into parent – toddler psychotherapy. Some parents complained that their child was unruly, "hopeless", hot-tempered, and impossible to educate. Others spoke of children who were sad and subdued.

I invited some such parents to embark with me on a joint therapeutic setting including the child. It was often the mothers who participated with their child of two to four years of age. Joint therapies with mother and toddler confirmed a suspicion I had, based on my PIP experiences: what the mother had described as a symptom *within* the child could also be found to reside within *their relationship*, as exemplified in Chapters 3 and 8. Certain emotional signals of the child unleashed anxiety or embarrassment in her. Since such reactions had various roots and manifestations that were unconscious to her, she could neither perceive them nor do much about them. But the child noted her distress and became confused, and a vicious circle started spinning.

I was also struck by other events in sessions, which today I would name the trace of the toddler's Infantile. In other words, the unruliness and temper tantrums of today's toddler could sometimes be linked with early trauma that the parents had not been able to contain sufficiently. Sometimes, the child could suddenly make a little game, a drama, or a gesture that seemed linked – and this interpretation was shared by the mother and myself – to the early trauma. I wrote two articles (Salomonsson, 2014b, 2015a) of which one (2014b) is presented here in a reworked form.

DOI: 10.4324/9781003640363-5

As for the differences in development between babies and toddlers, I must take them into account when handling the therapeutic situation and forming my conclusions. Toddlers have a large vocabulary and are often quite proud of it as well! Does this imply that when a therapist addresses him in joint therapy, interventions will simply affect him directly, as in traditional child therapy without the parent's presence? At this point, I disagree. True, the toddler interacts visibly and audibly with his mother, and the interactions can be enjoyable and beneficial or distressing and difficult. The child is also aware of me and my interaction with him and the mother. This is also the case if he is in the middle of a temper tantrum à la "the terrible twos". If the therapist upholds the analytic setting (Meltzer, 1967), the child will discover, sooner than later, that "this guy is interesting, worrying, curious, nice, and threatening". In other words, the child's transference to the therapist is soon established and waiting to be contained.

Expressions like "the terrible twos" are evidently used by the parent and not the toddler, who might see things completely differently. He might define that period as "the time in life when I discovered the power of my body and emotions, as well as the powerlessness when I related to adults. Nobody understood me, and they always thought the worst of me". My fantasised quotation elucidates that communications of mother and toddler are frequently vibrant and misunderstood – or let's say they are interpreted very differently by the two parties.

The therapist therefore needs to consider the behaviours and reasonings of both as well as their interactions. In other terms, we need to consider the entire *system* of mutual regulation and care-taking (Seligman, 1999). Second, the toddler will understand far from all of the therapist's or the mother's words – that is, in their literal sense. Yet such dialogues seem to affect him. How does this come about? Might communicative modes other than the verbal be crucial for therapeutic action? If so, which are these modes and how sensitive is he to them? These questions will be addressed and illustrated in this chapter.

Just as in work with babies and mothers, when I embark on a mother-toddler therapy I invite adult and child as active shareholders. I do not talk explicitly in such terms, but my way of talking, listening, and playing with them indicates it. I establish the therapeutic frame from the start by clarifying what is allowed and what is not and what is the aim of our work: to explore the conscious and unconscious urges at the root of the present disorder. These urges will manifest via play, words, body language, tone of voice, and so on, whether they emanate from the child or the mother or both. When the two note my interest in such communications, they begin to understand what therapy is about. They also note my wish to contain their frightening or embarrassing urges, but they will also defend against displaying what is pestering them. When I interpret such fears, the anxieties of both parties often diminish. It will clarify to the toddler that therapy is not "playtime" and to the parent that it implies something else than expert guidance or advice.

Interpretations may explicitly address an emotion or conflict that I assume motivates a certain behaviour, or they can be made indirectly through puns or games with the child and/or the parent. Though interventions of the latter type are spontaneous and unpremeditated, they are based on a psychoanalytic understanding of the situation. The importance of containing the child's anxieties is inspired by Bion's work (1962, 1970); O'Shaughnessy (1988) and its applications to infant work (Norman, 2001). My mode of addressing the child is influenced by the technique of Melanie Klein (1961, 1975). I am also inspired by Serge Lebovici (2000) and Lebovici et al. (2002) to foster an atmosphere that is playful and not threatening. Compared with Klein's work as it emerges in her writings, my address seems more relaxed, probing, and inquisitive. Furthermore, the interplay between external and internal objects – mother, child, and interaction – is visualised in the session. This sometimes gives interpretations a more solid foundation compared with individual child therapy.

The therapeutic process in these treatments often unfolds in steps or shifts. I may observe, for example, that the child is screaming or the mother is distressed. I will then make assumptions about the corresponding internal objects and ask myself why they urge the child to scream. Could it be a mother object he is disappointed in, angry with, or longing for or a father object whom he wants near him or wishes to get rid of? I may also guess which representations are causing the mother's expression of distress. This procedure is comparable to any other psychoanalytically oriented therapy. Specific to a therapy with a toddler and a parent is that the two will affect each other, and both will be affected by my interventions, too. A suitable analogy for this setting and technique is *couple therapy* – although parent and child are developmentally far from each other.

The fact that the chapter focuses on the therapeutic moment-to-moment interchange does not invalidate that I also uphold a developmental perspective on the child. Compared with an infant, a toddler has a more secure sense of self and no longer depends on the parent's constant physical proximity. The exclusive relationship with the mother has often, but not always, waned a bit, and the father has long since emerged as another central character. The child's omnipotence and strong will reflect strivings to handle "the context of emotional closeness and autonomy" (Lieberman, 1992, 573). The drive towards separation and individuation (Mahler, Pine, & Bergman, 1975) is at its height, which sometimes makes it easier for the toddler to discern the therapist as unique and interesting. If the mother is present, he may appreciate when he feels the therapist is standing outside of his power struggle with her. But he may also be aversive, petulant, or scared when he suspects the therapist discerns his scary fantasies and, so he fears, condemns him.

Despite the toddler's determination to carve out an autonomous existence, he is still dependent on the parent. This implies a technical challenge; on the one hand, he masters language well enough to take part in individual child psychotherapy. On the other hand, there are two arguments for joint treatment: one is the toddler's anxiety of being alone with the therapist. The other is the benefits to a therapeutic process when we enable parent and child to work together. We will now see how such work is performed.

Eric: almost three and almost unbearable

Barbara, a woman of forty, arrives with her two sons at my office at the Child Health Centre. Walter is five years old, and Eric will be three in two months. The boys are playing calmly, and Eric is imitating his older brother's games. Barbara speaks of Eric's strong emotions. His temper tantrums put a strain on the family, and she deplores that she cannot give Walter enough attention. Eric looks happily at me and says, "I never angry". In contrast, Walter looks sad. Without warning, he throws a building block towards his little brother's head. Walter looks terrified, whereas Eric has not noted any danger and goes on playing cheerfully. While still in a state of shock after the near-accident, I sense how hard Walter tries to quench his rage against his irascible little brother. I also see that though Barbara is abashed and pained by her sons' behaviours, she is notably vague and half-hearted in supporting them and setting limits. The episode indicates the extent to which Eric's mood swings put a burden on all family members. I suggest that the parents come for a consultation the next week.

When I meet with the parents one week later, they are at the end of their tether. They talk about Eric's earliest weeks in life. After a normal delivery, he started vomiting profusely. After four weeks, a pyloric stenosis was diagnosed. Barbara also suffered from this condition during her infancy; the upper orifice of the stomach is constricted and obstructs the passage of food. Eric underwent surgical intervention. All went well, but emotionally these were terrible times. The father says, "Eric's first weeks feel like a fog. I couldn't help but getting angry with him. There wasn't a clean set of sheets in the house!" The mother nods in agreement. She was able to maintain breast-feeding and Eric was weaned at six months. At about that time, his mood changed. He would yell during mealtimes and throw his head back. Later, his rage was directed towards every family member. Eric's mother described how, by the age of two, he was "almost unbearable".

Finally, a health visitor asked me to see the family. In the interview, the parents noticed my interest in Eric's infancy and realised that they had never talked much about it. I suggested that his strong feelings perhaps emanated from these times. There were several reasons why I suggested that Eric's mother, rather than his father, take part in a joint therapy. Barbara's anguish when talking about her newborn's operation was glaring. She also seemed to identify with him, emphasising that as a baby, she had the same malformation and operation. Finally, the impressions from our first encounter loomed in the background; Barbara was pained by Eric's violence yet ambivalent in putting a stop to it. The parents agreed to this plan.

The first joint session: the operation is still present

Barbara arrives with Eric. His mood is quite different compared with our first meeting. He sits in her lap with a dummy in his mouth, clinging to her and avoiding my eyes. Mother reports, "He had seven fits of rage this morning, and I don't understand any of them!" I bring out two dolls and let one be angry, while the other is shaking her head saying she doesn't understand. Eric looks with interest, but when I point out that he is sucking the dummy, he becomes sullen.

Analyst to Eric: "You didn't like when I talked about the dummy, Eric... Mum told me that you yell a lot at home. Maybe you think she doesn't like you because of it... Maybe you also think that I don't like you, and that we are angry with you."

My comment is based on the assumption that Eric has begun developing a specific relationship with me since, when he entered my office, he seemed frightened and avoidant of me.

Mother to analyst: "Funny, he seems scared of you now, but this morning he smiled happily when I told him we would meet you today."

Analyst to Eric: "Yes, Eric, people can have many feelings, all at one go. You like me and you're afraid of me."

Eric clings to Mum and reaches for her blouse to seek her breast. At first, the atmosphere is romantic, and I recognise in the countertransference similar boyish feelings towards my mother. But then he curls downwards in her lap and stretches one leg upwards to coil around her neck, a bizarre scene where Eric regresses to function far below his three years. Barbara says, "perhaps I don't see Eric in his own right". She was in psychotherapy years ago and now suggests she has "projected things" onto him since he was a baby. This strikes me as a slightly artificial confession, but I get a more genuine impression when she speaks of her feelings at the time of his operation.

Mother, crying: "All these tubes and machines, it was terrible. I was scared he would die!"

Until now, Eric has been silent while sucking his pacifier. Now he starts looking and nodding at me as if confirming Mum's story. I bring out a doll and point to its stomach.

Analyst to Eric: "The doctors cut your tummy here. Mum was afraid you'd die. But you're a strong and healthy boy."

As I compare his size with that of the doll, I add: "In fact, you're nine times bigger."

Eric: "Jonny's bigger than me! He's my pal."

Analyst: "Yes, there's always someone who's bigger. Mum was so afraid you'd die but now you're almost as big as Jonny."

As we compare our sizes, Eric adds: "You're bigger than me."

Analyst: "I am. I wonder how small you were when the doctors cut your tummy."

Mother shows how tiny Eric was at the operation. She notes his interest and tries to take out his pacifier. Eric protests and starts clinging again. This episode is the first of many to follow in which his emotional state oscillates in parallel to that of his mother or myself. When his mother authentically expresses feelings and memories from the hospital, and when I use the doll to explain the surgery and her feelings, Eric lets go of her body and becomes alert and curious. Nonetheless, her effort shortly afterwards at taking away the pacifier fails, and Eric regresses immediately.

Barbara explains how she has always felt sorry for him and now links this to the similar operation in her infancy. "This is why I've always felt close to him, much more than with Walter." She wonders if this has made her too indulgent with Eric. She moves on to describing her own childhood: a stern bourgeois life with mother, stepfather, and grandmother. Her father lived abroad, and the parents never lived together. She visited him regularly and describes the pain in commuting between two cultures with divergent values and habits.

By now I conceive of the psychodynamics of Eric's fits of rage and clinging as follows: Mother's congenital malformation and operation have always been part of her family canon. I think of it as a primally repressed trauma or an implicit memory in her. In contrast, her memories of Eric's operation are explicit and excruciating. As for the emotional experiences of her own operation, I speculate they are obscured in her Infantile. Combining them with her recall of Eric's operation, she has come to see him as a traumatised victim. The overall result is her overindulgence with him.

We discover another source: the acrimonious memories of her stern upbringing: "I want to give Eric love and warmth, instead of the admonitions my mother provided."

Eric relishes mother's affective intensity and protests when she hinders his efforts at separating from her. As for Eric's intensity, we might attribute it to the operation with the separation implied as well as the mother's difficulties in containing his anxieties at the time. Another factor is the father's panic and vexation with his vomiting son, which likely left mother distressed and missing his support. Could we conceive of Eric's Infantile as consisting of memory traces of him puking, pained, and scared? I don't know. I feel more certain that he grew up in a climate where his distress, whether we call it somatic or emotional, was met by an annoyed and worried father and a mother who was panic-stricken by the recap of her own infancy that she felt was going on. No matter how much the parents sought to comfort him in his panic of vomiting and tummy aches, their containing efforts must have been stained by their panic – and this would have affected Eric's ability to contain himself. This problem was clear to see: as soon as anything disturbed him, he could but yell and crave.

The second joint session: two lovers

Mother and son arrive for their second joint session. She is carrying him with his overcoat on and a pacifier in his mouth; once again, a rather bizarre scene.

Mother: "I've been thinking...I get into a state of alert as soon as he's whining, and I complain that he can't separate from me. But it's me who can't separate from him! Maybe he's angry because he wants to free himself from me and I won't allow it."

While his mother is speaking, the boy is peering at me cautiously. Mouthing his dummy, he orders Mum to make room behind her back in her chair. This leaves no space for her, and she moves to another chair. Now he indicates that he wants to sit in her new chair, and she lifts him over to her again. A sensual atmosphere develops as he fingers the buttons of her cardigan.

Analyst to Barbara: 'To me, that looks more like a husband tending to his wife.'

Barbara gives an embarrassed laugh and starts talking about her youth. She was in therapy and studied at university while living close to her father in his hometown abroad.

Mother: "What happened to my life? All my ambitions as a youngster, I just let them disappear! Today I live like a housewife from the fifties. It's not my husband who wants it like this. I guess it has more to do with my mother. She was a professional woman, but so inaccessible and intellectual. I don't want to be like her."

Analyst: "Eric, you're clinging onto Mum. You're fingering her cardigan, as if she belongs to you…You like her, but I think you're angry with her as well. You want to be a big boy like Johnny and the other guys at preschool, but Mum's holding you back. I think you and I should try to help Mum grow up. Do you want to?"

Eric nods eagerly.

Analyst: "OK, so what about you coming the next time without a dummy?"

Eric nods again.

The third joint session: struggling with the dummy

It is the third session with Mum, and Eric arrives without a dummy. Soon he starts yelling: "Dummy, dummy, I want my dummy!" After some minutes of unbearable yelling, Barbara says this is just like the temper tantrums at home. I suggest she give him the dummy, and Eric calms down while sneering at me.

Analyst to Eric: "I guess you're angry with me since I said you'd come without the dummy."

I get the impression that Eric is nodding. Barbara continues reflecting.

Mother: "Strange, not only did I study abroad. I also took painting lessons. Now my paintbrushes have all dried up. It's sad."

I bring out a sheet of paper and draw a line in the middle. On the right-hand side, I draw a big building and an easel. On the left-hand side, a dummy and a lot of threads, like a ball of cotton waste.

Analyst to mother: "You put your passions and interests in quarantine, especially after you became pregnant with Eric. Now you maintain your confinement by claiming he is a three-year-old baby, like when you carry him around with his overcoat indoors." I point to the right-hand side of the drawing: "University, art lessons, all is gone! The other, messed-up side in you, reigning at home, is flooding you. You don't know how to get out of it."

The boy listens as he watches mother reflecting. He lets go of his dummy and puts it in the pocket of Mum's jeans. After a while, he takes it out again and comments, "It's a dummy". Then he puts it back in her pocket again.

Analyst to Eric:	"When you came to me today, you wanted the dummy. You were angry with me. Now you let go of it and put it in Mum's pockets. Maybe you're done with it."
	Eric shakes his head at first but then nods in seeming agreement.
Analyst:	"You took out the dummy again. I guess you were angry with Mum and me about the dummy. You wanted it back but changed your mind again."
	Eric shakes his head while caressing Mum's hair: "I like Mum!"
Analyst:	"Yes, you like her – especially when you can rule over her and she does what you tell her to do... But when she's not like that you get angry."

The fifth joint session: Eric's mother is angry with me

Two sessions later, Barbara describes her emotionally restrained mother and her father abroad who wanted her to be chic and marry. Meanwhile, Eric is sitting in her lap. She is angry at feeling imprisoned in her two parents' homes during childhood. It was hard to commute between them, their atmospheres being so different. At present, she is about to apply for a job of organising aid and education for needy children.

At this point, Eric jumps out of her lap to sit on a chair higher than his mother's. He throws the dummy through the opening between its seat and back support, picks it up again, and repeats the game. Meanwhile, he is observing me and looking content and proud. He tells me that he and his family went to a party, and there was a clown and a ghost. The ghost was scary. "But it was cool, too!" Barbara adds that she objects to my suggestion that Eric let go of his dummy.

Mother to analyst:	"We agreed with Eric to give the dummy to Santa Claus at Christmas. We shouldn't let go of it for your sake but for Eric's!"

As the mother is criticising me, Eric makes thumbs up signalling, "I like this". He also nods as if agreeing with his mother's protest. We all smile at this scene. The hour is drawing to a close, but Eric says he wants to stay in my office, "till it gets dark, well no, the whole week!"

À la recherche d'un Infantile brouillé

Marcel Proust's novel *À la recherche du temps perdu* (*In Search of Lost Time*) occurs to me as a fit analogy for therapeutic work with Eric and Barbara and many other patients in the book. Importantly, in Eric's case, his Infantile had become *brouillé*, muddled by several factors. His mother had been unable to assume a more contained, as well as containing, perspective on little Eric and his operation. Probably, this was due to her own operation in infancy plus a corner in her personality where she had not managed to settle with her stern and conventional upbringing. Eric's father was also battered by the drama of the pyloric stenosis and annoyed with the tantrums.

Therapy with Eric and mother could not magically undo what had long since passed. But it could change the Infantile *brouillé* to something more of *éclairci*, clear. Several rapid shifts occurred in Eric's and Barbara's interactions. The first took place when she spoke about his operation. The second was when I suggested to Eric that we should help mother grow up so that she would not stop him from becoming a big boy. The third happened when I made a drawing to illustrate her resentment of having given up her interests in academia and art. The fourth was Barbara's disclosure that she was applying for a job and that she was angry with my suggestion about the dummy.

To phrase it as a paradox, *I helped Eric grasp and come to terms with his infantile behaviour, which helped him manage his Infantile much more clearly.* As long as he was yelling, clinging to mother, and insisting on the dummy, his Infantile was covered by layers of various defences. The outcome was incomprehensible to his parents and himself. True, memories of the operation during his infancy swirled in the mother's mind, but when we talked about them, they were of no help to her or Eric. What he did react to was something else. At first, he disliked my questioning of his regressive defence strategies, but he also became engaged when I suggested there was something in him that he could not get a hold of and that disturbed him. In such scenes, Eric stopped whining and clinging and became serious and listening, or playful and inventive, and his verbal and body expressions were easier to interpret. In short, he abandoned a regressive state and moved to a more advanced level of functioning. Parallel shifts took place in mother as she moved from her anxiety about his operation to her anger with her life as a housewife – and with me about the dummy.

If we wish to further theorise about the therapeutic interactions, we could conceive of them as unconscious communications between mother and son. According to Freud (1915b), "the Ucs. [Unconscious] of one human being can react upon that of another, without passing through the Cs [Conscious]". Two individuals in such interchange do not know what they are communicating or that they are communicating at all. As long as it is unconscious, words play a subordinate role – at least as bearers of lexical meaning. To understand the traffic, we might refer to concepts like projective identification and countertransference, but that would merely beg the question and force us to explain how such processes function. Analytic literature contains many references to unconscious communication, as when Rucker and Mermelstein (1979) claim that it is "the most basic and perhaps the most powerful level of human contact [...] the quality of any human interaction reflects a system of unconscious cues and counter-cues" (150). The question, however, is *how* this traffic of cues actually works.

True, it is not easy to decide more precisely which constituents in the therapy caused the shifts. In a broad sense, I understand therapeutic action as coming about through work with both Eric and his mother. The interventions had actually similar aims for both: to lift repressed notions and thus to make the participants become aware of feelings that are truer to themselves. A parallel aim was to help Eric and Barbara to express these feelings unequivocally. Thus, I addressed her about the incongruity when she complained she hadn't enough "integrity" in life while she accepted that Eric was coiling his leg around her neck. She "woke up" and got embarrassed since her infantile sexuality – a concept explored in Chapter 10 – was put on the table. She then became annoyed with her housewife life and said she wished to resume her youthful ambitions. Such a sequence reflects everyday therapeutic work, and its mode of action needs little further explanation. However, the action on Eric is harder to understand. As I addressed his sensuous beleaguering of Mum and anger when she barred him from becoming a big boy, he listened and nodded attentively – but why? What did he perceive in the therapeutic interchange and how did it affect him? The next section will focus on this question.

Therapeutic action in mother – toddler therapy – various perspectives

In the original paper on Eric and Barbara (Salomonsson, 2014b), I had tried to grasp how the prompt shifts in Eric came about. My model then included neuro-scientific and psychological research on emotional communication. I underlined that such studies were based on experiments rather than therapeutic interactions. Accordingly, they observed events from the outside and refrained from speculative interpretations. These caveats foreboded what was to become an important focus of my research, this time in collaboration with Tessa Baradon, Evrinomy Avdi, Michelle Sleed, and Keren Amiran in *The Layered Analysis Group*. Our assumptions and findings in our studies of the interactions in the PIP setting will be summarised in Chapter 9.

What follows is a sketch of my earlier efforts at understanding therapeutic action in joint therapies with babies and toddlers. Today, my views on the topic have developed. Yet I have included some earlier ideas below because they provide some interesting data that we can apply to the therapy situation.

What I did not realise in the original paper was that we must consider interactions with *every* participant in the session, and I now concede that I did not pay full attention to *the therapist's* communication. Also, I had only begun to appreciate videorecordings of parent – child therapies as an investigative tool. This changed with entering the Layered Analysis Group.

Let us return to Eric. The question remains through which channels his internal world was affected, such as when his mother voiced her vexation with me or when I spoke to her or to him. As for the literal meaning of my words, he understood quite a few. However, many terms and ideas in my comments to this mother were incomprehensible to him: university, painting class, housewife, and so on. Evidently, other communicative modes affected him as well. What were these modes and how did they manifest in the session?

To my knowledge, there are no detailed observational research studies on the interactions between toddlers and parents in joint psychotherapy. In contrast, adult behaviours have been studied experimentally, and there also exists studies on interactions between therapists and their adult patients. The experimental studies are, however, quite different from how therapy works. To exemplify, when adult subjects subliminally observe another person's face, they adjust their own facial muscles according to the emotion that they see (Dimberg, Thunberg, & Elmehed, 2000). When they perceive a happy face, smiling muscles are activated, and exposure to an angry face activate frowning muscles. It is almost as if the subjects become happy or angry for real. The face mirrors our emotions, and we become affected by others' faces though often without being aware of it.

Such behavioural observations are included in the Layered Analysis method as seen in Chapter 9. But the method comprises a crucial addendum: we must study the participants not only "from the outside" but also "from the inside"; that is, we need listen to the therapist's countertransference accounts and to combine the two perspectives to understand more deeply why and how changes in the emotional climate unfold in sessions.

If we want to find research studies to understand how Eric, Barbara, and I behaved in the referred vignettes, we are thus left in the lurch. But although Dimberg et al. do not explain their findings in psychoanalytic terms, I think we can rely on their results that facial reading relies on the capacity for empathy; people who are good at understanding emotions react to facial expressions in a stronger and more varied way. These researchers also suggest that "important aspects of emotional face-to-face communication can occur on an unconscious level" (Dimberg et al., 2000, 88). To repeat, these studies concern adults who were not in therapy, but I suggest that Eric and Barbara, who were close emotional partners since birth, were expert readers of each other's facial emotional communication. I propose he perceived when Mum's face moved from constrained cheerfulness to honest sadness about the operation or when she explicitly showed her anger at me about the dummy.

When her words, gestures, tone of voice, and facial expressions were clarified in therapy, they united to form a more consistent message. I further propose that this made him perceive her as less opaque and unintelligible. These moments diminished his anxiety and helped him make a progressive move.

These speculations would be better supported if psychotherapy research, rather than lab experiments, could demonstrate connections between facial communication and emotional experience in therapeutic situations. In fact, such research today focuses on patient – therapist facial interactions, and even how it is correlated with therapeutic outcome (Peluso & Freund, 2018). German and Austrian researcher-psychoanalysts have videorecorded interactions between therapists and patients (Benecke & Krause, 2005; Benecke, Peham, & Bänninger-Huber, 2005; Dreher, Mengele, Krause, & Kämmerer, 2001; Krause, 2010; Krause & Merten, 1999). Their research helps us to better understand therapy process, but since it concerns adult patients, it falls outside the scope of this book. However, one point is essential: Krause and Merten underline that it is the *unconscious* conflicts that are "dramatically choreographed in a condensed form" (107) in therapy. Unconscious communication seems to come about without passing the conscious system but rather via swift and subtle facial movements. Also, they showed that if facial interchanges in and between therapist and patient varied in a lively and complementary way and according to the emotional content of the conversation, outcomes were clearly better. Similar and extended results were found by a Swiss group (Paulick et al., 2018) emphasising the role of synchronous movements of therapist and patient.

Facial reading in infant and toddler research

We could now ask if the referred results on adult subjects are relevant to infants and toddlers. I suggest that swift and unconscious transfers of facial and bodily emotional expressions occur between therapy participants, as in sessions with Eric and his mother. Abundant research indicates how even infants can perceive and respond accurately to another person's affective state. From only a few months of age, babies differentiate between various facial emotions (Reddy, 2008; Nadel and Muir, 2005). Even very young children "experience emotions as shared states and learn to differentiate their own states partly by witnessing the resonant responses that they elicit in others" (Decety, 2010, 261). When this resonance is violated, as in the still-face paradigm (Adamson & Frick, 2003; Tronick et al., 1978), infants only a few months old often react aversively.

In contrast to babies, toddlers have developed a theory-of-mind-like processing, which allows them "to entertain several perspectives and a decoupling mechanism between first-person and second-person information" (Decety, 2010, 259). Eric, almost three years of age, can read many emotional subtleties in his mother's face and build a model of her as a separate person – even while being entangled with her. As stated earlier, he fails to fully understand many words in the interchange between his mother and me. But other components in our communication affect him.

Such impact was further investigated by a group under Joseph Campos (Campos, Walle, Dahl, & Main, 2011). In their visual-cliff experiment, 12-month-olds were subjected to a frightening situation: crawling across an acrylic glass shelf covering a precipice. If a mother at the other side of the cliff expressed joy or reassurance, most babies crawled across it to reach her. In contrast, if she posed fear or anger, very few babies crossed the cliff. A video is shown on YouTube (Campos, 2014). The baby by the glass sees mother's face as if she were indicating, "This is dangerous". He hesitates: "How am I going to act"?

Researchers (Walle & Campos, 2014) have registered a shift in the children's perceptivity at around 18 months: at this age, toddlers start distinguishing authentic from fake emotional displays. If the adult displays affects in an inauthentic way, the child gets into an emotional conflict. Thus, "emotion regulation involves the management of conflicting goals... between the goals of one person and those of another, and, on occasion, a conflict between the goals of a single person" (Campos et al., 2011, 28). To manage such conflicts implies arriving at a "negotiated outcome" (28). For this to come about, both participants need to communicate as clearly and unequivocally as possible. But when Barbara complained about Eric's tantrums and did little to stop them, or when he said he loves Mum while coiling his leg around her neck, their communication was muddled and confusing. In the therapeutic process, this kind of interchange must be clarified, and its unconscious determinants must be interpreted.

Summary of an unfinished puzzle

To understand therapeutic action in mother-toddler therapy, we saw that cure does not come about through mere interventions to the mother which then secondarily affect the boy. Direct therapeutic work with him is also essential, and the chapter investigated his assets for perceiving, interpreting, and progressing in sessions. I also brought out *unconscious communication* for understanding the "what and how" in the therapeutic communications. But unfortunately, this concept does not explain *how* messages from such levels of the mind are transferred to another person.

I therefore invoked research demonstrating that already babies react to alterations in the adult's emotional communications. These findings enabled us to bypass the objection that young Eric could not be affected by the adults' words because he did not fully understand them. Instead, he seemed to be affected by their shifts in facial, bodily, and auditory communication of emotions. My interventions, as well as the mother's emotional reactions, were thus perceived by Eric through these para-verbal channels and induced progressive shifts in him. Beyond this description of the impact on Eric, we should emphasise that mother and son interacted and changed according to the other's behaviour and to each other's present states of mind. In the child *and* in his mother, changes were elicited only partly through verbal communications. We must also consider the influence of gestures, sighs, laughter, frowns, crying, smiles, and so on that emerged in the session. Indeed, there is much for the therapist to consider in such a complex and elusive process.

As for the therapist, today I would also stress more that my influence, just like that of Barbara and Eric, ranged from the verbal to the nonverbal. As an example, take the scene where Barbara objected to my suggestion that Eric let go of his dummy. It mattered not only how *she* embodied her critique but also how *I* embodied my response. When Eric made thumbs up, he was perhaps signalling, "I like this, I want to keep my pacifier". In addition, he may have felt,

> I like how the two of you settle a conflict. You can talk about it without getting afraid. That's good to see, especially for a guy like me. Before, I saw no other way of settling clashes than by screaming.

Clinical epilogue

The treatment lasted fifteen sessions. In the last session, Eric asks, "Doctor Björn, why do you have a Band-Aid on your finger?" I answer that I happened to cut it. He recalls when we put a plaster on his finger during a session. He adds that Dad once cut his finger in the kitchen and that his big brother broke his arm. At this point, Barbara reaches for her own arm, indicating her deep identification with her sons. He sees my bike helmet and asks why it is there. I answer and he tells me proudly about his Ninja swords at home. The session continues on these lines: a world where castration looms but benevolent figures help him with guidance and plasters on his road to becoming a man. What Dolto called the symboligenic castration (Dolto, 1984) had now become accessible to Eric. It was fun, thrilling, and a bit creepy when we were sharing the dangers of castration, such as talking about cutting one's finger. To participate in this dialogue obviously made Eric proud and relieved. It was better to talk with me like this than to live in a world where he must avert concrete threats. I refer to the fears that when he was yelling, his parents would probably be angry at him.

In the context of our focus on the Infantile, this interchange shows the gains of analysing it as early as possible. After a normal delivery, Eric started vomiting due to a pyloric stenosis, just like his mother did in her infancy. Anxiety in the family was mounting, Eric became a fussy baby, and his parents were helpless. He became rowdy, screaming, and with endless temper tantrums. When the parents said that he was now "almost unbearable", this shows the extent of the family conflicts. They led to further escalations, because though the parents understood preconsciously that the stenosis and its aftermath played a role, they did not know how and thus could not tackle it. One way of describing the therapy gains is that it made Eric more conversant with his anguish and anger and more aware that there were adults who wanted to understand him and talk with him about it. This way, I think he avoided having a part of his Infantile becoming petrified into an attitude of quarrelsomeness or fear of his anger. I do not know if his Infantile contains such a trace even today, but I would hope – and even claim – that he is better equipped to deal with it than if he had not worked with his mother and me in therapy.

As the hour is about to end, Barbara watches Eric in amusement and warmth. She tells me it is time to leave. "One can go on in therapy forever, but that makes no sense," she says. I ask Eric what he thinks, and he responds clearly, "I wanna quit. It's boring here." I let him know that it is OK with me. His mother broaches another topic with me, and Eric gets impatient with her. Barbara tells him distinctly to calm down. I bring out two crayons and say, "Here are my Ninja swords. Wanna fight?" We fence a little with them. "My sword is the best!" he claims. His mother, who early in therapy claimed that Eric must not play with "war toys", now looks proudly at her battling son. As they leave, Eric wants to shake hands with me.

Eric: "I grab your hand hard!"
Analyst: "You sure do, Eric. Goodbye!"
Eric: "Goodbye Björn!"

Source

This chapter is a reworked version of a published paper, (Salomonsson, 2014b). I thank the publisher for giving permission to quote it in the book.

Chapter 6

When the Infantile disrupts intimacy

When people speak of intimacy, they commonly mean that they have reached and enjoyed the innermost of a loved one. The word can be defined as a "process by which a dyad – in the expression of thought, affect, and behaviour – attempts to move toward complete communication on all levels" (Hatfield, 1982, 271). But Klein (1975) stated that this is a chimera. "A satisfactory early relation to the mother... implies a close contact between the unconscious of the mother and of the child" (301) – but this does not imply a complete communication. Later in life, we love to

> Express thoughts and feelings to a congenial person, [but] there remains an unsatisfied longing for an understanding without words – ultimately for the earliest relation with the mother. This longing contributes to the sense of loneliness and derives from the depressive feeling of an irretrievable loss.
>
> (301)

Already in this quote, we grasp that intimacy and the Infantile have much in common. Both comprise mother-child relations, fusion, and nonverbal communication. This chapter will investigate how relational distress between mother and baby may hamper the development of intimacy in a child.

Intimacy, as I prefer to use the term, implies uniting with someone in understanding and love – but also accepting the loss and loneliness that a relationship inevitably entails. I conceive of it as a movement but not a state, a dance but not a fusion. As Klein also understood, intimacy builds up in infancy. But what happens if the intimate dance between mother and baby gets jagged and unrhythmical? How would that alter the child's development of affection, understanding, and other abilities? To tackle these and other questions, we first need reflect deeper on what intimacy means.

We are all fruits of intimacy as we are conceived – though far from always – in an act of love and hope. Once conception is accomplished, threats to the future parents' intimacy sneak into the marital bed. Seeds of jealousy, fears

DOI: 10.4324/9781003640363-6

of responsibility, and the threat of losing the foetus mingle with shared joyous prospects. The anonymous inhabitant is thus destabilising the internal worlds of the parents. They need to uphold the equilibrium between narcissism and libidinal love, autonomy and dependence, love of life and fear of death. The expectant mother must also adjust her image of a body that behaves in mysterious and sometimes also painful and even precarious ways. The father's narcissistic equilibrium is also endangered, but he may seek to deny this as long as the baby is "just inside her'". Later, such self-deception will crumble when the baby screams through the night, breastfeeding doesn't work, and he must change the diapers for the nth time.

The menace to intimacy is also posed by the awakening of infantile sexuality (S. Freud, 1905b). During pregnancy, the mother's bodily alterations challenged her autonomy ("Who's running my life, me or 'it' inside me?") and sexuality ("What does 'it' do to my body and my passions?"). Then the newborn comes crawling on her body; sniffing, licking, sucking, peeping, and pooing. There is little room for adult sexuality now that a tiny but insistent lover has appeared, and her partner has become a hollow-eyed guy googling at night-time on infant rashes. If intimacy is born in a close contact between the unconscious of mother and child, this implicates the infantile sexuality of both parties. As shown in Chapter 10 here and in studies by Jean Laplanche (1989, 1999b, 2007b), unresolved issues with infantile sexuality can disturb the child's development of intimacy. As presented in Colin's case in Chapter 1, upheavals in the father's infantile sexuality may also emerge and cause concern.

Another menace to the development of intimacy is postnatal depression, which is more common among mothers than among fathers, and which is often seen in dyads with infant distress and attachment difficulties (Field, 2010; Grace & Sansom, 2003; Murray & Cooper, 1997; Tronick, 2007b). The mothers can be low-keyed or anxious about the baby's well-being. They feel worthless, unable to love or feel intimate with the child, which makes guilt ever-present. They tend to be disengaged or intrusive with the baby (Cohn & Tronick, 1989), who may protest or look away. Their "primary maternal preoccupation" (Winnicott, 1956) has not turned out well, and this "very special psychiatric condition" (302) implies suffering and a decreased sensitivity to the child.

The sources of this chapter are three research interviews with a little girl and her mother who took part in an outcome study of PIP (Salomonsson & Sandell, 2011a, 2011b; Winberg Salomonsson, Sorjonen, & Salomonsson, 2015a, 2015b) followed by an account of a psychotherapy when the girl had started school. The mother-infant interviews were made by me, whereas the child interview at 4½ years and a later therapy with the child were made by Majlis Winberg Salomonsson. She is my wife and a child psychologist and psychoanalyst.

In 2005, I launched a randomised controlled trial that compared results of mother – infant psychoanalysis (MIP; Norman, 2001, 2004) with standard treatment at Child Health Centres (CHCs) in the families' neighbourhoods. The infants' mean age was five months at start. MIP sessions were offered more often than is done in PIP: a median value of 2.5 per week and a median of 23 altogether. The comparison treatment implied regular visits to CHC nurses. In about one third of these cases, nurses also instituted brief parallel psychological support and treatment, which thus was part of treatment as usual (Lojkasek, Cohen, & Muir, 1994). Results in favour of MIP were found (Salomonsson & Sandell, 2011a, 2011b) on mother's self-reported depression, general psychological distress, parental stress, and externally rated sensitivity to the child's signals. This led to a follow-up study when the children had reached 4½ years of age. Apart from collecting mother-report questionnaires of depression, psychiatric health, and child's social-emotional functioning, the children were now interviewed by Winberg Salomonsson and the mothers by me. Effects to the advantage of MIP on the children's social functioning and their interviewer's "ideal types" classifications – but not on the other measures – were now found at 4½ years.

One of the 80 participants was *Annie*, whom I met when she was five months old and then followed up until 4½ years. In the first interview, she and her mother were randomly assigned to the comparison group at their local CHC. Much later, at six years, her mother phoned me because she worried about her child. I understood the girl needed psychological help and because the study was over, I thought the best thing was to suggest that she contact an experienced child therapist. She replied that Annie, during one of her tantrums, spoke about seeing "that lady". After a while, Donna understood she meant her interviewer, Majlis WS. We agreed that the parents should meet with her for a discussion. This led to Annie's child therapy of one and a half years with Majlis WS.

A few years later, in 2017, we were invited as keynote speakers to the International Psychoanalytical Association (IPA) congress in Buenos Aires. Its theme was "Intimacy", and we thought our contacts with Annie and her mother would furnish excellent material for a discussion of that topic (Salomonsson & Winberg Salomonsson, 2017). The unique assets to the study were our videorecorded interviews with Annie and Donna at five and eleven months and at 4½ years plus the notes from her child psychotherapy at six to seven years of age. This enabled us to study how her object relations developed and how her behavioural and emotional problems could be understood and possibly relieved. The therapy laid bare threads of how Annie's Infantile were entangled and pestered her with unhappiness, loneliness, and tantrums. We could then, through recordings of the earlier interviews, follow the threads back to her prehistory. We also got glimpses of her mother's Infantile and indirectly of her maternal grandmother's.

Five months: first research interview

I'm no good at this parent-child thing! I don't like being off work, just rolling the pram. Guess I feel guilty. I know I'm not politically correct. I can't compensate by working even harder! I didn't feel well at the end of pregnancy. The doctor recommended a sick leave. I told him I don't have time. 'That's just your problem', he replied. Delivery wouldn't start so I had an emergency caesarean. The wound got infected, I was quite absent the first six weeks [laughs a little]. That 'immediate mother – baby-contact' never appeared. The girl never liked breast-feeding, throwing herself backwards like an angry starfish. I fantasized throwing her out of the window. Everybody is endorsing breast-feeding, but there's no scientific evidence that it's better than bottle-feeding! When my husband resumed his job I panicked. Being alone with the baby…

Donna claims her real problem is that she cannot fulfil societal expectations about maternal happiness. She switches between transitory depressive realisations of an agonizing relationship with Annie and lengthier periods when she, in a more schizo-paranoid (Klein, 1946) mode, accuses society of extorting erroneous attitudes in mothers. Yet she realises "that at one phase in life one has to go through this thing about someone being totally dependent on you". Donna speaks about her relationship with Annie. As said above, the interviewer is Björn S.

Donna:	"It's a functional relationship. I'm the one who understands her needs."
Interviewer:	"How do you think Annie would respond if I asked her?"
Donna:	"'I think she'd say Mum has too little patience, she is split and absent-minded [caricaturing her daughter] 'Mummy, I want attention ALL the time!'"
Interviewer:	"What about your relationship with your husband?"
Donna (tearful):	I'm very fond of him. I wish I had such emotions with Annie."

Donna's love for Annie surfaces only with difficulty. She detaches herself from the sensual aspects of motherhood and restricts it to a societal duty, which probably is an effort at ridding herself of guilt. When guilt becomes too weighty, she projects it onto society, stating that it is rigid and overly demanding. Annie is a child that was planned and longed for, but pregnancy came as a shock. If a mother needs to negate her own mind and offer the baby her "unimpinging subjectivity" (Gentile, 2007, 556), this clashes with Donna's worldview. Like every mother (Harris, 1997), Donna is quite annoyed with her "occupant" but cannot integrate such feelings with love and warmth that she also feels. She then speaks of her mother:

Donna: "We've a very close and frequent contact... Well, I've an academic education but my parents haven't exactly read Strindberg... My Mum is hasty and doesn't think things through. I asked her if she thought anything special when she had me. She looked at me as if I was a Martian: 'Was I supposed to think anything special? I just did what I did'."

Yet Donna feels that Mum's carefree attitude cheers up her own more sombre nature. I sense, however, that her quick-witted and chatty language rarely dips down into painful emotions.

Five months: first research video

Donna's emotional availability (Biringen, Robinson, & Emde, 1998) was assessed by "blind raters" from a 10-minute video, where I asked her to be with Annie like at home. It shows her limited sensitivity. Her tempo is too fast for a baby. Facing the girl's distress, Mum decides it must be due to "fart or poo-poo". One gets the impression of an intrusive identification (Meltzer, 1992; Meltzer, Milana, Maiello, & Petrelli, 1982), through which Donna seeks to depose unlovable and disgusting aspects of herself. Other such instances are her naming Annie "Plum-face" and asking, "Are you a Hawaiian who only knows vowels, Ouayah?" The girl wants to be held in mother's arms, but mother interprets this as appeals to sing or change the diaper. The up-tempo language that Donna used with me is also evident with her baby. As I review the clip, it is painful to see Donna's vain efforts at comforting Annie, whose distress is mounting throughout the recording.

After the recording, Annie starts crying and mother imitates her in an ironic way. As her screams intensify, so does mother's inability to soothe her. Meanwhile, Donna reports to me that breastfeeding was so-so until 2½ months, when Annie "refused the breast like crazy". Sleep was a constant issue, Annie was easily over-stimulated, and she could not be with her mother in a café. "All the time there has been something that didn't work". As said, they were randomly assigned to comparison care. Six months later, they arrived, according to the research design, for a second interview.

Eleven months: second research interview

Donna: "The filter between us is gone. The kind of transfer I have with my husband, now I can have it with her, too. I've got some distance now, I've entered a positive spiral. I didn't understand I was depressed. I felt like shit. Now I'm a mother with a job, not a professional who happens to have a child."

Annie has just learnt to walk. She seeks contact and offers me a toy. Donna says Annie also suffered during her depression. However:

Donna: "It didn't harm her. She still has food problems, but now that she's not breast-feeding anymore, I don't take it personally. The sleep issues are gone. She is intense, curious, lively, has never been sitting still for long but that doesn't matter now that she can move around on her own."

On the video, mother's sensitivity has improved. As I leave the room when the recording starts, Annie looks after me and the mother captures her emotions: "You got a bit sad as he left. Don't worry. He'll be back." Donna names various objects to the girl but does not notice when Annie is searching for her breast. She picks up a book to awaken her curiosity but does not note that she is uninterested. The tempo is still a bit up.

To sum up, Donna now realises she was depressed in the beginning of Annie's life. She feels better and is grateful for her husband's support. His contact with Annie is better than hers. She enjoys more being a mother and dreams of a second child. She tells herself that Annie suffered no harm but also reports food problems and a high level of activity.

Let us briefly return to the topic of intimacy. If it implies to dance together, this presupposes that one has a sense of rhythm, an ability to listen and pick up signals from the other, and a love of oneself and the other. To what extent can intimacy mature when a mother does not like rolling the pram and feels she has to go through "this thing" with someone who depends on her? What if a baby bends backwards "like an angry starfish" at the breast, sleeps badly, and cannot be with Mum at a café? These initial observations indicate this dyad's problems with upholding an intimate relationship. Six months later, Mum's filter is gone, perhaps because her depression healed, or Annie became more independent and her routines more established. But was Donna right that Annie had suffered no harm? New facts emerged in the third research interview at 4½ years of age.

Four and a half years: the third research interview

Donna and Annie came for a third research interview when the child was 4½ years old. We chose that age because children can use words, participate in verbal tests, and be alone in an interview. Majlis WS knew nothing about Annie's history, videorecordings, or treatment assignment. I interviewed the mother about her internal representations of the child (Zeanah, Benoit, & Hirshberg, 1996), and Majlis tested the child's cognitive functioning (Wechsler, 2005) and then gave a Lego toy, instructing, "You can put it together with Mum". Mother and child united, played with the Lego, and got cookies and lemonade. After separating again, I asked mother about health and life events since the infant study, and her child's behaviour and relations at home and at pre-school. Meanwhile Majlis assessed, in dialogue with Annie, scores on the Children's Global Assessment Scale (CGAS; Shaffer et al., 1983), attachment representations in the Story Stem Test (Hodges, Steele, Hillman, Henderson, & Kaniuk, 2003), and the drawings' indications of age adequacy and emotional regulation (Machover, 1949). Donna and Annie then reunited, and we said goodbye.

Afterwards, Majlis "filtered" her impressions of the children into "Ideal Types" (Wachholz & Stuhr, 1999). In brief, she created idiosyncratic epithets like "curious", "troublemaker", and "scared". In a second step, she distilled them into four types: The Open child was lively, confident, and open. The Orderly child was competent and kind but a bit inhibited. These two types were condensed into the *OK children*. The Anxious child was worried, inhibited, or shy. The Provocative child was spiteful or overtly aggressive. These two formed the *Troubled children*. All in all, a child could be either "Troubled" or "OK". Of course, these types were gross and square inductive types, but we thought they would function well as outcome instruments (Winberg Salomonsson et al., 2015a, 2015b). In brief, our hypothesis was confirmed in certain aspects: children who had been in MIP as babies now contained more OK than Troubled children. In reverse, children who had been in the control group contained more Troubled than OK children. The group differences were significant, with an odds ratio of 5.78, implying a large effect size. The CGAS scores also favoured the MIP group: the effect size (Cohen's d) was 0.69, indicating that these children had a better social functioning. As for the other outcome instruments, no differences were found.

Before her interview with Majlis, Annie had left her mother without problems. Now she focused on her tasks with Majlis. The girl looked silently at Majlis, a bit tense and shy. From time to time, she gave a little smile. The tasks were solved quickly and easily. She looked pleased though reserved and then prouder and more relaxed: "Wow, this wasn't that difficult at all". When asked to make a drawing of a person, she made a gruesome witch (Figure 6.1) that contrasted with her well-behaved manner. "She's making witch-soup with flies and mosquitoes", she said.

Suddenly, she needed to make poo and added confidently: "I can wipe myself". Majlis then asked Annie to complete so-called story stems (Hodges et al., 2003). The girl told of children who managed well by themselves, and all conceivable dangers were denied.

In the video with mother and daughter, Annie was talking about Majlis. Mother asked Annie in a mocking tone:

Mother to Annie:	"What did you talk about in there?"
Annie:	"We talked about what you need when it's raining."
Mother [laughing]:	"What did you answer, a swimsuit?"
Annie:	"No, I said rain hat and raincoat and rain boots."
Mother:	"Wouldn't a swimsuit fit just as well?"

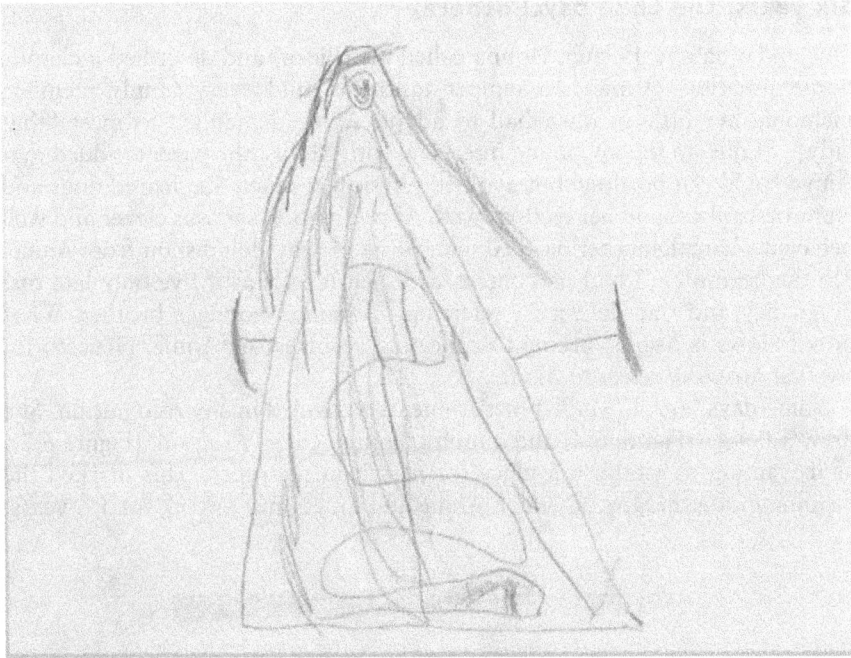

Figure 6.1 A witch.

Donna reported to Björn that Annie disliked new situations unless informed exactly in advance. She did not like playing by herself, and she wanted to control her peers when playing together. Fear of losing face was another issue. She was fond of pre-school with its rules and routines. She had always been fussy with food. Mother added: "Sometimes I wonder if she is still seeking that love I didn't give her unreservedly that first year."

Majlis' impression of Annie in the interview was of a gifted girl, restrained, inhibited, and task-oriented. She seemed self-propelled and used an "I-can-handle-myself" defence against anxieties, whose content Majlis could only ponder about in this situation. She assessed Annie as an Orderly child, thus belonging to the OK group. Majlis also wondered about the long glances, as if on the slant, at her. As for the countertransference in the interview, Majlis got curious and warmly affected by these looks. She recognised herself in this diligent, task-oriented, and overly independent little girl. Majlis also recognised Annie's pain of being lonely and not understood.

In retrospect, Majlis felt Annie got interested in her since the girl sensed her empathy. She showed her interest in the videorecorded dialogue with mother. In response to mother's inquisitive questions, the girl repeatedly said, "I wanna go back to Majlis again". Here, we note an embryo of a positive transference and, probably, the mother's negative transference as well.

Six years: the child psychotherapy

One and a half years later, Donna called me (Björn) and described a chaotic home situation. Annie had temper tantrums, and every family member, including her little brother, had to adapt. Annie demanded to meet "that lady": Majlis. In the upcoming interview with Majlis, the parents added that Annie could not be alone but avoided physical contact. She feared dogs and elevators and ground her teeth as well. At pre-school, she was clever and well behaved. Tearful, mother recalled that she had always felt distant from Annie: "In the beginning, I had no contact with her. It feels as if I've only had one pregnancy and one delivery", referring to Annie's younger brother. What now follows is Majlis' account of meeting and treating Annie. Henceforth, *the first pronoun refers to Majlis.*

Some days later I (Majlis) met Annie, who smiled in shy recognition. She drew a flower (Figure 6.2) and a multicoloured chair 'to sit on' (Figure 6.2), as if wanting to establish a place for herself in the office. This marked the beginning of a therapy, in which Annie and I met once a week for 1½ years.

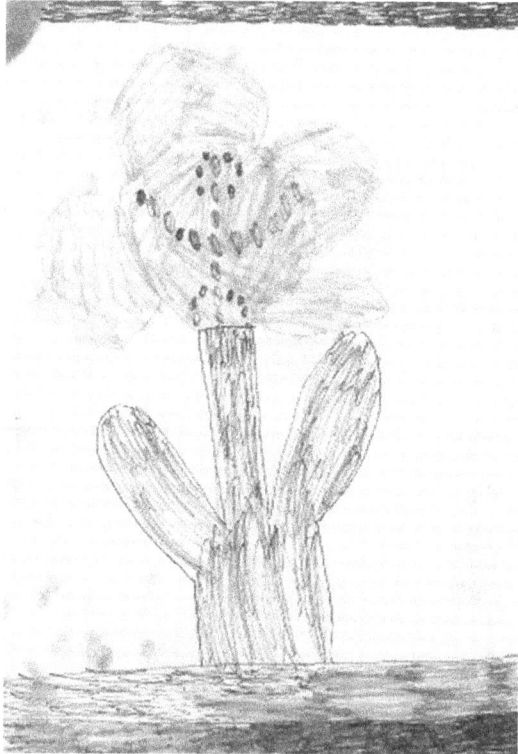

Figure 6.2 A flower.

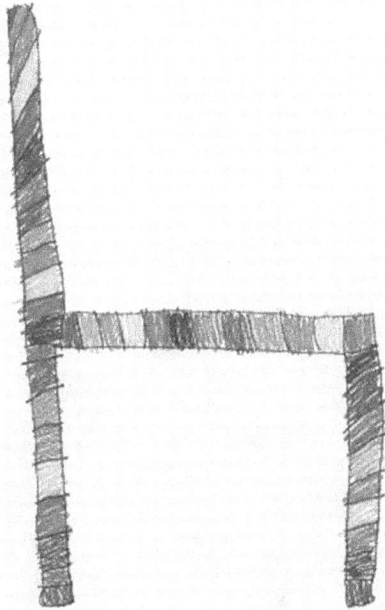

Figure 6.3 A chair to sit on.

I also saw the parents once a month. Annie was eager to come and seldom missed a session (Figure 6.3).

Annie soon abandoned her courtesy and consideration. She became spiteful, cheated in games, and wrote notes to me saying "Majlis is a shit, a fart sausage, a poo sausage". In Figure 6.4, everybody is laughing at Majlis. I said how hard it was to be treated that way and feel worthless. She got even more contemptuous and called me a "weak loser". This reflects Rosenfeld's (1971, 173) concept of a pathological organisation of narcissism, as the patient "withholds those parts of herself which want to depend on the analyst as a helpful person". Annie despised such parts in herself as well as those parts in me that were willing to provide help. Thus, both of us were "fart sausages".

In the countertransference, I felt a pull to both despise myself and seek revenge. This would correspond to Racker's (1968) concept of *complementary identification*. Here, "the patient treats the analyst as an internal (projected) object, and in consequence the analyst feels treated as such; that is, he identifies himself with this object" (135). In this identification, I felt like shit. Yet I also managed to reach a *concordant identification* with Annie's underlying pain and contempt of her poo-self. I thus could stay in containment and reflection or, in Racker's words, reach an empathy "that really reflect[ed] and reproduce[d her] psychological contents" (135). I told her it was not easy to

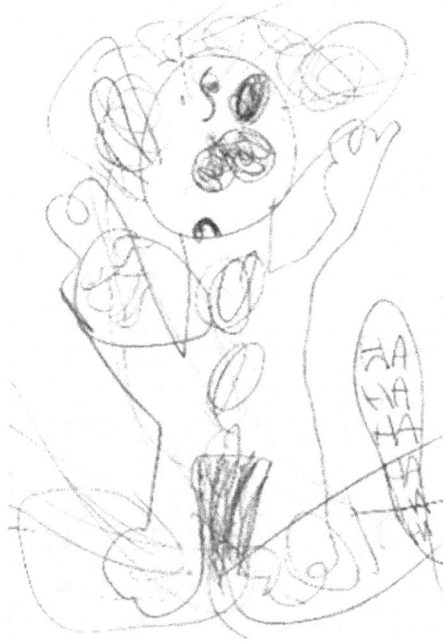

Figure 6.4 Everybody is laughing at Majlis.

feel left out and be afraid that others could be mean and laugh at her. My identification with this denigrated child self helped me taste what it felt like to be Annie. And it hurt.

Annie's attacks on me slowly decreased. One day, she said we should make a book together: *The tale of the perch who couldn't swim*. She dictated, I wrote it down, and she made the drawings.

Annie:	Once upon a time there was a perch who couldn't swim. The other fishes teased him (Figure 6.5). He slid down from the stone and got really sad (Figure 6.6). Another fish asked her:
The fish:	Do you want to play?
The perch:	But I can't swim so I cannot come and play. Can you teach me how to swim?
The fish:	Yes (Figure 6.7).

Annie pictures a green fish, who is alone and abnormal since he can't swim. A helpful object is introduced, the swimming teacher. In the last drawing, we recognise a formation like the chair returning from one of her first drawings. At that time, it merely indicated the hope of an upcoming frame to deal with her anxieties. This time, the drawing is more spontaneous and flourishing. The speech bubbles refer to a dialogue where the left fish says, "I can't swim.

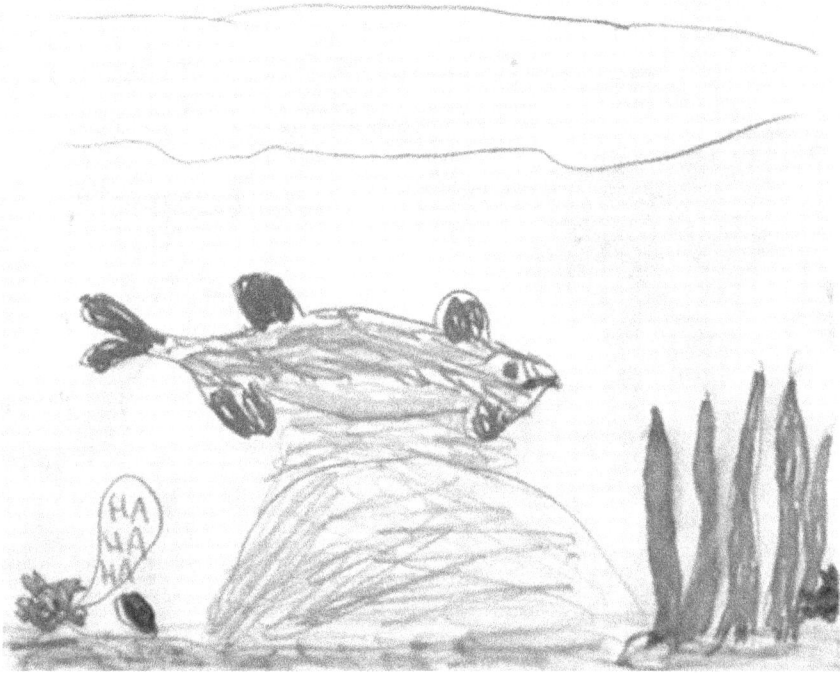

Figure 6.5 The other fishes teased him.

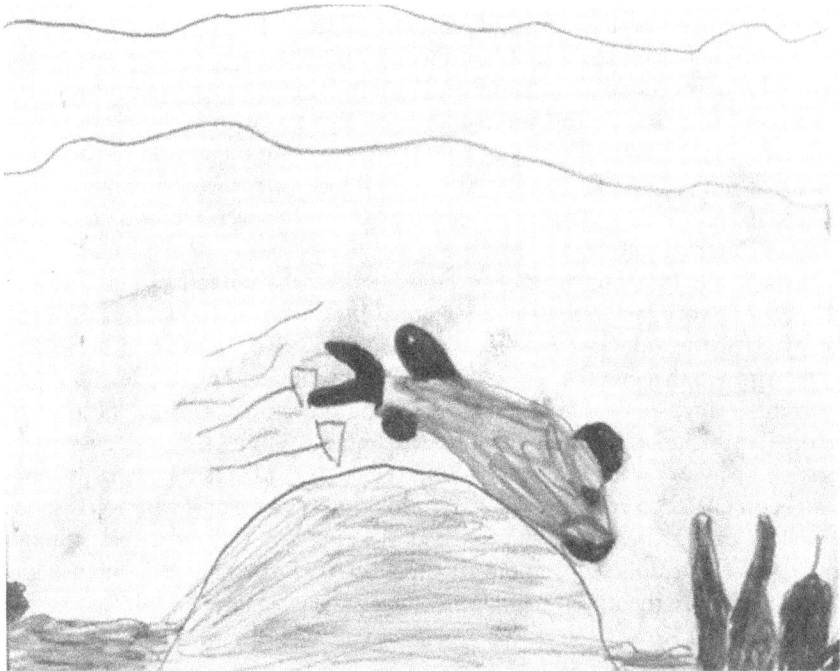

Figure 6.6 He slid down from the stone and got really sad.

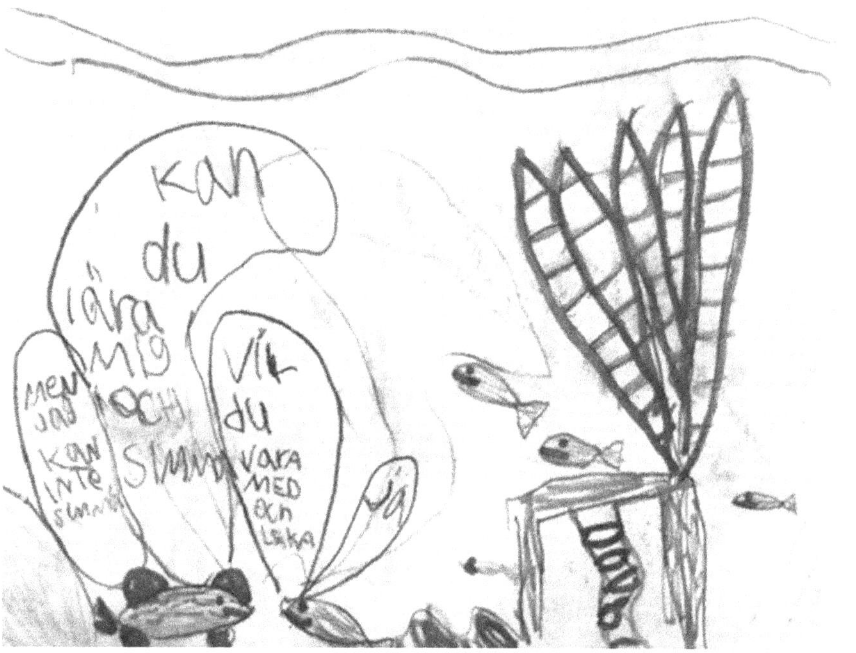

Figure 6.7 Can you teach me to swim? –Yes.

Can you teach me to swim?" The right fish answers, "Yes. Do you want to play together?"

I met the parents regularly to share information and take care of Donna's fluctuating self-confidence as a mother. At the time of the fish story, she reported a major change in Annie and a deepening contact. At bedtime, the girl burst into tears, saying she couldn't be nice to her family. Mother was surprised and thankful for this opening in their communication: "There are so many things in Annie's head that I had no idea of before. She always kept them to herself." Now Annie opened up, and mother received and contained her self-contempt and fear of not being loved.

At the same time, our contact deepened. Annie became more open, showed me her homework, and ceased attacking me. Also, her sadness was more overtly displayed. She wondered what she could do so as not to destroy an upcoming family trip with her usual angry comments and outbursts. After one and a half years in therapy, she wanted to end and spend more time with her playmates. 'Before, I thought I was only angry and bad, but now I think that inside me there is somebody who sometimes is happy and sometimes sad.' Her final words were: "Can I come back to you if I want to?" I took this as a sign of separation distress as well as of her confidence in me. Also, her question indicated that, though Annie and I had done substantial therapeutic work, perhaps this intense girl would need more therapy when approaching the challenges of adolescence.

Intimacy, the infantile, and transgenerational transmission

This was Majlis' account of her child therapy with Annie. We have followed her from five months to seven years of age. Initially, I (Björn) suggested that intimacy is like a dance with two people developing a closer relationship while yet maintaining respect for the other's integrity. This ability, I added, is rooted in the interchange of mother and infant. But in this dyad, intimacy had been thwarted from the start. Donna's pregnancy was wished for but also felt like a nuisance. The first videorecording and interview indicated several obstacles to intimacy. With her own mother, Donna said she had a relationship that was factual, benevolent, but not intimate. This left her unable to discuss her issues about Annie with her mother. The baby became a bright and diligent but bossy and anxious latency girl. She had difficulties in confiding her distress, and there was little of cuddling and trust in her. In brief, intimacy was stymied.

The three interviews and the therapy report raise two essential questions. Did the interviews contain precursors to what emerged later in the therapy relationship? Are character traits like Annie's transferred through the generations and, if so, how? As for the first question, I claim that the roots of projective defence strategies in this dyad could be seen already in the infant study. In the very first video, we saw the mother's evacuations (Rosenfeld, 1987) and intrusive identifications (Meltzer, 1992; Meltzer et al., 1982). If we recall Donna's comment "poo or fart, poo or fart" to the screaming baby, we see her depressed and negative image of Annie. Then, via Annie's introjection, this image was probably on its way to becoming the precursor of a bad internal object. In therapy years later, the girl sought to "export" this object – first when she needed to poo after having drawn a gruesome witch and then onto the therapist as a projection: "Majlis is a poo sausage". Annie's contempt and self-managing attitude can be viewed as her elaborations of early defence strategies in response to mother's way of handling her in infancy as well as her identification with comparable character traits in the mother.

As for the question of transgenerational transmission of character traits, we are investigating not conscious values or opinions but something more intangible and static. In other words, can the Unconscious – or at least facets of it – be transferred from generation to generation? As will be discussed further in Chapter 12, there is a close relation between the Unconscious and the Infantile, this book's major concept. Perhaps, the story of Annie and Donna and their issues with intimacy could help us in understanding how the Infantile in each of them has contributed to such a transgenerational transfer.

We recall Donna's way of talking about motherhood as just "rolling the pram". Motherhood wasn't "her thing" and "that immediate mother-baby-contact" never appeared. In the first video, she was insensitive when handling Annie's distress. Clearly, Donna had difficulties relating to Annie in an intimate way. However, she did not speak about her husband that way at all.

Why this divergence? I think the answer can be found in her ways of describing her own mother: a matter-of-fact, curt, and hasty person, who "just did what she did", as she used to reply when Donna asked her how motherhood had been to her. But in Donna's identifications as *woman and wife*, she felt much warmth and support from her husband. Clearly, there was love between them. But her identifications as *mother* were thornier. The harsh, gritty, factual, and restrained components in her ways with Annie resembled her descriptions of the relationship with her mother. The roots to these patterns were unconscious and probably related to unresolved ambivalence between mother and daughter. This being said, we must not forget that Donna was indeed a responsible and committed mother.

We are thus speaking of a transgenerational pattern of unconscious elements, a notion that is found already in Freud (S. Freud, 1933, 67):

> A child's super-ego is in fact constructed on the model not of its parents but of its parents' super-ego; the contents which fill it are the same and it becomes the vehicle of tradition and of all the time-resisting judgements of value which have propagated themselves in this manner from generation to generation.

This idea can be corroborated by the present case and by mundane observations, as when a parent complains that her child is cheating. "I cannot understand it. I always taught my girl to do the right things!" On closer inspection, one may find traits of a soft moral in the parent. This makes the child construct her superego not on what the parent *says* but on how she *acts*. The soft moral is transferred to the next generation, without anybody understanding why and how. Freud did not develop such ideas at length. The first analyst credited to such a perspective was Ferenczi (1949), who described the negative impact on his patients of their parents' behaviours of yore. Abraham and Torok (1984, 222) express such transfer vividly:

> The buried speech of the parent becomes a dead gap, without a burial place, in the child. This unknown phantom comes back to haunt from the unconscious... Its effect can persist through several generations and determine the fate of an entire family line. Could this be the "mysterious" primary repression hypothesized by Freud?

American analyst Jill Salberg (2015, 33) suggests that the vehicle of transgenerational transmissions is "ghostly attachments". She argues:

> Children are constantly observing their parents' gestures and affects, absorbing their parents' conscious and unconscious minds. In the shifting registers of attunement and misattunement, children adjust and adapt to the emotional presence and absence of their caregivers/parents, always searching for attachment.

This perspective on gestures and affects is akin to the one proposed in the Layered Analysis study in Chapter 9. We can link the case of Donna and Annie to another Salberg (2022) paper, where she focuses on such transfers in the lineage of mothers and daughters. Faimberg (2005) applies the term "telescoping of generations" to such transfers. Finally, in more Kleinian terms, Houzel (1996, 910) expressed transgenerational transfer this way:

> The dramas and traumas are repeated from generation to generation by the mechanisms of projective identification, identification with the aggressor and the repetition compulsion, unless there is a containing function that can transform them into thinkable elements.

The two last words, "thinkable elements", are crucial. Of course, Annie cannot explicitly understand that she feels something similar about herself as her mother Donna feels about herself, her daughter, or her mother. This is impossible because she is a little child *and* because these feelings are unconscious – in Donna as well. We are thus considering elements of the Infantile that can be neither thought of or talked about directly. Recall the metaphor in Chapter 3 of the futility in trying to perceive an object with the retina's blind spot. We must content ourselves with an indirect view and infer important details. And, as the astronomy metaphor indicates, we always infer the Infantile from afar and from ages ago. Accordingly, neither Annie nor Donna can explicitly disclose how elements of the Infantile were transferred to them by the previous generation. As outsiders, we can deduce that both of them have difficulties in being close to someone and that Donna's description of her mother matches such a pattern as well. This makes it easier to understand and empathise with Annie's mix of screaming, quarrelling, and loneliness – as well as Donna's tough ways of brushing aside her emotional pain.

How then is the topic of intergenerational transmission linked with our search for traces of the Infantile? This becomes clearer through the following example. I recall noticing in the first interview Donna's gabby, witty, and snappy way of talking about Annie and her mother. Only later, when I learnt about the child therapy and looked at the video interactions again, did I realise that Donna's account of her relationship with her mother contained many details of what I would call her own Infantile. I refer to her ironies about her mother and her sense of alienation. Likewise, I could better understand Annie's loneliness, anxiety, and recalcitrance by relating them to Donna's relationship with her mother. In brief, the Infantile of grandmother, mother, and young Annie were thus involved in an unconscious traffic across the generations, in which all participants were influencing and influenced by each other, whether directly or indirectly.

A child's lineage of parents, grandparents, and further back vanishes in the haze. The members in each generation can transmit traces of their Infantile to the next generation, which can affect the child now or later in development. We have seen other such lineages, such as in toddler Eric in Chapter 5, his mother Barbara, and her stern mother and distant father. Or Nicholas, his mother Theresa, and her matter-of-fact and brisk mother in Chapter 3. In a factual sense, the lineage is clear; for example, Donna is Annie's mother. But in a psychological sense, the lineage is much more hazy, entangled, and subtle since the most important contributor to this opacity is the Unconscious of each generation's members. This created a unique blend in Donna of not being sensitive with Annie – and yet wanting to do the best for her daughter.

In this way, the Infantile is passed on from generation to generation, and thus *the Infantile concept is closely linked with that of transgenerational transmission*. In PIP work, one meets with representatives of two generations, and the therapist thus gets glimpses of the transgenerational interaction and of the emotional pedigree. But when one is working with an adult patient, the sole present representative of the family tree and its history is the patient herself. In many such cases, therapist and patient embark on a journey we call reconstruction. In the next chapter, we will meet an example of such an endeavour. That chapter will also discuss the validity and truth of such reconstructions.

Source

This chapter is a reworked version of a published paper (Salomonsson & Winberg Salomonsson, 2017). I thank the publisher for giving permission to quote it in the book.

Reconstructing a traumatized Infantile in Laura

As I was writing up this book, I received a mail from a woman I worked with long ago:

> Several years before my daughter Beate and I were in therapy with you, I had ordered my records from the child psychiatry unit where I was treated as a child. I read them at the time but soon forgot about them, and I don't think I ever mentioned them to you. The other day, I was tidying up my desk and found them again. When I read them now, I reacted to other things than the first time. The first sentence spoke about a 'relationship disorder between mother and daughter', that is, between my mother and me. This theme recurred in the journal. I got quite chilly. Could this have affected my relationship with Beate? Do we repeat experiences without being aware of it? What is your opinion?
>
> Warm regards, Nadya

Reading Nadya's mail, I got amazed. "I'm writing about the Infantile, trans-generational transmission, emotional links in an individual between infancy, childhood and adulthood – and now Nadya, the mother in a mother – infant dyad whom I treated twenty years ago, approaches the very same questions!" Their case had started as a parent-infant psychotherapy (PIP) case when Beate was 16 months and continued into a child analysis from the age of two until three and a half years. Little Beate was unruly, restricted in her contact, and extremely clinging to her mother, including her breasts. In PIP, I managed to contain her anxiety and clinging, which gradually diminished. In parallel, mother Nadya slowly overcame her embarrassment and spoke of a profound depression when Beate was born. PIP led to a major improvement in their relationship, but first Beate developed a phobia of holes. She feared that mouth-less ghosts living in house ventilators wanted to devour her. Another phobic object was a shaft in an underground station where she had seen workers repairing an escalator. With these phobias came an insomnia and trouble at home, such as her being fussy and insisting on sleeping in the

DOI: 10.4324/9781003640363-7

parents' bed. We switched to child analysis, and the phobia had abated when Beate and I terminated our work.

The therapy inspired an article on how an infant might experience postnatal depression (Salomonsson, 2013a) and a book chapter (Salomonsson & Winberg Salomonsson, 2015). At first, the book appeared in Swedish, and some years later, Nadya contacted me after having read it. We met and she described Beate as today being a strong-willed young woman in her twenties with a bright personality, many friends, a boyfriend, and a decisive direction in her studies. Nadya also told me about her own recurrent depressions, for which she now had pharmacological treatment.

A few years later, and as I am writing these lines, Nadya's mail arrived with her question: her child psychologist had mentioned "a relationship disorder between mother and daughter". Could it have affected her relationship with Beate as a baby? And more generally, "Do we repeat experiences without being aware of it?" Of course, had my answer been no to her questions, I would not have written a book about "Traces of the Infantile". The challenge is, as we have seen throughout, how to find the traces concealed in present symptoms and to discern their roots backwards to childhood and infancy, and thus grasp better the transgenerational transmissions. The published texts about Beate and Nadya focused on the child and the mother-child relationship. In contrast, they contained little information about the mother's history, not the least since she was reluctant to talk about it. In connection with our questions on transgenerational transmission and the Infantile, I have included Nadya's mail since she is worried about the same questions: how are links forged between the generations, and could such an understanding yield knowledge about the past and about the future?

Nadya's questions will loom in the background as I introduce another adult patient alongside Colin, Simone, Bess, and Bianca. Their cases showed my efforts at linking the patient's Infantile with fragments of their infantile history. This led to some brief reconstructions linking past experiences and present suffering. As for my analysand Laura, the work of reconstruction needed to be more thorough because she was severely imprisoned by her past.

Reconstructing infantile trauma: the case of Laura

The text below was originally published as an article (Salomonsson, 2020). I had long since noted that PIP seemed to deepen my understanding of primitive despair, such as separation anxiety and wordless panic. I also thought I had come to better understand para-verbal communication such as tone, voice, tempo, body movements and posture, odour, and psychosomatic phenomena. Furthermore, I had needed to handle high-speed interchanges between container and contained in mother – infant interactions, which made me prone to improvise and become more volatile in analytic technique with adult patients. I had also observed a greater ease in acting as participant observer, thus taking a third position or a "helicopter view" on the transference-countertransference interchange. Another observation triggered my curiosity: my increased propensity to reconstruct, together with the patient, traumatic influences from infancy that I assumed was impacting on her present distress. Reflecting further on this last issue gave rise to this text.

Laura is 40 years old and seeks treatment with her second daughter Winnie, 2½ years. She is severely depressed and has been on antidepressant medication for several years. Winnie appears bossy and up-tempo, and Laura feels she "never really made contact" with her. She also realises that she projects her own dismal self-image onto the girl. PIP lasts some months, and we see how the girl reacts promptly and anxiously to mother's sadness. Laura has mentioned an abortion between the births of her daughters; a CUB (Combined Ultrasound and Biochemical screening) test revealed a chromosomal aberration. Laura is addressing her guilt while Winnie is running around the room. I tell Winnie, "Mum is sad. She had another child before you were born. He was sick and died." Winnie retorts, "No! Mum's HAPPY!" Laura is taken by the girl's sharpness and manic denial of Mum's sadness. She constantly worries about her girl, who is also her "comfy blanket". During PIP, the girl gets calmer, and Laura feels more competent as a mother. We then decide to end PIP and Laura begins a personal therapy with me, which is soon transformed into psychoanalysis four times a week.

Laura is not consistently depressed. She can also be heated, humorous, and censorious. When her dependence on me emerges and I address it, she gets enraged. After some months in analysis, she observes that she tends to feel worse when returning on Mondays after the weekend vacations. Once, she returns gloomy after my week-long vacation and complains of a tough week with the children. I suggest it might also relate to my absence. She retorts, "So you think I'm a sick jerk!?" Later, the dependency theme emerges on a Monday session. She relates a dream where she marvels at a dazzling moon (Monday is "Moon-day" in Swedish). A fire breaks out near her childhood home and the bystanders neglect it, but a fireman extinguishes it. Now she accepts my suggestion that she has been longing for Moon-day to return to me, the fireman, to extinguish her panic. But the night afterwards she dreams of being with a male colleague at a conference centre. There was fire and smoke, so they must escape. They went down to the kitchen, where the smoke was less disturbing. The bottom floor contained dormitories, like in a prison, where guards were watching the conference participants.

Now that I have interpreted her fear of depending on me, psychoanalysis feels like a choking fire smoke, says Laura. She is terrified of fires and always checks the fire exits in hotel buildings. The kitchen in the dream reminds her of a family visit at a restaurant.

It was so nice and welcoming, and the food was good. But I couldn't help asking the staff if they had a formal permission of allowing our children into the kitchen. Why did I come up with that censuring comment!?

The basement dorm she associates with her cloistered life. I interpret that she has transformed yesterday's theme of the fire that was extinguished by me, the fireman, into a catastrophe. She runs to the dormitories seeking help, but the staff down there turn out to be prison guards. The kitchen is turned from a good and nurturing place to a courtroom where she displays her moralising attitude. Life itself is a prison with no possibilities of penitence or consolation.

Laura defends against dependence in various ways. She asks about my personal life and when I respond by asking about her fantasies, she gets furious. "I know nothing about you, but you expect me to trust you!" One day, she reveals that she checked me up on the Internet and mentions my mother's maiden name and date of death. She is terrified that I will get enraged. "You must think I'm prying into your privacy". I interpret that since she cannot directly receive from me what she believes is real care – because she feels I am rejecting and callous – she must look me up on the Internet. However, the web data provide merely sham comfort, not vital containment.

Another defence against dependence is her idealizing strength and self-reliance. A friend speaks of his employees as "dead meat". Laura laughs in unison with his contempt but feels like dead meat herself: "In the mirror, I see my mother's dead eyes. You must feel the same when you see me." She has few close friends, since confiding in someone means divulging her misery. She thinks my true pleasure is bringing her case to congresses and laughing at her with my colleagues. She feels her husband despises her but she cannot imagine living without him.

As for Laura's history, she is an "afterthought child" born many years after her siblings. Her father still dominates the family with bigoted statements about people who, for example, do not share his dietary philosophy. He idealizes his wife but seems to covertly despise her ignorance and social ineptitude. Laura identifies with his values and contempt. Her mother seems poorly equipped intellectually and emotionally and has only briefly taken up jobs outside of home. Laura cannot recall any interesting or intimate chats with her.

Psychoanalytic formulations of Laura's case

Laura's condition does not exactly match that of melancholia in Freud's sense (S. Freud, 1917). She is interested in the outside world, has a dry sense of humour, and is not suicidal. Yet her mood, guilt, and self-denigration do match Freud's description. One part of her ego has set "itself over against the other, judges it critically, and, as it were, takes it as its object" (247). Now, if her self-accusations "fit someone else, someone whom the patient loves or has loved or should love" (248), who is – or was – that object? Who was involved in what Laura perchance experienced as "a real slight or disappointment coming from this loved person" (249). Freud suggests that, owing to such setbacks, the object loss leads to an "ego-loss". This results in "a cleavage between the critical activity of the ego and the ego as altered by identification" (249).

If we follow Freud's model, with whom does Laura identify? Many signs point to her mother. Laura is terrified of becoming similarly weak and narrow-minded. Her parents' marital balance is displayed in the transference, where she views me as superior and omniscient thanks to reading my "psychiatry books". I am like her father, who preaches his opinions to the family members. Laura's ways of relating vary, from adopting the role of a neglected housewife and a helpless Mum to an enraged woman feeling oppressed by my "know-it-all" attitude.

To Laura, her professional work is the main source of maintaining her shaky self-esteem. During the CUB test and the abortion, she allowed no time for reflection or relaxation. Before Winnie's birth, she collapsed with a burn-out condition and has been unable to work since then. She handles the malignant introject that Freud speaks of by identifying with her father, developing a rough and superior attitude towards "helpless nerds". Yet, as a mother to her daughters, she is responsible and caring, and she is desperate not to repeat the relationship with her mother.

Reconstructing the impact on Laura of her mother's depression

Laura is deeply attached to her mother though in a special way: she takes care of her mother but never confides in her. "I outgrew her when I was ten years old", she says sadly. She brings up childhood memories when mother's cookies came out scorched from the oven. Yet Laura was expected to praise them. Today she tells her parents that her life is great, but they do not ask about details, such as why she cannot work. She also accuses me of having no genuine interest in her. These stories and impressions assemble in my mind – and here I am clearly inspired by my PIP experiences with depressed mothers and their infants – to an image of a dejected baby in mother's arms where the contact contains annoyance, hopelessness, avoidance, and a mutual sense of incarceration in a gloomy dungeon. We will now follow the fate of this budding idea.

One day, I suggest to Laura that her mother seems depressed nowadays. She agrees but not when I add that mother perhaps was in a similar condition when Laura was a baby. Later, I extend my reconstruction: "Your father, who despises feeble people, can hardly have been of much support to his wife." The family culture is to sweep flaws and worries under the carpet. This attitude plus the description of herself as an afterthought child make me daresay: "Maybe you were an 'accident', as you've hinted, and maybe mother never worked through her feelings about your arrival." I also base this painful and risky interpretation on how she experiences our relationship: she is convinced that I think it is a mistake to have her in analysis but now I cannot back out. She is an "afterthought" patient, whom I can offer only mock containment and a view of her as an idle yet "interesting" case.

I ask myself if I am closing my eyes to a part of the countertransference where I do look at her as interesting – but from a detached, disdainful, and superior position. Yet I cannot recognize this in myself. What I sense, rather, is deep empathy with her pain. But there are also instances of vexation and fatigue: "Nothing that I do is of help, anything I say is rejected by her". Such feelings remind me of depressed mothers' interchanges with babies, accompanied by shrugging shoulders, a flat tone of voice, and annoyed comments like, "However much I offer him the breast, he won't take it".

Laura receives these reconstructions with disbelief, scorn, and sometimes wrath: "You know nothing about my infancy!" From one perspective, Laura is perfectly right. This important objection will be considered later in the chapter's theoretical sections on reconstruction. She continues dreaming about fires, dungeons, warlike scenes, and so on. Then one day, she brings a photo album with some excruciating mother – baby pictures. Her mother, with a frayed appearance, slouched posture, and unhappy expression, is looking away from her six-month-old baby Laura, who seems unhappy and limp and is looking in another direction. There are similar pictures up to some years of age. Laura bursts out, "Why did they put such pics in the family album!? Didn't they see anything?" I comment, "This looks like a very unhappy couple". Laura reports that her mother recently gave her some cartons, one containing her Child Health Centre records. "I read that my breast-feeding was interrupted at two months. I asked Mum and she pretended she didn't hear me."

Why did Laura bring the album to the session? One answer is that she wished to confirm my reconstruction of the mother's depression and its effects on her. Did she yield to my persuasions? I find this improbable since Laura only slowly ceased to attack my "baby fixation". Another answer – and, in my view, more correct – was that she felt relieved when I paid attention to her suspicions about the relationship with her mother. Over the months, the album became the basis of a shared reconstruction of the climate during infancy and its links with her present gloom and the torturing transference. Further, it provided a refreshing look at the countertransference/transference interplay. One day, she spoke of her "dead eyes" and accused me of avoiding them when I greeted her. I responded: "You're right. I now realise that I'm sometimes scared of your eyes and look away." Of course, she felt repudiated but became interested. "We two are looking away from each other, like in the photos." This interchange revealed another aspect of the countertransference: my identification with a scared baby who gets scared and confused when looking at mother's (here, Laura's) still face (Tronick et al., 1978) and thus avoids it.

In periods, Laura crouched on the analytic couch under a blanket and dozed away, as she did at home after sessions. This provided a psychic retreat (Steiner, 1993) from her depression and anxiety about resuming work. It was cosier and more comfortable to stop time and doze off, though only to wake up again in distress of wasting her life. Analytic progress was thus thwarted, and I finally suggested she sit up. Now I could see the pallor, despair, and embarrassment in her face. She hid her eyes with her hands or looked at me on the sly, like a terrified child.

Laura: "I'm embarrassed… looking at you… I realise that you're a human being. Other times, I feel you're a monster. I can't stop thinking that you hate me and that you're evil, yet I know you aren't."

Next day, she sat down and slowly, her gaze became warmer, curios, and playful. We spoke of the previous session. "Nothing happened afterwards. I took the girls to their sports, had a migraine attack, drowsed in bed as usual." Yet she had been wondering at length what to do about her present confinement. She also discovered that "I can't stop distorting my image of you." Now and then, she looked at me with open, childish, confidential, and curious eyes.

Analyst: "I'm thinking of those photos with you and Mum looking away – like you're turning your eyes away from me now and then."
L: "Because I'm scared of looking at you!"
A: "You fear the hatred, both mine and yours, yet we can speak about it. But when hatred remains unacknowledged by everyone involved, it makes for a sham contact. Maybe this happened between you and Mum back then."
L: "Also between me and my Dad! In another photo, I'm lying alone on the carpet, yelling. Shouldn't he pick me up rather than photographing me? He seemed delighted the other day when we were looking at those pics."

Clinical emphasis was now on our combined visual contact and dialogue and a transference switching between fear, hatred, object hunger, and warmth. She toggled between shunning and imbibing my eyes. I confirmed that she probably felt, and probably also was, rejected and silently detested then – and that today she often tends to hate me in lieu of seeing me as helpful. I thought it was important for her to look at me now for some time as we worked through her dread of me.

PIP as source of inspiration in work with Laura

How did my PIP experiences with mothers and babies influence the clinical approach in Laura's analysis? As I now recall the years of work before my PIP experiences, I would then probably have interpreted her accounts of previous and present family life more as *subjective experiences* than as *credible renditions of events.* I might, for example, have focused on her pathological narcissism (Rosenfeld, 1971), with which she sought to maintain her self-idealization and quench the pangs of dependency on me as an object she both desired and envied. Such focus is visible in my work from "the pre-PIP days" with Bianca in Chapter 4. I focused on this theme with Laura as well since she indeed was ruled by what Rosenfeld called a Mafia-like internal gang. But my PIP experiences helped me now to keep a simultaneous and constant eye on what I'd call "baby Laura with her depressed mother". Earlier, I had come to sense a certain hesitancy in myself and other analysts from the post-Kleinian tradition to utilise what we had been told by the patient to reconstruct the baby's experience – then as it emerged and now in the transference. As said in Chapter 4, I think this hesitancy is a heritage from Klein, who did not spell out in detail how a mother interacting with a baby can contribute to future pathology. She addressed more how the child's drive conflicts instigated scars in his or her internal world that could lead to emotional disorders later in life (Aguayo & Salomonsson, 2017). This probably diminished an interest in reconstructing the mother – infant *interaction.*

To sum up, I do not claim that my PIP experiences were a sine qua non for reconstructing Laura's mother's depression. And, of course, neither does PIP help a therapist understand all instances of depression. One may also ask if the previous mother-toddler therapy with Laura and Winnie propelled my fantasies about a depressed mother and her baby and yielded the reconstruction. My answer is yes and no. Laura was certainly depressed with Winnie in the initial sessions. Thus, she might have provided me with a template of a depressed mother. Yet Laura was talking in a dedicated way with Winnie, who responded actively. She told Winnie about how she felt and was also eager to grasp what went on inside Winnie. In that sense, Laura was cognitively and intuitively much more alert than her mother had been – as I imagined her. Further, my visions centred on a suckling infant, not a 2½-year-old toddler girl. Thus, I think the major impact on my fantasies and reconstruction work – apart from the transference – countertransference interplay – came from experiences in PIP that sharpened my acuity of how babies pick up and react to a depressed mother's state of mind. This inspired me to persist, despite Laura's initial rejections, to reconstruct links between relationships now and in infancy.

Reconstructions: historical or narrative truth?

The following sections are perhaps a bit cumbersome and dry, but the topic is essential in our quest for the traces of the Infantile. We recall Florence Guignard speaking about the Infantile, this "strange *historical/ahistorical* conglomerate, the *crucible* of primal fantasies and sensorimotor experiences that can be stored as memory traces". She does not tell us *how* these fantasies and experiences are stored as memory traces. I have argued that "traces of the Infantile" are anything but insignificant relics in our adult personalities. Like Guignard, I think of them as keystones in forming our character and our emotional suffering or wellbeing, in short who we become and why we suffer or enjoy life.

In this and other chapters, I have linked the patient's present plight not with their "real" infancy but with my reconstructions of its fundamental emotional traits. My argument would be more credible if I could dissect these links' logic. One could start with an objection to Laura's case:

> We understand that PIP experiences show you first-hand the intensity of mother – baby interactions. We also agree with Freud, Guignard, and others that our character is based on memory-traces of early and repressed impressions. If Laura's mother was depressed during her infancy, we concede that it might hamper the baby's development. But you must tackle two questions:
>
> • Are you sure that Laura's mother was depressed long ago?
> • And, if she was depressed, was it a major factor explaining Laura's present suffering?

Donald P. Spence (1982, 1986, 1989, 2000) has disputed the validity of our conclusions drawn from case work. He argues that our conjectural interpretations often masquerade as veridical explanations. He says we must submit case presentations so that the reader can judge whether our interpretation is the most plausible one – or whether other data point in alternative directions. He warns that our "satisfaction of finding a narrative home for the symptom, dream fragment, or piece of behavior completely overshadows any doubt as to the credibility or validity of the explanation" (Spence, 1986, 7). Spence thus cautions against muddy science and argues that our narcissism might make us avoid assessing the validity of our conclusions. He recommends that presenters clarify how they (1) link past and present events ("rules of inference"), (2) formulate their hypotheses, (3) have compared them with other possible explanations, and (4) argue that unconscious processes are transformed into manifest behaviour and reasoning ("rules of transformation").

Spence has been criticized for a one-sided empiricist and positivistic view of psychoanalysis (Morris, 1993; Sass & Woolfolk, 1988). Morris argues Spence has misunderstood Freud's (1937) archaeologist metaphor for reconstructing the patient's repressed memories. Freud claimed the analyst's job is easier than the archaeologist's because patients display their reactions dating from infancy in the *transference*, and "even things that seem completely forgotten are present somehow and somewhere" (260) in the psyche. Freud did not imply that these "things" can be dug up in their original form. Rather, events become experiences and take on traumatic meaning only *nachträglich* or in a deferred way after a lengthy process, which may start as a traumatic experience and then, in psychoanalysis, can be discerned as enactments, atmospheres, and relationships.

Such phenomena can then be *reconstructed* as traces of the past, a work that "involves two people, to each of whom a distinct task is assigned" (S. Freud, 1937, 258). One example is my idea about Colin's yearning (Chapter 1) for his preschool darling as an *après-coup* of the much earlier and vaster trauma of his hospitalisation and separation form his mother. Another example is the analytic work that Laura and I did at length. When Freud writes that reconstructive work involves the work of two people, he thus includes the analyst's subjectivity. This topic will be addressed in the section "Reconstruction: one-way or two-way procedure".

As to the confirmatory value of a patient's reactions to a reconstruction, Freud is cautious. Her plain "Yes" is "by no means unambiguous" (S. Freud, 1937, 262). It can also be meaningless or hypocritical unless it is followed by indirect confirmations, such as "new memories which complete and extend the construction" (262). When Laura brought the photos, I felt that my reconstruction began to be meaningful *to her*. She agreed that they gave a gloomy and lonely impression. Thus, the construction did not result in a "recaptured memory" (266) from her childhood. But it achieved a similar therapeutic result in that she recognised "its kernel of truth [that] would afford common ground upon which the therapeutic work could develop" (268). Freud's "*common* ground" points again to his view that reconstruction work is a joint effort of patient and therapist.

One question and one challenge await us. The question is what a patient might gain from a reconstruction. I will discuss this in the final section. The challenge is imposed by Spence's critique. I might object that his view of psychoanalysis downplays its two-person hermeneutic method (Gadamer, 1975/1989). I might also claim that there is nothing wrong if a clinical interpretation "might be true, [though] not necessarily… is true" (Spence, 1986, 6). But it is harder to dispute when Spence urges us to make the grounds for our interpretations transparent – especially since I argue that my PIP experiences of stressful interactions of *other* mothers and infants have provided such ground and support for reconstructing Laura's present depression from similar interchanges in her infancy. I will now approach this challenge.

Rules of inference and of transformation

Spence might ask which rules of inference made me suggest the links between past and present events in Laura's case. I begin by stating that she describes her mother *today* as a depressed, listless person. She rarely participates in family conversations, finds little joy with her grandchildren, and complains much. However, this does not prove she was depressed with baby Laura. So, on what do I base this inference? One answer is her childhood memories: "My mother was like invisible back home. I was afraid of looking into her eyes, like dead. I can't recall ever singing a song with her. Some folks say she was lively, but I never saw anything of that."

These memories intimate that the mother was depressed during Laura's childhood. As for the indications of an even earlier depression, I refer to Laura's breastfeeding records. Swedish mothers rarely stop breastfeeding at two months. When it happens, one would expect a note in the records about the reasons. This, plus mother's silence about it, indicates its emotional charge. Finally, it is hard to detect any happiness, playfulness, or eye contact between mother and baby in the photos. One photo is no proof, but we are talking about many pictures with a similar atmosphere.

Spence also asks us to compare our hypotheses with other possible explanations. One obvious candidate would be Laura's Oedipus complex. We have spoken a lot about her father in his role of a husband who grasped little of his wife's depression. My view is that the relationship correlates sparsely with a classical Oedipal configuration. Laura is attached to him in a peculiar way: she thinks his ideas about the dangers of coffee, wine, tomatoes, and so on are weird, but it took her years in the analysis to gain courage and have a glass of wine in front of him. She likes talking with him: "He is smart and knows a lot, unlike mother". He thus functions more like an *antidote to mother's depression* than as an "ordinary" Oedipal father evoking desire, admiration, and disappointment.

Following the reconstruction of the maternal depression, I even claim it would have been disastrous to interpret Laura's sense of dejection as mirroring the disappointment of a little girl enamoured of her father. There is too little of a viable triangle in this family for Laura to feel the full impact of Oedipal love and dethroning. Had I interpreted, for example, that she was disappointed in me because I rejected her advances she would most certainly have felt not only that I was putting her off but also that I felt she was presumptuous in believing that she would have such an impact on me. Laura rather corresponds with Britton's (1989) description of patients who experienced an "*initial failure of maternal containment* that made the negotiation of the Oedipus complex impossible" (93, italics added). For them, encountering "the intercourse of the parents, in phantasy or fact, without having previously established a securely based maternal object through the process of containment" (Britton, 2000, 54) can be detrimental. This is why an unfounded Oedipal interpretation can have such dire consequences.

Another question by Spence is how I assume the mother's postnatal depression had been transformed into Laura's present depression. My answer is built on how Laura's transference developed. She experienced me as sarcastic, foppish, aloof, and malevolent. She also felt strongly that I found her loathsome, boring, and despicable. I infer that this analyst persona is moulded on repressed memories of a depressed mother who cannot master her ambivalence towards the child, feels fettered, and fulfils her duties with scant enthusiasm or pleasure.

Another hypothesis of how mother's depression infiltrated Laura's psyche stems from her hatred of her dependence on me and from her elitist values:

if one is weak and dependent, one is worthless. She feels she must get back to work; however, this is impossible due to her present abilities. The only alternative is to stay home. There is no room for compromises or an easier job. I understand her narcissistic organization as partly nourished by an identification with her father's expressed contempt of frailty in general and, I assume, his latent condescension of his wife. Importantly, this organization is also nourished, from infancy onwards, to defend against the pain of being with her mother. It helped her stay unperturbed by mother's rejection and maintain her self-esteem. In Hurley's words (2017), if a parent fails to be "sensitively involved, mirroring and emotionally responsive... the baby is thrown back on his own resources" (194). This can result in "illusions of self-sufficiency and pseudomaturity, and by evading the need for dependent relationship" (204). Laura was probably not depressed in infancy or childhood, but in adolescence she was sometimes low-keyed. She left home late, married soon, and became a hardworking professional. Depression set in as she aborted a foetus with congenital malformation and had a second child but little joy in motherhood. Her self-contempt overwhelmed her, and she sought help.

What about my "transformational rules" in this reconstruction? Here, Spence (1986) demands a lot to assert validity: "So long as the link between latent and manifest content follows an unknown transformation rule, there is no way to predict from a given piece of latent content, A, to its manifest content, A'" (9). If we accept that Laura's mother was depressed and that this affected the baby, how was this transformed into the suffering of a 40-year-old woman?

To answer, I emphasise that psychoanalytic speculations about early interactions and empirical infant research are two different fields of investigation. Therefore, no approach to understanding the child's inner world and its repercussions later in life can be all-inclusive (Aguayo & Salomonsson, 2017). Deep-reaching analytic speculations can be fascinating yet lack empirical grounding in the more positivistic sense of the term. Experimental or population-based research can also be intriguing yet unable to reach beneath observable phenomena into their unconscious roots and implications. In my belief, the more we can join these two perspectives, the more comprehensive, vast, and deep our notion of the patient will be.

I conclude, in contrast to Spence (1986, 5), that transformational rules of "evidence and logic" are not applicable to psychoanalytic theory. Even if we claimed to know with absolute certainty some latent content, we would be unable to predict how it would be transformed into overt behaviour – not because we were ignorant of any rules but because *no such rules exist in psychoanalytic theory*. Thus, little Laura might have had experiences with her parents as described earlier and yet developed in another direction. Instead of rules, we have to content ourselves with searching for *correlations* that endorse the existence of those transformations that we assume occurred during development.

I find three such supportive correlations: (a) findings from population research demonstrating links between postnatal depression and distress in childhood and adolescence, (b) observations, in PIP and in experimental research, of babies' swift reactions to shifts in the mothers' emotional state, and (c) therapies or research videos with babies and depressed mothers, where the child was followed up in individual therapy. As for (a), population studies have demonstrated the prevalence of postnatal depression (Gavin et al., 2005; Parsons, Young, Rochat, Kringelbach, & Stein, 2012; Petersen, Peltola, Kaski, Walters, & Hardoon, 2018) and its links with child and adolescent distress (Chronis et al., 2007; Field, 2010; Murray et al., 2010; Olson, Bates, Sandy, & Schilling, 2002; A. Stein et al., 2014). Interaction studies have shown that depressed mothers exhibit more negativity towards the baby (Field, Healy, Goldstein, & Guthertz, 1990; Tronick, 2007a) and regulate their babies' affects less well (Reck et al., 2004). They also have less optimal affiliative behaviour, attachment representations, and distress management (Leckman, Feldman, Swain, & Mayes, 2007). Their infants have less social engagement and play (Edhborg, Lundh, Seimyr, & Widström, 2003), less mature regulatory behaviours and more negative emotionality (R. Feldman et al., 2009; Moehler et al., 2007), and less propensity to develop secure attachment patterns in early childhood (Toth, Rogosch, Sturge-Apple, & Cicchetti, 2009). When we infer correlations between maternal postnatal depression and distress in the developing child, we stand on solid ground in the general case. In an individual case like Laura, we need to analyse if our suggested correlations are plausible or not.

Point (b) implies that babies studied in therapy and experimental research react to shifts in the mothers' emotional state. In one experiment (Murray & Trevarthen, 1985), babies interacted with mothers via TV. If the contingency between mother's image on the screen and the baby's communication was artificially disjointed, the baby reacted with confusion, distress, and avoidance (Nadel, Carchon, Kervella, Marcelli, & Réserbat-Plantey, 1999). The Still-Face experiment (Tronick et al., 1978) can be seen as a micro-depression that provides a snapshot of the effects on the baby once the mother is continuously depressed. She and the baby then have a hard time forming a "dyadic state of consciousness" (Tronick, 2005), and the baby reacts with protest or avoidance.

Selma Fraiberg (1982) discovered babies who avoided the eyes of mothers who were "psychologically absent for a very large part of the infant's day" (616). Such behaviour was "always associated with discord in the mother–infant relationship and with avoidant patterns in the mother herself" (618). Other clinicians have noted gaze avoidance and linked it with maternal aversive, indifferent, distressed, or guilt-ridden behaviour and emotions (Cowsill, 2000; Kernutt, 2007; Salomonsson, 2021). For more examples, see the cases of Simone, Bess, David, Eva, and Chloe in Chapters 1, 2, 8, and 9. I conceive of it (Salomonsson, 2015b) as a psychological defence against an interaction that the baby feels to be discontingent: the mother's caretaking does not integrate her ambivalence towards herself and the child. I assume similar processes have been active between little Laura and her mother and continued into a longstanding alienation between the two.

Today, eye contact is pivotal for Laura. Looking in the mirror makes her think of mother's "dead eyes". She experiences my eyes as hostile or feigned. When I introduced the parameter that she sit up, the impact of eye contact emerged even stronger: her shame of looking into my eyes alternated with a fear of damaging me with her "bad eyes". We also noted her shy imitation of my gestures and her "eye hunger" to help establish a good introject. The correlation between infant studies and Laura's behaviour in therapy can be summarized thus: Like a baby in the Still-Face paradigm, she panicked due to any perceived aversion or lack of life in my facial expression. And, like a baby in Fraiberg's study of gaze avoidance, she shunned my eyes and wanted to protect me from hers as well. What differed from Tronick's and Fraiberg's babies was that she, simultaneously, sought to actively imitate and introject a friendlier version of that object, namely me.

Point (c) refers to therapies or research videos with a baby and a depressed mother, where the child was followed up in individual therapy. The research video in Chapter 6 shows how five-month-old Annie avoided her intrusive depressed mother's eyes. The mother demonstrated negative attributions (R. Silverman & Lieberman, 1999) of her daughter, such as "poo-poo or fart" or the "Hawaiian ouayah". Six years old, Annie likened her therapist to "poo-poo sausage" and "shit", expressions quite similar to the mother's expressions. As suggested in that chapter, the girl had introjected the attributions into her self-image, which she tried to get rid of by projecting them onto her therapist. In brief, she had internalized her mother's negative projections, identified with them, and set up a negative self-image. Such chains of psychological events can shed light on Laura's childhood and present transference. I assume that an unintegrated maternal ambivalence was projected onto Laura, who identified with it and felt worthless and rejected. This she has tried to "export" into me by belittling and caricaturing me as a fake and cynical analyst.

Reconstructions: one-way or two-way procedure?

Peter Fonagy (1999) also casts doubt on the rules of inference in analytic reconstructions but from another vantage point. A therapist who seeks to recover the patient's repressed memories, especially those that are implicit and pathogenic, is pursuing "a false god" (220). Fonagy argues against Freud's archaeological metaphor. "The only way we can know what goes on in our patients' mind, what might have happened to them, is how they are with us in the transference" (217). This is because although our implicit memories, including their defensive distortions, greatly influence our "experiences of being with" (Stern, 1985) others, they are irretrievable after all.

As analysts, we encourage them to be played out in the transference – counter-transference, with the "aim of modifying implicit memories… [and an] active construction of a new way of experiencing self with other" (Fonagy, 1999, 218). In contrast, the aim is not to achieve "relatively superficial changes in autobiographical memory" (218).

Another critic, Hoffman (2018), argues that "reconstruction may say more about the analytic present than about the patient's historical past" (473). He asks, "how much change occurs as a result of the analyst's communicating the meaning of the patient's communications, and how much occurs as a result of the nature of interaction between patient and analyst?" (476). The "relational turn" in psychoanalysis implies that we pay greater attention to the analytic couple's modes of functioning, but surprisingly, "the traditional view of reconstruction (and reconstructing) seems largely to have remained untouched by the new perspective" (Gottlieb, 2017, 307).

In terms of Laura's analysis, a suspicion arises: did she change in a positive direction because I imposed on her my eruditions about depressive mother-infant interactions? Was she my "token case" to prove the value of PIP? If we join this suspicion with Fonagy's caution that nobody can recall memories from infancy, this would risk collapsing the entire reconstruction as an imposture. Whereas I agree with his point about implicit memories, another factor facilitates traffic between them and memories that are explicit. This factor blurs the strict division by the two. As argued in Chapter 6, every generation transmits to the next atmospheres, personal labels, and family myths through ambiences, gestures, sighs, mimic expressions, or cues when talking about specific topics. Or they emerge, simply and subtly, as brief sentences in family conversations. They exert their effects as shadows of an irretrievable infantile past, as when Bess in Chapter 2 says that "certain themes are never brought up in my family, like the escape from our home country and what happened after my birth". In line with Fonagy's argument, Bess cannot recollect her neonatal separation, but the family stories about it have puzzled and intrigued, and underneath also scared and unsettled, her and the mother.

I suggest that Laura gave similar cues from her childhood, such as the memory about mother's scorched cookies that Laura must praise. This can be interpreted as a story about a delicacy (the breast) being destroyed by the mother's negligence (her depression) and then followed by denial of it and a demand that Laura should submit to it (close her eyes to her mother's depression and its scary effects on Laura). The mother's reticence in speaking about breastfeeding is another example. A third cue is Laura's impression of mother being "invisible at home" and her fear of mother's "dead eyes" and the absence of memories of singing or playing with her. Fourth, Laura reports that her father took care of his weeping wife every night but that nobody ever talked about it. There seemed to be a family consensus that one could not communicate with the mother as with others. And there is much to indicate the father's helplessness and perhaps even hesitation in getting in intimate contact with his wife and her suffering – which left Laura alone with a downcast contact with her mother.

To once again argue against myself, I might have admitted that I imposed on Laura my experiences with other depressed mothers and babies – as well as my ideas about their consequences later in life – to claim that her baby relationship with mother had the effects we now saw in analysis. Maybe, I only did it to prove the value of my PIP experiences and thus wanted her to buy my reconstruction? Well, here I might defend myself by bringing up the baby photos, but there is a better argument for the clinical value of the reconstruction. It is based on a condensed statement by Blum (2003): "Reconstruction is synergistic with and may substitute for memory retrieval, and provides a developmental context for genetic interpretation" (500).

Reconstruction does not, as Blum cautions, replace the analysis of transference or countertransference. Remember that my reconstructions were no unequivocal proofs of Laura's infancy. Furthermore, I did not force her to believe in them as "false gods", to paraphrase Fonagy (1999). Rather, they enabled us to talk about her present ailments and their possible, or plausible, connections with the earliest relationship with her mother. And, although I do not contend that one must have PIP experiences to believe that our earliest experiences can be of crucial importance later in life, they do provide vivid examples of how a baby can be impacted when mother is depressed or anxious. This is not more farfetched than to say that an analyst who has been facing death, loss, or severe illness may develop a deeper empathy with patients who are living in such situations.

The therapeutic gain of reconstructions

Freud suggested that reconstructive work consists in liberating historical fragments from their distortions and attachments to the present and leading them back to the past where they belong. That sentence contains the seed of possible therapeutic gains: the reconstructions liberate Laura from the idea that she has caused all her suffering and that she is a bad person. She can indeed do something about her elitist values, her unrealistic expectations of a suitable job, and her view that she is doomed to be a copy of her depressed mother. True, she cannot magically undo the relationships from her infancy, with a mother whose depression was denied and not taken care of. The therapeutic gain emerges when Laura realises the difference between areas where she is an agent or a victim – and that this sorting out is done with an analyst who strives to reach "the kernel of truth" (S. Freud, 1937, 268) in a frank, compassionate, and non-condemnatory way.

Arguably, I cannot prove more clearly the links between an assumed postnatal depression 40 years ago and Laura's depression now. Actually, Spence (1989) does not demand more of us. "What passes for reconstruction is largely narrative truth", but Spence does not reject such truth as being useless.

Quite the contrary… all therapies… provide a framework within which certain sets of seemingly disconnected life events can be placed. Each therapist establishes his or her own narrative truth, and in the right hands, it has the power to heal. But this should be kept separate from the true recovery of the past – and separate from the scaffolding we like to call theory.

(520)

To illustrate the link between reconstruction and therapeutic gain, I end by submitting a brief vignette. During a recent session, Laura has pre-ordered a taxi to pick her up afterwards because she feels weak and tired after recovering from a flu. She gets anxious that there might be problems with the taxi. Her cell phone just broke down, so she cannot reach the taxi service. She glances at my cell phone on the table, says nothing, and continues voicing her worries about the taxi ride. After some waiting, I ask her: "You're worried about missing your cab, your phone is down, you look at mine here…" She responds, "I wouldn't ask for your phone, because you'd say no or be angry at me for asking". She turns silent, hesitates, and then asks me if she can borrow it if needed. I say yes. At that point, she becomes annoyed with herself for creating this negative scenario. I link it with the relationship with her mother, where Laura always expected an indifferent or negative response, feeling that she did not have a right to disturb mother. Now she sought to push me into the position of a hostile mother but then changed it into a friendlier object whom she could ask for the phone.

To quote Spence (1989, 520), "seemingly disconnected life events" were brought together for Laura. To paraphrase Freud's ideas about reconstruction, we liberated a fragment of plausible historical truth (mother as depressed and rejecting) from its distortions (me as rejecting) and its attachments to her life today (I won't lend her my cell phone) and led it back to the past where it belongs. This enabled her to handle the situation as an agent. The reconstructions contributed by making such situations more comprehensible. Britton (2000) suggests that if maternal containment fails, the infant's "unformulated fear of death" is transformed into nameless dread. When fear does not become identifiable, something even worse occurs: "the *uncomprehended* has become the *incomprehensible*" (62, italics added). I'm quoting Laura here:

Laura: "That photo album, I had it at home for ages, but I never thought anything special about the pics. Now that I think of it, I was often anxious from childhood up to adulthood. Every time it happened, I mumbled to myself: 'My mum, my mum'. I never grasped why I did this."

Laura's comment implies that our work of reconstruction has helped her transform a phenomenon from being incomprehensible to becoming comprehensible and even comprehended.

Addendum

I end the chapter by with returning to Beate's mother Nadya and her questions. Could the "relationship disturbance" between little Nadya and her mother as mentioned in her child psychiatry records have affected mother Nadya's relationship with her little daughter Beate some 30 years later? Would Nadya be prone now, in her fifties, to negatively influence Beate once she would become a mother? Rephrasing Nadya's questions in impersonal terms, do we repeat such experiences without being aware of it? Thus, does the Infantile play any role in our adult lives? Through Laura's case and my discussions of reconstruction – how its kernel of truth can be ascertained and doubted and how we may conceive of its value in psychoanalytic therapy – I have arrived at answering yes to Nadya's questions. To emphasise, it is a qualified, complicated, delimited, and far from dead-certain yes; nevertheless, it is a yes. It is similar to saying that traces of the Infantile may be vague, subdued, and subterranean – but they are there, and they affect us, whether in pain or pleasure. There is, however, a window open for change. Nadya is now seeking my help to understand better the transmission of the Infantile through the generations. Thus, she hopes to become better equipped to break the transmission chain with Beate. This work is ongoing with Nadya and me.

Source

This chapter is a reworked version of a published paper (Salomonsson, 2020). I thank the publisher for giving permission to quote it in the book.

Chapter 8

Language concealing and revealing the Infantile

A recurring proposition in this book is that parent – infant psychotherapy (PIP) can inspire therapists who wish to grasp even better why and how their adult patients suffer and how they can contain their patients' calamities. As our cases have illustrated, I refer especially to anxieties about separation and lowered self-esteem, mishaps in intimate relationships, excessive quarrelsomeness, and so on. I do not claim, however, that all such hardships are "caused" by the Infantile. Several developmental levels and psychic structures, grounded and solidified over a lifetime, are always involved in psychological distress.

Since I put forward PIP as a major support in understanding certain patients and/or some clinical situations referring to their Infantile, I must also approach some critical questions. First, is PIP a *psychoanalytic* therapy, or is its focus more on rectifying derailed interactions and behaviours in the dyad? Second, is the baby a patient – or is the mother the sole receiver of the therapist's interventions? Third, if I claim that the baby is a patient as well, how do I explain that he or she cannot comprehend my verbal interpretations?

I have responded to these questions in publications (Salomonsson, 2007a, 2007b, 2011, 2014a, 2018, 2021, 2022, 2023) and here in Chapter 3. From early on, I applied a semiotic perspective to conceptualise what was going on in PIP therapies. It highlighted that when we talk to somebody, so many other modes of communications are running in parallel. I used C.S. Peirce's theories (Kloesel & Houser, 1992, 1998; Misak, 2018) to account for these modes. See Chapters 3 and 12 in this book. I also argued that while babies do not understand the lexical import of words, they are expert readers of other communication forms.

Many analysts, especially those who had seen my PIP videos and experimental videos such as the Still-Face paradigm, agreed that the PIP baby was affected by my attention to his or her words, gestures, tone of voice, eye contact, and so on. As seen in Chapter 9, such interactions may also take a negative turn, as when I intervened to help the baby – but my Infantile pushed me into a contradictory embodied communication that seemed to make the baby distressed.

DOI: 10.4324/9781003640363-8

Still, I was not satisfied with merely stating that a baby could grasp my intentions, ideas, and containing comments but *not* comprehend its lexical content. There was too much of "not" in my argument. Was it true that the baby did not understand spoken language at all until one day an aha experience hit him? This sounded rash and simplistic. Furthermore, it did not answer an essential question: During the time when babies understand no literal meanings of words, why do parents speak to them anyway ("You're a sweetie" or "The phone's ringing, maybe Dad's calling")?

Could we dismiss these examples by, "They just express the mother's feelings. It's an outlet *from* her, not a message *to* the baby!" I am not content with these arguments since parents talking to their babies seem to believe that there is a receptive partner on the other side of the line. To learn more, I began studying neurophysiological and developmental literature on these topics until I could rephrase the questions. Although the baby does not understand "sweetie" or "phone", she might grasp that the mother's smile, stress reaction, or longing for her husband was accompanied by another specific component. We, who know how to speak and understand it, call it "language". It issues from the same body parts, from our pharynx and mouth, as do babies' screams and babbling. Yet it is a specific communication mode. Might the baby grasp the specificity that we attach to it?

To compare: I neither speak nor comprehend Chinese. But if I hear a couple talking, I might think, "They are probably speaking Chinese. I don't understand it, but I'm quite certain he wants to convey something gentle to her". Babies often seem to hark when parents are talking to each other, as if they grasp it is different from singing or humming. But how and when do they begin to get it that spoken language is a specific and rich mode of conveying all kinds of information? These questions became important as I was writing a paper, "The function of language in parent-infant psychotherapy" (Salomonsson, 2017). It addresses a paradox: The basis for psychotherapy is *verbal* dialogue, but many phenomena that I subsume under the concept of the Infantile stem from *nonverbal* experiences and memories. Thus, how can you *talk* with an adult about traces of an epoch that was "untalkable"? Likewise, PIP consists, largely but not solely, in talking to a "non-talker". Is such a method reasonable? To get food for thoughts, let us start with an everyday encounter.

Nicole's baby daughter Valérie won't fall asleep

Nicole is a young doctor and mother of nine-month-old *Valérie*. She just started a new assignment at a hospital and tomorrow, she will make a case presentation. Tonight, she must study relevant literature. But Valérie won't fall asleep. Nicole picks her up, cuddles and feeds her, walks around with her saying, "It's time for bed, darling, it's dark outside and all babies are asleep". Nothing helps. Valérie keeps whining and seems restless and unhappy.

Finally, Nicole tucks her to bed again and says, "Now, really, Valérie. Mum's got to be on her own. I must read my books to help a sick lady become well again". A minute later, the girl is asleep and sleeps through the night.

Nicole states that in her final address to the girl, her more decided tone of voice sprang from an attitudinal change: from pleading with the girl to fall asleep to recognising her own vexation and wish to prioritise her work duties. "Still, I wonder what made Valérie fall asleep instantly at that point. Because my tone of voice became sharper? Or was it rather that inside, I felt more determined? Or because I told her explicitly *why* I wanted her to sleep?" Nicole meanders between three explanatory models:

1   A change in the nonverbal and emotional layers of her communication
2   An internal change of balance in her priorities
3   The explicit verbal explanation about the sick lady

All three models contain enigmatic factors. Model (1) can be corroborated with experimental research on infants. Their sensitivity to emotional communication is well demonstrated (Bornstein, Arterberry, & Mash, 2004; Carver & Vaccaro, 2007; Kugiumutzakis, Kokkinaki, Makrodimitraki, & Vitalaki, 2005; Leppänen, Moulson, Vogel-Farley, & Nelson, 2007; Sorce et al., 1985; Tronick, 1989, 2007b). When Nicole got in emotional contact with her own desire to prioritise her job, how did this materialise in her nonverbal communication? When considering model (2), we must also acknowledge the concept of unconscious communication (S. Freud, 1912, 1915b). Freud (1912) provided a metaphor: like a telephone receiver that converts the sender's electric signal into sound waves, the analyst's Unconscious is able, "from the derivatives of the unconscious which are communicated to him, to reconstruct that unconscious" (116). If the analyst fails to remove the resistances "which hold back from his consciousness what has been perceived by his unconscious" (116), he cannot fully grasp what the patient told him. In brief, when the analyst is unable to look into his Unconscious, he cannot do a good job. In parallel, at first, perhaps Nicole resisted listening to her unconscious anger and frustration. This transformed her into a Gestalt in which conscious and unconscious communications intertwined in a muddled way. Valérie could not decipher mother's communications and went on whining.

Model (3) is problematic since it presupposes that the lexical content of verbal language would be explicitly comprehensible to little Valérie. She would thus discern the differences between mother's words, "It's time to go to bed, darling" and the ensuing "Valérie, Mum's got to be on her own". If we apply another perspective, could we agree that her differential reactions did relate, at least in some way, to mother's verbal address – without insisting that she understood the literal content of Nicole's communication? If we retract from the latter claim, then what constituents of language did Valérie grasp?

Sometimes, parents report that the baby seems affected by the words per se, though they cannot pinpoint how. They do not need to attend to these theoretical issues, but PIP therapists must ask if there really is a distinctive point in using language with a baby. Many therapists (Cramer & Palacio Espasa, 1993; Fraiberg, 1980; Lebovici & Stoléru, 2003; Lieberman & Van Horn, 2008) go beyond talking to the *parents* about how their painful feelings are connected with the baby's disorder. They also speak to the *baby* about her internal state and its connection with her behaviour and mother's emotions. One, Françoise Dolto, will be covered further down. Another analyst was Johan Norman (2001, 2004) and myself (Salomonsson, 2007a, 2007b, 2011, 2012a, 2013a, 2013b, 2014a, 2015b).

The focus of Norman and myself has mainly been on models (1) and (2) to explicate how our address might impact on the baby. I will summarise the two and move on to other objectives. One is to investigate whether model (3) conceals a further argument for speaking to the baby. The hypothesis is that when the analyst speaks to the baby, he makes evident to him/her, not only that a *symbolic order* exists in the form of language but that *the way he uses it differs from the parents' use and this will help the baby handle the distress more efficiently*. Another objective is to examine *if neuroscientific studies warrant such an address*, namely if they support that the baby's brain can register verbal communication as being different from other modes. The story of Nicole comes from everyday life. It is time for a clinical vignette to illustrate the discussion.

Clinical material: Irene with her son David, seven months

Forty-year-old Irene tells me that David, seven months old, was born by caesarean delivery due to a breech presentation. She fears this has affected him negatively. Two months old, he got a viral infection and was hospitalised with her. "I hadn't understood how ill he was! All these tubes and machines were terrible." After some days, they returned home and David was fine – but at four months, he began avoiding her eyes while looking at his father and Benny, his three-year-old brother.

During our first encounter, David is breastfeeding while playing calmly with mother's hand. He never looks into her eyes but gives me long happy smiles. Irene speaks sadly of her pain, guilt, and stress with her children. She fears that her concerns about Benny during pregnancy might have harmed David: "He was born with a frown on his forehead." As he avoids her eyes again, she exclaims: "What did I do wrong to you!?" We start therapy twice weekly focusing on her guilt, frustration, and humiliation, and his gaze avoidance. From the third hour onwards, the sessions are videorecorded upon the mother's consent.

During the fifth session, the mother reports that Benny was crying when arriving at preschool. "It was excruciating, I felt so guilty. Already during my pregnancy with David I had such a bad conscience about his brother. *He* looks in my eyes, and *David* looks at everyone but me!"

Analyst to David:	"I see that you avoid Mum, David. Let's work with this, shall we? Mum doesn't dare move her head closer to yours."
	(As she lifts him up towards her, he avoids her eyes insistently. She tries to kiss him, but he recoils).
Analyst:	"When you, Mum, hold David it seems you're approaching and rejecting at the same time."
	(He climbs on her, avoids her eyes and cries).
Mother:	"I can't fling myself at him, he must want to do this, too!"
Analyst to David:	"Well, David, I think you really want to come close to your Mum. But you're terribly afraid!"
	(He whines more).
Analyst:	"Now it's getting scary for you."
	(David stands on her lap, whining, and avoiding her eyes).
Analyst:	"You're hurling yourself backwards from mother, looking at me. 'Björn, help me with this monster looking at me'."
	(He looks away briefly, laughs a little, and folds back into mother's lap without eye contact. He grabs her décolletage).
Analyst:	"You want Mum's breast? The usual solution... You're thinking of breast-feeding him now?"
Mother:	"Yes... but it doesn't really solve the problem."
Analyst:	"It's like getting a fix."
Mother:	"Yeah!"
Analyst:	"David, you needed a fix when you got afraid, coming close to Mum."

During the remainder of the hour, David often screams in despair. Yet Irene also says that the past weekend was "like magic. I was breast-feeding and for the first time he looked into my eyes at length. It really gave me hope! Still, it's so hard to forgive myself."

Analyst:	"Shouldn't you be given a second chance, Irene? What kind of love is that? (David smiles at me). And you David, you need to forgive Mum... Maybe you, Irene, need to forgive David as well. Perhaps you're thinking: 'You silly kid, avoiding my eyes! Yes, Mum's angry with you as well, David. Now you calmed down."

The atmosphere becomes serene and calm. She caresses his hair and there are some brief moments of eye contact. At one point, she says to him, "I love you".

Therapeutic work dealt with Irene's sense of rejection by David, her guilt of accommodating him without feeling she abandoned his brother, and her vexation with the husband. I also clarified to David his disappointment and anger with Mum, his repudiations, the fear of her eyes, and his yearning for her. My countertransference paralleled many of Irene's emotions. When he avoided her eyes, it was humiliating to her and bewildering to me. When he smiled at me, I felt favoured at Mum's expense, which disconcerted me. As he avoided her eyes, I felt sorry for him but also annoyed and curious at the same time.

Perhaps David had noted Irene's conflictual feelings in her ways of holding him, tone of voice, and so on. This hypothesis would go along with models (1) and (2) in the previous section on Nicole and Valérie; David had been affected by mother's changes in communicating nonverbally her affects and priorities. What might be contentious is the extent of my talking to David and the assumption that it might help him, which would have followed model (3). But David did not understand "terribly afraid" or "this monster looking at me". Instead, it was perhaps *the mother* who listened and understood my words. We could then discard all three models and state that *she* was the sole patient. Through my words to him, she grasped his internal situation and changed her behaviour, which made him calm down. So why did I speak to both of them? This faces me with a crucial question: to what extent was David affected by my words – if at all?

Babies and signs: a brief summary

To account for the various communicative levels on which humans produce and understand verbal or nonverbal signs, I have applied semiotic concepts of C.S. Peirce (Kloesel & Houser, 1992, 1998, Misak, 2018). Put very briefly, his model suggests that all signs may be interpreted as *icons, indices*, and *word symbols* in various combinations. This perspective runs throughout the book, especially in my accounts of PIP work. Today, many analysts working with adult patients also apply semiotic theory to conceptualise their work (Chinen, 1987; Gammelgaard, 1998; Goetzmann & Schwegler, 2004; Grotstein, 1980, 1997; Martindale, 1975; J. Muller, 1996; J. Muller & Brent, 2000; Olds, 2000; da Rocha Barros & da Rocha Barros, 2011; Van Buren, 1993). Now if, as Olds (2000) states, life "requires the presence of systems in which signs function" (507), we could assume that a very young baby is fit for reading the signs that the family conveys: smiles, frowns, sighs, kisses, and so on. He also produces signs that the family members capture: screaming, cooing, smelling, smiling, and so on. Mother – infant interaction is thus an intercourse of signs, and semiotic terminology can help us conceptualise what goes on inside and between mother and baby.

A reader unfamiliar with semiotic concepts might feel at a loss here. Allow me then to formulate this perspective in Winnicottian terms and to do it with a focus on the young baby who comes with the mother to the PIP therapist. In his paper "*Ego integration in child development*" (1962), he differentiates a baby governed completely by his or her Id from a slightly older one who is also influenced by a nascent Ego. There is "no sense in making use of the word 'id' for phenomena that are not covered and catalogued and experienced and eventually interpreted by ego-functioning" (56). An "Id-baby", someone Winnicott compares to an anencephalic baby, can perceive but not represent. Gradually, Id-functioning is "collected together in all its aspects and becomes ego-experience". In a formula, as long as Id = 0, the analyst has nothing to say. But when Id combines with experiences that are made with the help of the mother and the child's nascent Ego, we PIP therapists have work to do. This implies that, as Winnicott states, we can study the Ego – and thereby influence the child – "long before the word self has relevance" (56).

The tools that enable such work are the signs that the baby's mind produces. When I saw Nic in Chapter 3 fretting at the right-hand breast and I heard about the mother's previous sore nipple, I took his behaviour as a sign, like "I'm not feeling well here". His mind had evidently created a representation, a sign, that sucking at this breast was linked with distress in mother and thence in him. This was due not only to the mother's pained nipple but also to other reasons for her distress, which disabled her containing capacity. As for Nic, it prevented his Ego from integrating the various components of breastfeeding into a nice and calming experience.

Now to our questions: Do the therapist's words only reach the *mother* to increase her comprehension of the dynamics behind the disturbance? And/or is the *baby* able to grasp our verbal address on an iconical and indexical level and feel contained by it (J. Muller & Brent, 2000; Salomonsson, 2007a)? Might it even convey to the infant that the analyst is *using the symbolic order in another way* and with another intent than the one he or she is used to from his mother? Perhaps, her use of words has been obfuscated by conflicting affects that she does not dare to acknowledge? If the analyst speaks in a different way, what are the characteristics? And does the baby react differentially to them? If so, would it affect our argument if we could demonstrate that a baby not only perceives the emotional import of nonverbal communication but also perceives *language as a specific mode of communication?* Specifically, does speaking to a baby concur with modern neuroscience and developmental psychology? Does David's brain register words differently from my other sounds?

Parler vrai to babies

After having formulated the questions at the end of the previous section, we need to account for neuroscientific studies. Yet there is still much that needs our attention regarding psychoanalytic theories of how a baby receives and processes language. Let me first insert a literary quote to portray our topics in focus. In Antoine de Saint-Exupéry's (1946) novella *The Little Prince*, the fox is teaching the boy in order to tame him and create a bond. He says: "Sit down a bit from me, in the grass. I'll look at you from the corner of my eye and you'll say nothing. *Language is a source of misunderstandings*" (80, italics added). I interpret the fox as stating that our interpretations of verbal communication may be contradictory at various sign levels. The way our words are understood also depends on the emotional climate, the tone of voice, and so on. For each emotional situation, we can find appropriate ways of pronouncing the words: with gratitude, warmth, coldness, embitterment, rancour, irony, ecstasy, and so on. Such "hyper-semiosis" applies to all verbal communication. Babies don't understand words literally, but parents use them to help their baby regulate affects and solve conflicts. They can say "Thanks" with warmth when he gives them a lovely smile and with vexation when a splash of poo stains their clothes at the diaper changing board.

It is important to consider if a speaker is conscious or not of her affects and if the verbal and nonverbal facets of communication coalesce or diverge. Irene was enmeshed in guilt vis-à-vis her sons, anger with her husband, and panic at recalling the stay at the hospital. In her state of primary maternal preoccupation (Winnicott, 1956), the border between her Unconscious and Preconscious was more permeable, and we saw a "re-emergence of previously repressed fantasies into pre-consciousness and consciousness" (Pines, 1993, 49). One example was her idea that David was born with a frown because she had worried about his brother. This created a jumble in her which, I speculate, made David confused and uneasy. My aim with speaking to him was to indicate that words can be used to *parler vrai*, namely to say loud and clear what is the matter, as did Françoise Dolto (1982, 1985, 1994a, 1994b) when she addressed infants in a plain and truthful manner. Her argument proceeded from Lacanian theory, some parts of which we need review briefly with examples from David and his mother.

In Lacanian theory, David's whining expresses various *demands*, behind which *desires* lie concealed. "Desire" is "a function central to all human experience, [but it] is the desire for nothing nameable" (Lacan, 1991, 223). Its kernel is always inaccessible, and no object can fully satisfy it. Irene becomes its first protagonist in her role of the Other whom David demands, cries and yearns for. Importantly, at bottom, he covets the unreachable "desire for her desire" (Lacan, 1966/2006, 462). Irene's desire is directed both towards her son and backwards towards her own infantile objects. Desire thus roams forever, within and between mother and baby, as in a hall of mirrors.

The analyst teaches the patient "to *name*, to articulate, to bring desire into existence" (Lacan, 1954–1955, 214). But since desire cannot be named, no interpretation can cover it accurately. Therefore, one cannot re-find "the original *jouissance* with the Other" (Dor, 2000, 192). We must thus qualify Freud's (1905b) idea that "the finding of an object is in fact a refinding of it" (222). In fact, such refinding is as futile as capturing one's shadow, a point I brought up in Simone's case in Chapter 1. We seem to have reached an impasse: our interpretations aim to describe the patient's desire but can never pinpoint it. Like an asymptotic curve, our words approach the X-axis of desire without touching it. A second problem, specific to PIP, has been mentioned: babies will not grasp the lexical meaning of interpretations. Is there any way out of the deadlock?

Dolto insisted on *parler vrai* to infants because "we only exist by being linked with others through words" (Ledoux, 2006, 188). And, if her verbal address was not *vrai* to herself, she would express a jumble where melody, facial communication, and literal content conveyed contradictory meanings. Dolto said things to the infant that his parents had been silent about, "for his own good" as they reckoned. When I told David that he was hurling backwards from Irene as from a monster, I described an emotional truth I believed both avoided. Her eyes represented an internal reality that he was struggling to comprehend and integrate: her vexation, frustration, guilt, love, and concern. Maybe, in David's mind, her eyes had also been "infected" by his vengeance and anger – or in other terms – the projections of "bad feelings" and, thus, he had better shun them.

Parler vrai to mothers

We need to also ask if *parler vrai* with the mother is just as important. My briefest answer is, yes, it is both important and difficult. Parents in PIP are loaded with painful feelings:

> What is wrong with my child? What did I do wrong to her? Doesn't she love me? Is she autistic? Did I harm her by drinking that glass of wine after the pregnancy test? I did want a child but now, I don't know. She's the sweetest and loveliest child in the world. Sometimes I feel it, sometimes I don't – and then I hate myself and feel so ashamed and afraid of talking to anybody about all this.

Such maelstroms probably occur momentarily in most mothers. But a vast majority can keep them at a distance or call on their partner or parent to talk and get comfort. The parents we see in PIP are precisely those who did not succeed in keeping the torrents at bay. When they meet a therapist, they may view him as someone to talk with and get comfort from. But there is also a fear that he shall be condemning, moralising, partial, or simply uninvolved. This sprawling transference includes the mother's fear that PIP would harm her child or their relationship. "We shouldn't poke into my history. Our child is born now, and it's time to start a new chapter in my life". Well, I wouldn't be a psychoanalyst if I thought that dust should be left under the carpet for eternity. PIP experiences have taught me that it is often crucial to take seriously mothers' questions cited above – but to do it gently, with good timing, and without any know-it-all attitude.

Thus, *parler vrai*, with both infant and parent, is essential. Here is an example from the second session. Irene talks with disappointment and anger about David's father. At the same time, I sense that she is comparing her partner and me to my favour. Her idealising transference is unsettling since I am quite certain that David won't give up his gaze avoidance instantly – and when Irene realises that we will need much time to work this through with him, her idealisations of me might crunch. This would be healthy in itself but could also rebound into more resentful attitudes towards me and our joint work.

Irene:	"A big crisis yesterday! The climate between me and Mike, my partner, was tense. Then David tried to roll toward Mike and refused to be near me."
Analyst:	"That's why you sound tense today?"
Irene:	"Maybe. It never happened that he didn't allow me to tuck him to bed."
Analyst:	"Perhaps you think, 'what the hell is Björn doing!?'"
Irene (laughing a bit sourly):	"Well, yeah, but I'm prepared this can take time."

The *vrai* or truthful element is about her negative transference, that she fears I don't know what I'm doing. A week later, Irene criticises her partner again. She also hates nagging at him, which makes her feel like a vixen.

Analyst:	"You sound like you're possessed by a devil inside."
Irene:	"Well, not possessed but... unrestrained."
Analyst:	"Unrestrained sounds nicer than possessed, but I believe you are afraid of that harpy inside, especially when you feel something similar about David, although you don't yell at him as you do with Mike."

The milieu of this dialogue is that David is screaming and avoiding mother's eyes since the session started. Our dialogue is therefore doubly taxing to Irene: David is yelling, and she fears her frustration and hostility towards Mike – and towards David too. I use horror story–like words such as "devil" to capture the strength of her feelings and the fears they evoke in her.

In connection with the book's focus on the Infantile, this dialogue exemplifies that when we want to detect its traces, we must often use interventions that are *vrai*. Irene and I needed to talk much about her "internal hag" that caused her guilt in relation to David and rage in relation to Mike. After having traversed such battlegrounds of witches, devils, and harpies, Irene realised she could not kill those internal objects but had to acquaint herself with them. Then the scene calmed down, as when we discovered that Irene is also a timid person.

Analyst to David:	"Before, I thought Mum was depressed and that's why you couldn't look at her. But maybe Mum was shy? Maybe she didn't dare look at you? (To Irene:) You were looking at me, you looked sad, it was a straightforward look. To be depressed is being closed, restrained. To be shy is more like stopping up the flow of one's feelings."
Irene:	"I'm both timid and not timid. Once, a teacher asked me to represent all students in a seminar. 'I don't dare, I'm too shy', I replied. 'But Irene, all sorts of people are needed in this world!' I loved that teacher forever!"

I did not learn more about Irene's timidity. Neither did we work much on the internal "harpy" object, which I assumed had many links with the relation with her mother (H. C. Freud, 2011). But her memory of the sensitive teacher brought forward a tender facet in her that she could embrace and perceive as a valuable asset. I think this timid girl inside helped her in the relationship with David: when he was in a bad mood, the timid girl could function as a counterpart to the bitch.

Language substituting for desire

It is time to focus again on David. One may agree with my description of his internal dilemma without supporting Dolto's idea of *parler vrai* to him about it. Her claim that a baby can capture the lexical meaning of words has been criticised by analysts (Anthony, 1974; Axelrad, 1960; Bacon, 2013). It is also contradicted by common sense and research studies (Karmiloff & Karmiloff-Smith, 2001; Bergelson & Swingley, 2012). Yet nobody would question parents who talk to their babies or deny that it is better to speak warmly than harshly. But is it even helpful to the baby if *the analyst* is practising *parler vrai* with her, especially about excruciating matters? Our answer depends on how we envisage the baby's external and internal situation and our prime task as therapists. In Dolto's view, the infant cannot hold together and make meaningful his self by an inside sense of truth, but rather, "like words in a sentence, by law or grammar or force ... [a baby] is continuously being *formed in* and *informed* by language and speaking" (Bacon, 2002, 260, italics added).

In a second paper on Dolto, her proponent Bacon (2013) goes beyond saying that the infant builds up his self *like* words in a sentence. Words are now viewed as the very building blocks of the baby's Preconscious. He becomes a subject by immersing himself in the parent's speech. In Dolto's words,

> By speaking with her child of what [the baby] would like but which she is not giving to him, [the mother] makes known to him the absence of an object or the non-satisfying of a demand for partial pleasure, while at the same time giving value to... this desire.
>
> (Dolto, 1984, 63–65, translated by Bacon, 2013, 524)

A parent might tell the child: "I know you want to be with me all the time, but I want to speak with Grandpa on the phone now. Then I'll be back with you again."

In everyday life, parental speech contains "ambiguities, shifts, and transformations" (Bacon, 2002, 260). Recall Doctor Nicole, who at first used *parler faux* with little Valérie. As long as she blocked her vexation from awareness, she kept pleading to Valérie in vain. Not until she told the emotional truth did the ambiguities dissolve, the girl's distress vanish – and the girl fell asleep.

Can we apply these ideas to the clinical situation? Are *the therapist's words to a baby* of any help? Dolto would answer yes: "Speaking to a baby and putting words to what he is experiencing participates in founding his [psychic] structure" (Ledoux, 2006, 189). Parents need to "talk about [the baby's desires] because they are always justifiable, even though one does not want to help him with them" (Dolto, 1994b, 108). In my view, this position applies to the analyst too. David has been closing his eyes to a mother whom he loves, fears, resents, and reproaches. Irene has avoided speaking clearly with him about the desires she intuits in him and in herself. She does realise that breastfeeding does not remedy David's ongoing whining, but she cannot address him about how their desires are clashing. At this point, I comment on his wish for a "fix" and the need to forgive his mother. I am thus acknowledging his desire of the breast *and* comparing it to an impossible panacea or what Dolto calls a "short-circuit satisfaction" (97).

There is an austere element in Dolto's conception of *parler vrai*, such as when she speaks of subjecting a child to *symboligenic castrations* (1982). Only through them can the child gain access to sublimation and the symbolic order. Readers familiar with Winnicott's thinking may find this hard to accept. Dolto would deny neither that there exists "an intermediate area of experiencing, to which inner reality and external life both contribute" (Winnicott, 1971, 2) nor that "psychotherapy has to do with two people playing together" (38). But she did caution that the transitional object may prevent a child from "addressing his pain and give him the illusion that he is still at the breast" (Dolto, 1994b, 143). Her words to infants aimed to counter this illusion.

I agree with Bacon (2002) that Winnicott viewed the identification of mother and baby as "the sine qua non of good-enough mothering", whereas to Dolto it was more like "a dangerous realm of imaginary relations which is and has to be subject to castration in order for a speaking subject to emerge" (260). These two emphases lead to different techniques. Dolto focused on truthful words of frustration that should inspire the child to embrace the symbolic order. *Language should substitute for desire*. Winnicott focused on how a child maintains an illusion that the breast is part of him and under his magical control. This illusion is kept until the child is ready to drop it and then create a new game or jingle.

The baby's response to *parler vrai*

Let us stop for some questions. Do I contend that David responds to the lexical meaning of the analyst's words? No! Do I claim that he pays attention to me as someone who "parle vrai"? Yes, I do. Does his attention differ from the one he pays to his mother? Most probably, because I speak differently than her. Then why would he appreciate truthful speech? First of all, I do not think babies automatically and always appreciate *parler vrai*. Like older persons, they are caught up in conflicting desires and maladaptive defences and vote for a conservative line, so to speak. Still, when David encounters my persistent address, it catches his attention and even curiosity. What distinguishes Irene's from my ways of speaking, and how and why would David react differently to them?

As to how the analyst's and the mother's communications differ, I have mentioned the extent to which our verbal and nonverbal communications coalesce or diverge. Here, I would add my elaboration within the countertransference. When working with the two, I sensed their agony, I identified with them in feeling helpless, incredulous, empathic, and frustrated myself. I also observed how they countered their agonies with maladaptive defences. Finally, I put words to these intra- and inter-personal conflicts: "David, I think you want to come close to your Mum. But you're terribly afraid". In other words, I first immersed myself in the quagmire of his helplessness and Irene's despondency. Then I exited from that state and took up courage to speak out. Freud (1912) compares the analyst to the surgeon, "who puts aside all his feelings, even his human sympathy, and concentrates his mental forces on the single aim of performing the operation as skilfully as possible" (115). I certainly do not put aside my feelings, but I stay with them and then take the next step: to pluck up courage and "operate skilfully", namely to *parler vrai* about painful matters.

The second question could be split in two: does the child *confirm* that he has been impacted by my words, and does he listen to them *differently* than how he listens to his mother's communication? As for the first, I am at odds with Dolto (1985); babies do not give unequivocal confirmations to analytic interventions. When I intuit that my address indeed has affected a baby, what signs do I rely on? I need to answer tentatively: sometimes, I cannot discern any reactions in the baby at all to my words. At other times, as in David's case, the child seems to be slowly captured by my address. With other babies, there are moments when they suddenly look earnestly at me, after which an affective change ensues; they might start sobbing or, in contrast, become relaxed.

These impressions might seem like weak confirmations that the intervention has any substance to it and that the child has received and processed it. But this uncertainty applies, more or less, to analysands of any age. Children in analysis rarely provide a "yes" or "no" to an intervention. Instead, they may change the play or create a new fantasy story. And as for adult patients, how often can we claim that their response to an interpretation confirms it was accurate? I believe our work is more about containing their anxiety and confusion, to which they may respond with relief and a sense of being understood, which enables them to move a bit from a locked and unfruitful functioning. Importantly, we cannot exactly discern *what* in our intervention helped the patient budge: its lexical content, our tone of voice, rhythm, gestures, or something else. To quote Bion (1962), in psychoanalysis "the criterion cannot be whether a particular usage is right or wrong, meaningful or verifiable, but whether it does, or does not, promote development" (iii).

Let us now return to David. I have already suggested he paid attention to my words due to their assets that we adults call sincerity and truth. What does their veracity consist of? As said, verbal and nonverbal communication coalesce; that is, there is no dissimulation. Second, I address his *psychic conflicts*, and this – or rather the earnest way with which I speak to him about them – will capture his focus because *he wants to develop*. True, David wants to short-circuit his internal conflicts by craving for Mum's breast and avoiding her eyes. But he also suffers, he is stuck and cannot progress. A child has a strong "wish to be grown-up and to be able to do what grown-up people do" (S. Freud, 1920, 17). It is as if every child intuits that "Who does not grow, declines", as Rabbi Hillel formulated it in the Talmud.

Parler vrai can be seen in the light of this developmental drive. My address is poignant and clear, which David registers. He distrusts it at first but then intuits that I want to help him realise his wish to move on. To extend Freud's metaphor, perhaps he thinks of me like we think of a surgeon: we do not necessarily love him, but we would be foiled if he did not lance the boil. David's "boil" is the covert conflicts in him and mother which need to be opened up. In another framework, we can say he is on the verge of developing an insecure attachment. Note, however, that I don't seek to directly promote attachment, encourage him, or scaffold the mother-infant relationship. I verbalise his inner conflicts, which have thwarted the building-up of a secure attachment.

Parler vrai to adults in psychotherapy

By now, a therapist who is familiar with adult patients but not with infants is probably asking how the philosophy and method of *parler vrai* relates to one's daily work. In brief, I believe it is as important in work with adults as with babies. I will return to a dialogue in Chapter 1 between Simone and me:

Analyst: "You cling to Martin, it's all about his lips and devotion of you, and you only. It's like a baby who searches her mother's eyes and breast and cannot come to rest until the two are re-united. But why this unrest when Martin and you are apart? Why is it only the kisses you long for? You never speak of his male body."

I conceive of this as to *"parler vrai"*. Simone wants to convince me that her relationship with Martin is wonderful and unique. She speaks of their encounters as moments of bliss and salvation. However, as I listen to her, I get neither any internal images of Martin nor any idea about what makes him so desirable. My take on their relationship is thus different from Simone's and, of course, this is hurting to her. *Parler vrai* means being not blunt but honest and communicating something that is helpful to the patient.

At this point, one might ask why Simone, madly in love, continued talking about it with me, especially since I shared my doubts whether this was love or "addiction" as we called it. Here, the word "madly" is key. She relishes being with Martin but also fears her passion because there is something "mad" about it. Not only because it can topple her marriage and family life. There is also a hunger-like feeling in her to get a text message from Martin NOW; otherwise, she despairs. "It feels as if I'm possessed though... actually I don't know much about him", she says with embarrassment and anxiety. This answers our question. Simone intuited that therapy would be not a honeymoon but an encounter with someone who was thinking and talking to her in a respectful, empathic, and truthful way. She wanted *parler vrai* and she got it. The next chapter will show that *parler vrai* is essential to the therapist as well.

Language development: findings from neuroscience

We will now touch on our second investigation: whether the technique of speaking to a baby gains support from neuroscience. Thus, *is the infant brain capable of discerning language as a specific mode of communication?* If not, the concept "verbal communicatio with babies" would be a *contradictio in adjecto* since they would actually listen to the sounds of spoken words as they listened to any other sound in their milieu. The original paper underlying this chapter (Salomonsson, 2017) accounted for neuroscientific and developmental research, though not because I hoped that it would confirm the *psychoanalytic* validity of an intervention. Such a confirmation can be reached only in the analytic situation and not in the neuroscience lab. I rather wanted to investigate whether such research might show if the baby is capable of differentiating *language as a special mode of communication.*

Neuroscientific research ages quickly and – though fascinating – it veers far from our study of the Infantile. Thence, I will be brief in this section and start by bringing in a finding that allows for some reflections from an object relational perspective. It has been known for long that babies prefer their mother's language to others (Moon, Cooper, & Fifer, 1993) and her voice to that of other women (DeCasper & Fifer, 1980). These effects are probably instigated *in utero* (Moon, Lagercrantz, & Kuhl, 2013). But even if one would summarise this into "Mum's voice is the best", this does not prove that babies perceive language as a specific communication mode. Yet we know that two-month-old babies prefer words from a human voice to similar but artificially produced words (Vouloumanos & Werker, 2004).

The grand question is *"whether evolution has endowed humans with a genetically determined cortical organization* particularly suitable to process speech or whether fast learning quickly specializes the auditory network toward speech processing during this initial period" (Mahmoudzadeh et al., 2013, italics added). Indeed, the hemispheres of three-day-old premature babies of 28–32 weeks' gestational age react differently to a change of voice quality (female vs. male) compared with a change of phoneme ("ga" vs. "ba"). All these stimuli elicit a higher response from the *right* cortex, which simply reflected the auditory stimulation. Thus, this finding does not answer our question. Remarkably, however, only the ga-ba paradigm led to a response in those *left* areas that are known to process speech. The conclusion relies on the fact that differentiating "ga" from "ba" has more to do with processing *language* than whether the speaker is male or female. Thus, there probably exists "an early organization of the immature human brain into functions useful for deciphering the speech signal" (4850). Similar findings were published by Teinonen et al. (2009).

Newborns also detect simple speech structures (Gervain, Macagno, Cogoi, Peña, & Mehler, 2008) and primitive artificial grammar. Three- to four-month-old babies grasp that words have a specific function too, like categorising toy animals and other objects (Ferry, Hespos, & Waxman, 2010). The underlying neuroanatomy is well mapped (Sato et al., 2012; Clarke, Tyler, & Marslen-Wilson, 2024; Januário, Bertachini, Escarce, de Resende, & de Miranda, 2024).

To sum up, a PIP therapist talking to a baby should know that though the child perhaps imitates his facial expressions and pays attention to his nonverbal communication (gestures, tone of voice, rhythm, smiles, frowns, etc.), she cannot understand any lexical meaning. But she does perceive speech as a specific input and not only as a "voice melody" (Fernald, 2004; Vouloumanos & Werker, 2007). The therapist can also feel confident that the infant can discern some emotional meaning of words, such as approval and disapproval (Fernald, 1993). To conclude,

> Infants may analyze speech more deeply than other signals because it is highly familiar or highly salient, because it is produced by humans, because it is inherently capable of bearing meaning, or because it bears some not-yet-identified acoustic property that draws the attention of the rule-induction system. Regardless, *from birth, infants prefer listening to speech over listening to closely matched control stimuli.*
>
> (Marcus, Fernandes, & Johnson, 2007, 390, italics added)

PIP therapists can thus feel certain that a baby's brain has been wired to register speech as a special form of communication.

Final comments about verbal interventions to babies in PIP

Distressed babies often face communications that are coloured by parental "ghosts in the nursery" (S. Fraiberg et al., 1975), "negative attributions" (R. Silverman & Lieberman, 1999), or "projective distortions" (Cramer & Palacio Espasa, 1993). This may be a heavy burden, as shown in PIP reports (Anzieu-Premmereur & Pollak-Cornillot, 2003; Beebe, 2003; Emanuel & Bradley, 2008; Jones, 2006; Likierman, 2003; Pozzi-Monzo & Tydeman, 2007; Thomson Salo, 2007; Tuters et al., 2011; von Klitzing, 2003; Watillon, 1993). If words meant only their lexical content, such babies would have fewer problems. If David's mother's words, "I love you", were *vrai* in the complete emotional sense of the word, they would not create distress. But "the sounds and rhythms of language systems are much more than signals. They are *indices or addresses to information about affect states and relationships*, as well as about concepts and objects" (Litowitz, 2014, 299, italics added). Thus, Irene's "I love you" comprises that she loves David, feels guilty about his older brother, worries about his relationship with her, is mortified by his gaze avoidance and angry with his father, and feels bad about herself as a mother. In Dolto's terms, Irene's "I love you" is not to completely *parler vrai*. Rather, from an emotional perspective, it is a very mixed message.

As Litowitz notes, everybody uses language to deceive, as when a parent tells the baby, "It's bedtime, darling", when he wants to watch TV. This is everyday life. The question is to what extent such deceptions permeate the interaction and how far the parent's affects and wishes are conscious to him or her. Interpreting and communicating with a baby compound distortion and clarity. Distortions arise when a parent's conceptions of the baby are more motivated by *her* desire than that of the child. A paradoxically good outcome arises when the baby manages to set aside the pleasure principle and slowly learn the symbolic order to express himself more clearly. Conundrum arises when a boy like David cannot grasp the varying meanings of Irene's verbal and nonverbal communications and then "solves" the problem by avoiding her eyes. A negative spiral is set in motion: he becomes incomprehensible to the mother, which frustrates her and makes her renewed words of "I love you" appear even more bewildering to him.

We can sum up the arguments for an analyst speaking to a baby: (1) His speech contains a lexical word-stream. The baby is neurologically prepared to grasp that this sound is specific to "talkers". She may even intuit that adults speak when they want to convey something they cannot express by a mere gesture, mien, or change in vocal tone. (2) The nonverbal components in the adult's talking can affect her emotionally, such as being calming or distressing. (3) The baby pays attention to an analyst who attends to her, and she may notice emotional alterations in the clinician, and (4) the baby becomes interested in an analyst who tries to *parler vrai* about her distress.

David and his mother Irene were in PIP therapy for 35 sessions covering four months. She then wanted to continue in personal therapy. I had no slots, so I referred her to a colleague. One year later, she sent a photo of David. She wrote that their contact was warm, joyful, and relaxed and that the gaze avoidance was gone. Sometimes, she still struggled with not feeling good enough in her contact with David. He had become a happy, active boy, playing football, dancing, and so on. Irene noted in surprise that her two boys had developed into different personalities. "It's totally natural, don't know why I had other expectations". This shows, in my view, that PIP had achieved another aim as well. Reducing her projections onto David enabled her to see him *vrai*, namely as a boy in his own right.

Source

This chapter is a reworked version of a published paper (Salomonsson, 2017). I thank the publisher for giving permission to quote it in the book.

Chapter 9

Layered analysis of the traces of the Infantile

The previous chapter described how we can use language to deceive and to clarify – in psychotherapy and other human interchanges. It also extended the meaning of verbal communication, considering all other things we do when we talk: we make gestures, raise the tip of the nose to mark disbelief or contempt, tighten an angle of the mouth to emphasize irony, lift our eyebrows in surprise or attention, and so on. New studies emerge using facial action coding systems. They show that the human face has around 50 muscular "action units" that cooperate to signal various emotional expressions (Haritha et al., 2024). We thus "speak" with our face as well as our fingers, fists, buttocks, and more. We can use the sound world in just as many ways by changing voice tonality, dynamics, tone colour, glissando, and so on. The purpose is the same, to bring out or cover up our words' emotional meanings.

Should we name these nonverbal or paralinguistic "accompanists" to our words? When we listen to a singer and her accompanist or band, we tend to regard her as the Number One performer though she may rely heavily on the musicians. Afterwards, we hum the tune and its words rather than the accompaniment. But as for verbal and nonverbal communication running in parallel, I prefer calling the two "teammates", each in their own wright. Adults rely on the lexical and, sometimes without reflection, they exalt words as the most important teammates. But it was different when we were babies – and much less so than we think when we try to understand adults in therapy. As therapists, we need comprehend all "teammates" – the lexical, emotional, and structural – in a communication. We focus on the lexical, because a patient's words can divulge many peculiarities and incongruencies. We need also to focus on its emotional "colour", as when a patient says "please" with a glimmering smile, a sneering mouth, or a dejected sigh. Highlighting the structural aspects can help us decide if a communication is closer to our Conscious or Unconscious and what are its cognitive peculiarities.

These considerations extend the meaning of the term *parler vrai*. As said, it is not a mere method of being outspoken with the patient. The therapist's verbal address to the patient must also be *vrai* to himself. If not, we'd express

DOI: 10.4324/9781003640363-9

to the patient a jumble in which melody, facial communication, and literal content convey contradictory meanings. But to *parler vrai* is easier said than done since every human act is a compromise between conscious and unconscious urges. In Chapter 8, Nicole got nowhere with tucking little Valérie to bed as long as she repressed her professional ambitions and her vexation with her child. The watershed was her words, "Now, really, Valérie. Mum's got to be on her own" as she got in contact with hitherto unconscious negative emotions. If you speak out her words as if you were in that situation, you may discern the musical difference when you are deaf to, or in contact with, your irritation.

Nicole asked what made the girl fall asleep. Had her tone of voice become sharper? Or did she feel more determined? Or was it that she told the girl explicitly *why* she wanted her to sleep? Her conjectures thus covered many "teammates" and not only the verbal. This brings us back to our main focus: the Infantile and the traces that reveal its existence and content. We cannot expect to find them merely in the verbal domain – because many infantile elements of the Infantile (mind the small and capital letters) were *never* verbal. As babies, we did not literally understand our parents' loving words or admonitions. But we did perceive an atmosphere, a gesture, a sound, an odour, and so on, and we sought to grasp the emotional nuances.

Once we realise that human communication goes far beyond the lexical meanings of words, we realise that this includes therapists as well. We need highlight our emotions vis-à-vis the patient, Freud's "countertransference" (1910), which he insisted was an obstacle to analytic work. As we saw in Chapter 2, this mistrustful view has changed substantially today, and it is now regarded as a central "instrument of research into the patient's unconscious" (Heimann, 1950).

Like Heimann and Gabbard (2001), I use countertransference in this broad sense, covering both conscious and unconscious emotions in patient work. But there is a problem: as every therapy student knows, when we tell a supervisor about our clinical work, the experienced colleague can intuit our emotional tones, prejudices, anxieties, predilections, and so on. What we present is not an exact account of what took place in the session, but rather our later recollection of it. The student may be perfectly honest but cannot help being partially unconscious of his Unconscious. This can emerge in his ways of presenting the clinical dialogue, unconsciously concealing the "teammates" in his interaction with the patient, such as how he himself looked or sounded when addressing the patient.

This circumstance when we present our clinical work is a well-known and inevitable aspect of therapeutic work and of supervisions. Lately, some authors have taken up a broader look at countertransference with the help of video technology (Beebe, 2000). Their idea is to scout for visual and auditive signs of countertransference and to see how they affect process in psychotherapy. Such methods have not always been well received by the psychoanalytic community. Bion (1962) is one example. He knew that when we report a clinical experience, it always implies some falsification. He claimed that his terse writing style contained "immeasurably less" falsification than a photo. "Despite a superficial accuracy of result, [the photo] has forced the falsification further back – that is into the session itself" (ix). He claimed a photo contains even more falsification in that "it gives verisimilitude to what has already been falsified". Bion's epistemological perspective is strict, but I recall having agreed to his scepticism about photos. I guess he would have been just as sceptical about filming.

However, when I started with parent – infant psychotherapy (PIP), session events passed by quickly, communications in the room were hard to survey and comprehend, nonverbal communications were paramount, and my session notes seemed not to capture what was "really going on". I thus began videorecording sessions upon the parents' consent. Another input was my research on PIP outcomes (Salomonsson & Sandell, 2011a) described in Chapter 6. Videorecorded interviews with mothers and babies offered me insights into divergencies in the dyad between verbal and nonverbal communication, and conscious and unconscious content. As an extension, I began videorecording my own PIP sessions to understand more about the therapeutic process.

My colleague Tessa Baradon in London then invited me to a group of researchers with herself, Keren Amiran, Evrinomy Avdi, and Michelle Sleed. They were psychoanalysts, psychology researchers, and a cinematographer (Avdi et al., 2020; Baradon, Avdi, Sleed, Salomonsson, & Amiran, 2023). It sounded exciting to get multiple perspectives on clips from my own or others' clinical practice. Some of them came from other fields than my own. Taking part in the group, I began realising that a comment that I had often heard from analysts, "One cannot film the Unconscious", is overly simplified. If a clinician takes part in a group, he can speak about the countertransference in specific clinical moments, and they can assemble the puzzle together. I already knew that discussing psychoanalytic sessions in a group can be enriching (Norman & Salomonsson, 2005; Salomonsson, 2012b). Now, videos were added to these experiences.

When I viewed my own clips with the group, it was a bit like when you suddenly see yourself in a store front in the street. You are looking at and interpreting other people, but you are also being looked at and interpreted by others and, last but not least, by yourself. I had assumed I would focus on the dyad in the session, but the "store front phenomenon" amazed me. I was now looking at myself in the videos, discovering details of my conduct in the session that I had been unconscious of. I had been aware of my emotions in the session, such as fatigue, vexation, sadness, and shock – but I had not known when and how much I *displayed* these feelings through my *embodied communication*. Thus, I had focused considerably less on how my behaviours impacted on mother and baby.

I will use our findings to complicate the remark "one cannot film the Unconscious". What do we see in those clips? In my terms, we see *traces of the Unconscious* as they emerge in observable behaviours in the therapist and the patient(s). These traces are observable – *and* they need psychoanalytic interpretation. Without this combination of video observation in the group and the dialogue with the therapist, these traces will be left to our hazy conjectures. I emphasize that one needs to look at the videos, again and again. This is because we, patient(s) and therapist alike, emit signals without being aware of them, and they may also have multiple meanings.

The following text is based on a paper (Baradon et al., 2023) starting with a scholarly survey of the field. That part and some others are abbreviated here to arrive at the vignettes, a discussion of PIP, and the link with the traces of the Infantile. Our major question for now is this: In the group, we picked out details from PIP videos to scrutinize their course and speculate on their meanings. Could these details, which we thought were significant, be conceived of as "traces of the Infantile"?

Studying clinical process in detail

What happens within a therapeutic encounter? What may contribute to change, stalemate, or harm? What dynamics are introduced by each participant and how do they affect the system? One approach to these questions is to study patient – therapist interactions in detail. We will examine embodied and verbal micro-transactions in PIP sessions, especially moments of *rupture* and how they relate to the therapists' countertransference. We are also focusing on how *repair* comes about. We believe these foci are relevant to clinical practice and training.

Another key source for understanding psychotherapy process is therapists' countertransference, which is pivotal to how they understand and handle the analytic process. Unavoidably, their narratives are limited by biases of memory and defence. Also, most nonverbal communications are excluded from their accounts since they are rarely fully conscious of them – and they are not always aware of how the patient responds to these communications. Countertransference is thus a necessary yet insufficient source for understanding clinical process. By combining video observation and dialogue about the countertransference, we hope to expand our understanding of surface and extend it to more hidden aspects of the psychotherapeutic process.

Infant researchers such as Stern (1971), Trevarthen (1979), and Tronick (1989) have shown how participants co-construct interactive processes in micro-events of interaction. Their methods reveal brief (less than a second. Beebe, 1982) shifts of gaze, vocal response, facial expression, and body orientation. They can rarely be perceived in real time. These authors have also argued that the participants' key relational dynamics can be discerned in such brief interactions (Beebe & Lachmann, 2002; Stern et al., 1998).

Clinical microanalysis uses such methodology to study therapy process. It has been extended from infant research to the study of psychotherapy process (Boston Change Process Study Group, BCPSG, 2002, 2007; Lyons-Ruth, 1998; Stern, 2004; Stern et al., 1998). It was applied to adult and child psychotherapies (Avdi & Seikkula, 2019; Harrison & Tronick, 2007; Vivona, 2019), music therapy (Suvini, 2019), dance therapy (Houghton & Beebe, 2016), and PIP (Beebe, 2000, 2005; Cramer & Palacio Espasa, 1993; Downing, Bürgin, Reck, & Ziegenhain, 2008).

We pose our detailed observations of parent-infant-therapist interactions in dialogue with the therapist's countertransference. The method used, Layered Analysis (Avdi et al., 2020), is of particular interest to PIP because embodied, nonverbal parent-baby communications are central in sessions (Baradon et al., 2016; Lieberman & Van Horn, 2008). This is in line with research on how parents and babies co-construct patterns of interaction and defence (Beebe & Lachmann, 2002) as well as with discussions of how psychoanalyst and analysand co-construct their analytic space (Lyons-Ruth, 1999; Ogden, 1994). Videorecorded PIP sessions thus enable us to include the therapist as a subject of study in ways beyond psychoanalytic supervision (McWilliams, 2021; Yerushalmi, 2019).

In every relationship, including the therapeutic, interactions move between states of "match", "mismatch", and "repair" (Cohn & Tronick, 1989; Tronick, 2007b). Sometimes, mismatches can lead to deep connection and change in the end (Cavelzani & Tronick, 2016; Eubanks, Muran, & Safran, 2018). Other times, they create ruptures – that is, sudden and distressing breaks of contact. They are often accompanied by poorly modulated emotions, whose origin and meaning may be hard to comprehend. Ruptures can negatively influence the course of therapy and sever the therapeutic relationship. Conceiving of interactional rupture this way has many similarities with research on therapeutic alliance (Eubanks et al., 2018; Safran & Muran, 2000).

We examined ruptures at the micro-level in PIP sessions, including the therapist's role and how ruptures related to countertransference. Also, what happened when therapist and patient then reached towards repair – or failed to achieve it? There is research into parental contributions to rupture and its impact on the infant (Barbosa, Beeghly, Moreira, Tronick, & Fuertes, 2021; Tronick & Beeghly, 2011), but to date, research has not focused on the therapist's part.

The method of Layered Analysis

We studied brief video clips from PIP sessions and analysed the clip's cinematic qualities, such as movement, timing, rhythm, affective tone, and narrative. "Layered" reflects how image-editing software works, where an image is composed of an unlimited number of layers. Each layer can be seen separately, or a few together. A clip was always first studied in its original form.

We then layered different inputs in a non-hierarchical order. All of them contributed to the picture and the meanings we discerned. We could add or reduce elements, the whole as a structure was not solely dependent on any one of them, and there was not a preference for one over the other.

Four mother – infant PIP cases were studied, all with girls of one to six months. Mothers had sought help to improve the relationship with their baby, and they also reported difficult attachment histories or conflicts with their parents. Therapists were psychoanalytically trained, experienced in PIP, and were working in Europe. We had asked them to select a clip where they felt that something troublesome, worrying, or incomprehensible had happened between them and the patient(s). The clips, 3–6 minutes in length, were shown to and discussed with the Layered Analysis group: five researchers plus the therapist of the studied case. The heterogeneity of the group helped layering our observations and co-constructing a multifaceted description of clinical process.

The Layered Analysis process involved repeated viewings back and forth in time. We observed both verbal and embodied communications, and our interpretations of the dialogues took into account both their conscious and unconscious levels. Sometimes, we studied micro-moments frame by frame. We might zoom in on a participant, a behaviour, a movement, an expression, and so on. We often moved beyond interpretations of *one* expressive mode to focus on multimodal perceptions of the therapy process. For example, instead of building an interpretation on solely the verbal therapist-mother dialogue, we could create meaning by layering words, vocal tone, facial expressions, bodily movements, and emotional expressions of the therapist, parent, and baby. We could thus move from linear causal interpretations ("he said X and she replied with Y") to global, circular ones ("he said X, moving his body forwards, while the baby grunted, and the mother replied with Y"). When viewing the clips, we used the following tools and methods:

1   Discourse analysis is a qualitative, interpretative approach to studying dialogue (Avdi & Georgaca, 2007). It can illuminate details of how meanings are reconstructed in therapy (Georgaca & Avdi, 2011). We paid particular attention to linguistic evidence of reflective function in the adult, since mentalization is pivotal in infant psychological development and therapy process.

2   The Atypical Maternal Behavior Instrument for Assessment and Classification (AMBIANCE; Bronfman, Parsons & Lyons-Ruth, 1999) is used to study parental behaviours associated with infant attachment disorganization. Researchers trained in the coding system identified markers of disrupted communication in sessions, such as incongruent or contradictory messages and behaviours that were hostile and intrusive, frightened or disoriented, role-reversed or withdrawn. We used not quantitative ratings but a qualitative analysis of the behaviours alongside other layers of meaning.

3 Clinical microanalysis. This technique of analysing segments of interaction frame-by-fame was pioneered by Stern (1971) and developed by Beebe (1982) and others. It enabled us to distil elements that make up the broader picture. We viewed each tiny part of the clip backwards and forwards so that communications preceding and following each other could be discerned much more clearly. We thus saw subtle and rapid affects and behaviours that could not be seen in real time. This tool was also valuable for answering questions such as "What came first?" or "What led to that reaction?" or "What emotional state is being communicated?"

4 Clinical narrative and countertransference report. This layer drew upon the therapists' narrative. It was based on case notes of the therapy and therapists' reconstructions when viewing and discussing the clip with the group. Being both observed and observer, the therapist could integrate countertransference and affective experiences with the new layers of meaning, such as the embodied unconscious behaviours that the research group observed.

Findings

The therapists' clips, selected due to their sense that something bewildering or disturbing had happened, were seen by the group as displaying interactional *ruptures*. The therapists' unease and/or puzzlement paralleled the researchers' observations of dysregulation in one or more of the therapy participants. Sometimes, the therapist had been aware of the negative affect, whereas in others, the Layered Analysis revealed subtle nonverbal responses by the therapist, such as pulling away, freezing, or displaying a stunned facial expression. They had not been reported and were presumably unconscious. Some therapist behaviours could be codable on the AMBIANCE. This implied that the therapist unknowingly contributed to heightened negative affect and mutual dysregulation. The therapist then seemed to be a transient source of threat to the patient.

We observed the following key characteristics of rupture and repair processes in the therapies and organized our findings in three key areas:

i   Characteristics of ruptures: Ruptures were manifest in the structure and flow of the interaction and in the relationship between the verbal and nonverbal domains.

ii The therapist's role in ruptures: Therapists could be strongly affected by, and contribute to, interactional ruptures.

iii Processes of repair and the therapist's role: Repair relied on the therapist re-establishing self-regulation, and it was most often initiated by the therapist.

Characteristics of ruptures

Smooth, affectively attuned, coordinated, and coherent interactions differed from those where rupture occurred. True, coherent interactions could include disruptions, but they were transient and not interrupting the flow. In attuned interactions, markers of mutuality (fluid turn-taking, appropriate length of pauses, affiliative tone of voice and gaze regulation) predominated. Verbal and embodied expressions complemented and reinforced each other, with overlapping rhythms. The two also accentuated each other's meaning. In addition, nonverbal modalities (for example, tone of voice and gaze) cooperated to form a specific emotional contour.

> Dora and Daphne. The clip is from the first PIP session with mother Dora and baby Daphne, age 3 weeks. Dora and therapist are on the floor with Daphne lying on her back between them. Daphne is gazing calmly at the therapist and both adults are looking at her. The therapist bends down facing Daphne. Daphne is looking at the therapist, who shifts her gaze between mother and baby. The therapist looks at the girl, smiles, and says gently: "And she has your *very* blue eyes". She looks back at Dora, who, upon hearing the therapist, recoils subtly but abruptly away from Daphne and the therapist. Less than a second later, the therapist recoils from mother and baby. Mother leans back slightly, her head turning away from Daphne and shifting sideways towards the therapist. She points to the baby and states categorically in a questioning tone: "Is it my- hhh I can't see *nothing* in her (.) in me". The therapist mirrors Dora's movement away from Daphne, looks at Mother, and says in an interested, modulated voice: "Oh *really*? Ooh, I'd say she looks like *you*".

Dora's response to the therapist's comment about baby Daphne looking like her was unexpected and out of sync with the conversational flow. From a discursive perspective, the adults' views diverged and the therapist's proposed link between mother and baby did not develop further. The therapist described to the group feeling surprised at Dora's reaction, since in his/her experience linking baby and mother often brings about a softening in the mother. The therapist was intrigued by Dora's denial. He/she also worried that the baby was rejected by the mother. Dora denied, both verbally and nonverbally, their alikeness, perhaps because she felt threatened by the therapist's remark for reasons unknown to us. The therapist registered and mirrored Dora's recoil, creating a matched response. The therapist's verbal and nonverbal response was affiliative and interested, and this presumably cued Dora that this was something they needed to think about and that it was safe to do so. This way, the therapist could explore Dora's perspective on her baby and their relationship to foster mother's mentalizing. What seemed like a nascent interactive rupture was thereby avoided.

Judging from this and other clips, disrupted interactions were often jerky, the narrative lacked coherence, and communication seemed to reach a dead-end. Turn-taking was interrupted by overlapping speech or long pauses, and the tone of voice was sometimes raised or inauthentic. In such situations, therapist and parent did not construct meaning jointly. Instead of a true dialogue, there were two monologues. Affects often erupted intensely and unexpectedly. Also, disrupted AMBIANCE behaviours were sometimes displayed by participants. Furthermore, the messages in verbal and embodied communications often seemed divergent and thus undermined each other.

The therapist's role in ruptures

Dysregulated parent-infant interactions could "get into" the therapists and transiently disrupt their self-organization. Therapists described countertransference as feeling "confused" or "off balance", which differed from their habitual therapeutic stance. When they viewed and discussed the clips, it added to their understanding of these situations as they manifested in observable embodied expressions. When such behaviours evoked shock, confusion, or withdrawal in the other, including the therapist, such reactions seemed to be disorganizing and traumatising in the therapeutic relationship. Thus, the therapist could unwittingly contribute to further dysregulation in the triad. These processes of therapist and triadic dysregulation are illustrated through two examples below.

> **Clara and Chloe.** The interaction takes place with 3-month-old Chloe and her mother, Clara. Chloe rarely initiates eye contact with either adult. Clara sits on the floor, holding Chloe on her knee, and recounts a recent swimming session. She makes a sudden "PSHSHSH" sound to illustrate how Chloe reacted when going underwater. Chloe responds by signs of interest and positive engagement (looking at mother and vocalizing) and of negative affect (she startles, her smile turns to a grimace, she flails her arms, her arms and torso tense up). Chloe's behaviour suggests she was confused and frightened by mother's loud tone. The therapist responds quickly in a loud and high-pitched voice "Oh yeah, what did mummy just DO?" and then laughs in a high-pitched, prolonged manner. Here, Chloe frowns and averts her gaze from both adults.

The therapist's response to this dysregulated interaction was both aroused and arousing. He/she described picking up on Chloe's expression and putting baby's shock into words. The aim was to offer a possibility of finding meaning in the interaction. The therapist unconsciously linked mother's response with her expression when she had previously talked about sexual abuse. He/she thus responded to Chloe's startle, put words to her experience, and invited Clara to reflect upon her baby's experience and mental state. However, there was a discrepancy between her words and her laughter, and both were expressed in an aroused affective state. The therapist's affective arousal was thus also arousing for mother and daughter, as evidenced in Chloe averting her gaze.

> **Flora and Fleur.** Fleur is sitting on mother Flora's lap facing her chest and avoiding eye contact with both adults. Flora comments on her distress about diaper changes during the night. When she exclaims they feel like an "assault", Fleur whines briefly. Simultaneously, the therapist recoils rapidly away from mother and baby in a big body movement but with a neutral face and then leans forward into a collapsed posture. Mother Flora mirrors the therapist's back-and-forth movements, and then, as the therapist freezes, she turns abruptly to Fleur, says "You wanna dock in?", and starts breastfeeding. Flora continues to talk, facing her baby now, while the therapist has a frozen and blank facial expression for 16 seconds.

The therapist's nonconscious communication of what seems like a chaotic retreat (recoil, still-face) seemed to have cued mother and baby to threat; in response, they withdrew into self-protective manoeuvres. The therapist reported having felt thrown and perplexed by the sudden use of the word "assault" – it felt like a breakthrough of violent unconscious material in Flora. But in the session, the therapist was aware neither of the bodily cue of retreat nor of the momentary freezing.

To sum up these examples, when unconscious traumatic material emerged in parent-baby or parent-therapist interactions, they dysregulated the therapist. This was reported by the therapists and reflected in their behaviour as well, leading to further dysregulation in mother and baby. Mothers might turn away from the therapist, display facial withdrawal, become still, and show signs of disorientation or hostility. Babies might be frightened or display active defences (gaze avoidance, twisting body away, withdrawal) as well as disengagement with bewildered facial expressions and bodily tension. All in all, the threat was moving between the triad members, each one potentially acting as trigger to the other.

Repair and the therapist's role

Interactive repair emerged as a gradual, cumulative process, whereas rupture was more abrupt. Like rupture, repair processes also started with bodily cues. In some instances, the therapist made embodied invitations to resume contact. In other situations, it was more like a mutual cueing by mother and therapist who each wanted the relationship to continue; baby then settled into the changed atmosphere and joined the interaction.

We found that the therapist's capacity to register, reflect, and respond to the rupture was crucial in determining whether repair would come about – or if a dysregulated dynamic would continue. We identified four inter-related elements of interactional repair after a rupture: the therapists' capacity to self-regulate their affective arousal, emergent meaning-making as the therapist began to make sense of the interaction, the therapist's actions towards re-establishing connection, and the time needed for these reparative responses.

For repair to come about, the therapist needed to work internally to restore self-regulation or, expressed in another terminology (Bion, 1970; Ogden, 2004), to contain himself/herself. This was often seen in the therapist's pause before responding. Their reports did not always document this pause, so it was not necessarily conscious. Pauses could be observed in the therapists' transient withdrawal from the interaction, through a preoccupied look, silence, and in facial or bodily stillness. Whether or not such pauses reflected disorientation or self-regulation was deduced from the actions that followed: when the therapist exited the pause with a gesture or a comment indicating resolution and understanding, we assumed that he/she had moved from a disrupted to a more coherent state.

Therapists' reports also emphasised the importance of meaning-making in the process of repair. Ruptures may signify not only the loss of joint meaning-making but also the therapist's confusion, expressed as "What is happening? I don't understand". Regaining a sense of understanding moved the therapist towards self-regulation and empathic openness to the other.

When self-regulation or self-containment returned and led to mutual regulation, the therapist's embodied knowledge often preceded conscious symbolic knowledge and verbalization. Embodied knowledge was seen as slowing down or stilling, nodding, and leaning forward. In successful repairs, the therapists often commented on or invited explicit exploration of the underlying feelings.

Eliane and Eva. Baby Eva often averts her gaze, which worries mother Eliane. As they settle on the floor, the therapist waits for Eva to look at her, and after a moment, Eva turns her gaze to the therapist, while mother Eliane watches. Eva moves her head away, lowers her face, and shuts her eyes. Eliane says, "Oh DEAR" in a high-pitched voice and laughs eerily, with a frightened facial expression. Eva still looks away and twists her torso away from the adults. The therapist's face becomes still, with a frozen smile. Eliane then looms in towards Eva, and the therapist leans in and asks Eliane how she is finding Eva's gaze. Eliane looks up at the therapist with a startled expression and then engages with the therapist and begins to talk about her feelings about Eva.

At first, this shows a mutual traumatization in the triad. Eva's turning away triggered a dysregulated, frightened laugh in her mother, which seemed to "get into" the therapist, who transiently froze. The countertransference report indicated confusion and shock. In a reconstruction of the event, the sense was of rejection ricocheting between the triad. As Eliane started to loom over Eva's face, which the group interpreted as a hostile behaviour, the therapist interrupted this by looming into the girl and inviting mother to talk about her relationship with Eva. Frame-by-frame examination of this micro-interaction revealed that the therapist's intervention came mid-way through Eliane's loom. The response was too fast to be the result of conscious processing. We suggest that, during the brief pause, the therapist regulated her arousal and dysregulation that had been triggered by Eliane's tense behaviour with Eva. She then reconnected with Eliane and invited self-reflection. The rupture was repaired, and Eliane and therapist could begin to explore Eliane's experience in relation to Eva.

Discussion

Clinical process in psychotherapy is complex, multidimensional, and varying. Many things happen in a session, and we need tools to register, comprehend, and interpret what occurs on all these levels. Layered Analysis combines clinical insight and report by the therapist with microanalytic approaches by a research team. Both countertransference and observation are sources of information.

We found a concordance between the therapists' reports of surprise and/ or unease about a specific micro-interaction and the researchers' observations of embodied expressions of rupture and repair. This suggests that observations and reported countertransference capture similar phenomena but from different perspectives with different assets and shortcomings. The reported countertransference reflects what arose, on the spot and *après-coup*, in the therapist: thoughts, fantasies, feeling states and bodily reactions. During the session, the therapist could not be aware of all of this while simultaneously trying to capture what went on in the others' minds in the session.

The researchers had even less access to the therapist's feelings and thoughts, but through careful viewing of the clips, they could perceive markers of rupture and repair that were unregistered by the therapist and thus unavailable as information about the countertransference. This refers especially to bodily markers of countertransferential feelings, manifested in displeasure, annoyance, or a feeling of being "assaulted". Therapists had selected clips based on their unease about specific interactions. They thus had some awareness that something "wasn't quite right" in these interactions. Careful observation along the Layered Analysis method added detail and depth to their unease. Observing bodily expressions also showed how they affected the patients, consciously or not. In our view, countertransference reports and researcher observations are complementary perspectives that enable a "binocular vision" (Bion, 1965, 66). This enabled us to simultaneously study interactive events, conscious internal experiences, and embodied communications.

Ruptures are heralded for the therapist as experiences of unease, confusion, shame, or other negative emotions. Such feelings can be transmitted to the patient through anomalous behaviours such as withdrawal, freezing, or interactive errors, of which the therapist may be unaware. Although we did not have access to *the patients'* self-reports, the observed behaviours in mothers and babies (withdrawal, avoidance, hostility) suggest that they may at times have felt the relationship with the therapist to be aversive or threatening. The researchers' countertransference when watching the videos offered additional insights, such as when they reported "a sinking heart" or "tension" or realised that they were holding their breath while watching. Such countertransferential "resonance" (Salomonsson, 1998) and "tuning fork responses" (Stone, 2006) helped us further understand the patients' experiences.

The therapists' reports and the behaviours we observed in the clips indicated that, in tandem with the interactional disruption, their self-organisation was disturbed. Similar phenomena occurred in mothers and babies. Perturbance thus seemed to roam about in the triangle of therapist, baby, and mother who mutually influenced each other's behaviour (Butner et al., 2017). Disruptions thus occurred in the self, in the dyad, and in the therapeutic system. They occurred so rapidly that it was impossible to establish a linear causal chain. We assume that these parallel and inter-related trajectories are fleeting, embodied cues of disorganisation, split-second chains of movements that are taken in subliminally (Boston Change Process Study Group, 2002, 2005).

In such situations, the participants' expectancies are disrupted. The ordinary frame of working together, which always includes ongoing mismatch and repair, is abruptly thrown off course. Such situations occur in all therapies. In PIP, the therapist may witness interactions that are especially disturbing and challenging since infantile affective states are primary and raw. Probably, such interactions violate the normative expectancies of the therapist's attachment and caregiving systems. They may also trigger memory traces of perhaps only partially resolved states in his/her own past. This may cause the therapist to lose one's habitual therapeutic stance and become threatening to the patients. Being dysregulated and challenged in one's capacity to mentalize and make meaning in the here-and-now, the therapist cannot move towards interactive repair with the patient. Something needs to take place in the therapist to regain a sense of self-regulation and capacity to think.

Moving towards repair and restoring the therapeutic working relationship are underpinned by the therapist's internal "metabolizing" or containment (Bion, 1962). By this term, we mean the emotional and mental digestion of the raw elements that imploded the interaction, emotional regulation, and meaning-making (Grotstein, 2008; Ogden, 2004). We observed that such metabolizing often started with a physical response, such as stilling or recoil, which indicated that the patient's communication had been taken in. We suggest that the therapist may unknowingly have paused briefly to carry out the required internal work. This embodied aspect of metabolizing arguably preceded more conscious mental work in the therapist.

In other words, meaning-making is not only a conscious process of symbolized understanding and mentalizing. It is also an embodied, implicit response that gives meaning to the other's actions. Sletvold (2016) suggests that the psychoanalyst's listening to their body is the foundation for analytic thinking. He acknowledges the importance of reflective thought but sees it as "resting on the analyst's ability to become aware of her unconscious bodily relational experience" (186). At this point, the disturbance lodges inside the therapist's body. Often this is accompanied by an expression such as stilling or "turning inward". These behaviours differ from disrupted (AMBIANCE-codable) behaviours, such as withdrawal or dissociation, in that additional cues are given that contradict threat. For example, the therapist may still maintain eye contact, physical proximity (leaning in), and vocalisations ("mm"). Another aspect of such pauses is that the therapist "comes back" to the patient but in a subtly different manner. Then the therapist seems inclined to a more nuanced affective joining-in with the patient and, from a mentalizing point of view, tends to a state of mind associated with and enabling genuine inquiry (Fonagy, Campbell, & Luyten, 2022).

The therapists reported that such metabolizing allowed them to self-regulate and regain their habitual capacity to think. This is a prerequisite for interactive regulation, which concurs with Beebe and Lachmann's (2020) proposition that "self-processes may be even more organizing than interactive processes" (313). This may result in a successful interactional repair as the patient and therapist resume collaborating on the work of therapy with a strong affective bond (Eubanks et al., 2018). This was confirmed in our study. While the internal work of the therapist seems to be a condition for repair, a mutual wish for resumed emotional connectivity is equally necessary, whether this is conscious to the patient or not. In the clip with mother Flora and her daughter Fleur, Flora actively cued her wish to restore the therapeutic work through glancing rapidly at the therapist. In the case of Eliane and Eva, mother responded to the therapist's intervention, albeit with negation of the content. The therapist continued with interested reflection and quite quickly the rebuff was left behind, and regulated turn-taking and collaborative reflection took place again.

Layered analysis – a method of discerning traces of the Infantile?

The original study (Baradon et al., 2023) showed that Layered Analysis made therapists more aware of their unconscious bodily experiences, affective states, and countertransference. They learnt to see themselves a bit more from the outside, as in the "store front look" mentioned earlier. They became more sensitive of how they behaved, how the other perceived them, and how the bi-directional influences in micro-events took place. We also learnt that when they had not sufficiently metabolized the patient's emotions and/or their own countertransference, they could be more susceptible to interactive errors. In this sense, the method is somewhat like holding a mirror to the therapist's Unconscious. The study clinicians were surprised at the extent of negative emotions that their bodies conveyed. Thus, the patient is not the sole trigger of ruptures: the therapist may also prompt them. This might seem evident, but the Layered Analysis showed it more explicitly.

It is time to ask how this method relates to tracing the Infantile in psycho-therapy. To begin an answer, we will not find such traces by merely looking at clips "from the outside", as if they were specimens in a microscope. No, we need invoke the therapist and the Layered Analysis group *in interaction.* They should all be perspicacious and meticulous about behavioural details and emotions. The group found that the therapists were deeply involved in sessions and that such involvement was often unconscious and embodied. Group members also recognized how involved *they* were when seeing the videos and listening to the presenter.

What did researchers and therapists see and hear? What was clearly most concealed to the therapists were their embodied communications: the recoiling torso when Fleur's mother compared a diaper change to an assault, the therapist whose voice got high-pitched in response to Chloe's mother's loud voice. All these were unconscious and embodied reactions to sudden changes in the emotional ambiance. The archetypical situation to find such shifts is baby-parent interaction. Babies don't talk, argue, or discuss – and they don't dissemble their feelings. They communicate with us through their "soulbody" (Salomonsson, 2011), implying that "soul" and "body" are one entity (Winnicott, 1949). Affects do have *some kind* of representations in their mind, but they are also "some thing" inside their body. This merger recedes gradually – but never completely – as the child grows to being an adult person.

Does Layered Analysis help display the Infantile in the participants? I think so. Flora's and Fleur's therapist felt disconcerted and pained by the mother's comparing a diaper change to an assault. The recoil was an embodied variant of a baby's startle when she's frightened. The ensuing "Still-Face" mirrored a shutting-down described by Fraiberg (1982) as "freezing". The therapist reported thinking for a long time about what mother meant by the comparison. But evidently, the therapist was emotionally overwhelmed and shut down. It is safe to say that a part of his/her Infantile was dislodged by mother's comment, which in turn overthrew the flow between the three participants.

The novelty of this method is not to reveal the evident, that embodied communications exist and may be rooted in the Infantile, but that they *move so quickly, so much passes under the radar of the participants, and that the therapists' embodied communications can affect mother and baby.* I hope this clinically important finding can inspire other therapists – whether they videorecord sessions or not and share them or not in a peer group – to increase their awareness of these strands in their interactions with patients of whatever age.

The parallel between a therapist and an astronomer, mentioned earlier, still yields new insights. If anybody sees a therapist's position as static, like sitting behind a "telescope", Layered Analysis reveals this to be utterly false. In a session, there is no immobile Infantile on the firmament for the therapist to register. Things happen at once, quickly, simultaneously, and they are discerned only partially by the therapist. Even more fascinating, and disturbing, is that the therapist is part of the very system he is studying with the aim of helping the patient. Astronomers studying the movements of a celestial body know how to calculate their position on Earth in motion. But at least, they can rest assured that their telescope is fixed to the terrestrial ground. In contrast, no therapist can claim that his position is fixed in the sense that he, and only he, perceives the Truth in an object called "the patient". Such claims were effectively dismantled when the concept of countertransference began to be taken seriously. But what may be even more unsettling in this study is the following: despite therapists' efforts at discerning the countertransference, we move about more imperceptibly, unpredictably, and quicker than we are able to perceive. Thus, we know less than we imagine about how we conduct ourselves in sessions. On the other hand, this makes our job all the more fascinating.

Source

This chapter is a reworked version of a published paper (Baradon et al., 2023). I thank the publisher and my co-authors for giving permission to quote it in the book.

Chapter 10

"What do his lips want from me?"

Infantile sexuality in PIP

Many chapters in the book make a backward-forward journey. The tours backwards went from my adult patients to their prehistory as babies. They also went forwards when we imputed from babies and mothers in parent – infant psychotherapy (PIP) to understand emotional sufferings in adult therapy patients. The book thus offers return tickets between the experiential worlds of infancy and adulthood. This does not refer to the kind of historical journey we make when browsing the family album and grandmother confirms when and what happened. In psychoanalysis, the only fixed point is the present, namely what happens and is interpreted in sessions. The past is reconstructed backwards, as Laura and I did in Chapter 7. The future may be speculated forwards, like Simone in Chapter 1 worrying what will become of her marriage. Freud followed his patients' to-and-fro motions as they told of their present suffering and associated to their childhood and infancy. He forged links and ideas, not to prove causality in the strict sense of the word but to uncover junctions between their experiences throughout life.

How does an idea emerge in the analyst, perhaps an idea that will develop into a concept, an article, or a book? The titles of many analytic texts refer to a theoretical concept, such as "repression", "countertransference", or "intersubjectivity". Often, they also contain a case vignette or history. Does this imply that the analyst started with the thought, "I wonder if this patient is expressing concept X or theory Y". I think this is rare, actually. Analysts rather start with clinical observations, events, and feelings that arouse their curiosity to understand deeper and connect the clinical atmosphere with the theoretical apparatus. Such connections are easier to make with certain concepts. Others are more ambiguous and imprecise. A most haunting and elusive concept in analytic theory is *infantile sexuality*. Already its phrasing is ambiguous. One would think it means "sex in babies". This is only partly true and in a specific sense. It also covers "sex in adults" since analysts assume that all adults possess what we call infantile sexuality. We even speak of a confluence of, or a conflict between, adult and infantile sexuality in the adult. We might criticise analytic theory for being contradictory and confused, but we will see that this conundrum is inevitable and even fertile.

DOI: 10.4324/9781003640363-10

This chapter is in line with the analytic tradition of selecting a clinical event and looking at it with psychoanalytic spectacles and from many points of view. What differs from that tradition is that it was not something the analyst had noted in the session. Rather, he – that is, I – noted it when reviewing a video clip with the Layered Analysis group: the case of Flora and Fleur in Chapter 9, where I was the therapist. Upon my perhaps thirtieth (!) viewing of the clip, I discovered that when I was frustrated by baby Fleur avoiding my contact efforts, I made a kissing lip movement twice. Neither I nor the group had seen them before. I was taken aback, not only because it had taken me so many viewings to perceive them but also because they seemed out of place and misguided. It made me reflect if they could have some unconscious sexual connotation to be subsumed under concept of infantile sexuality. This led to a paper (Salomonsson, 2025) of which the following text is a revised version.

The link between the chapter's topic and this book's focus on "traces of the Infantile" is as follows. We will see that the modern usage of the term infantile sexuality is much more relationally oriented than in Freud's time (S. Freud, 1905b). The analyst Jean Laplanche rephrased it into a phenomenon that emerges when the baby is interacting with the parent – and this emergence comes about also via the parent's infantile sexuality. As said earlier, it is a complicated concept! Contributions signalling such unconscious infantile sexuality may come from any adult, thus also from the analyst. Based on what happened between me, Flora, and Fleur, I argue that such inputs are also observable, not in a simplistic sense but when we combine concrete observations with psychoanalytic interpretations. Used together, *they sometimes enable us to see what I call the traces of the Infantile.*

The chapter applies three perspectives on how infantile sexuality can emerge in PIP. The methodological angle accounts for the Layered Analysis method as in Chapter 9. The clinical perspective brings forth stressful moments when my behaviour changed in a direction that had been unconscious but was now observable on the video. The theoretical approach investigates if these behaviours correspond to what Laplanche called the traffic of *enigmatic messages.*

Many of my writings have investigated if it is possible and fruitful to apply classic Freudian concepts to – and thus reach a deeper understanding of – the clinical process in PIP: infantile sexuality, transference, primal repression, defence, and verbal interpretations (Salomonsson, 2012a, 2013b, 2014a, 2015b, 2017). This goes for the present chapter too. My assumption has been that a psychoanalytic theoretical view adds to our understanding of what occurs on unconscious levels in parent-infant interactions as described by other clinicians and by infant researchers. These studies complement those that rely on attachment theory and infant behaviour research.

Almost all of my PIP cases in the published studies were supported by videorecorded vignettes. As argued in Chapter 9, interest among analysts with classic and object-relations orientations in using videorecordings of therapy sessions has been rather tepid. But in PIP, things pass by rapidly for the three persons in the room, nonverbal communications are paramount, and session notes seem not to capture what is "really going on in the session". This was my first reason to begin videorecording sessions. My PIP mentor, Johan Norman (2004), *audio*recorded sessions to help grasp and demonstrate the clinical process. These recordings were valuable, but they also left room for speculations about the process, which I did not always find to be well grounded.

When we began evaluating outcomes (Salomonsson & Sandell, 2011b; Winberg Salomonsson et al., 2015a), all interviews were *video*recorded. Videos offered clinical insight into how verbal and nonverbal communication, and conscious and unconscious content, varied in the dyads. They also enhanced my understanding of countertransference. The observational scope and depth of the recordings were surprising, and I concluded that videorecording PIP sessions would help to understand the therapy process. When I then compared my videos with those of infant researchers like Beatrice Beebe, Ed Tronick, and Joseph Campos, their skills in perceiving speedy changes in dyadic interactions were impressive and inspiring. They immensely improved our comprehension of the baby's development and interactions with the parents. But a conceptual challenge remained: they conceived of findings in terms of attachment theory (Beebe & Lachmann, 2014) or other theories (Tronick, 2005), whereas classic psychoanalytic concepts were sparse. This "transmission gap" between Freudian and attachment theories of the infantile mind and behaviour was perplexing to me. After all, both rely on precise observations as well as on intuitive conjectures, attachment researchers more on the former and psychoanalysts more on the latter.

This chapter uses Layered Analysis to further our understanding of *infantile sexuality*. I had suggested earlier (Salomonsson, 2012a) that when I addressed a crying baby girl in PIP, my words had a parallel unconscious sexual connotation when I exclaimed "I'm totally charmed" when she finally gave me a beaming smile. They reflected "my conscious effort at containing a screaming baby" but also "an unconscious fantasy about adult sexual relations" (93). I conceived of the passage in Laplanche's terms (1989, 126), as a primal seduction where "an adult proffers to a child verbal, non-verbal and even behavioural signifiers which are pregnant with unconscious sexual significations". In my interpretation then, "totally charmed" related to my own unconscious sexuality.

I then noted that the paper did not ask if *infantile sexuality may manifest as observable behaviours in the clinical situation and also influence the therapy process*. In brief, its conceptions of the clinical passage relied too much on verbal communication and too little on nonverbal and embodied expressions like gestures and intonations. The Layered Analysis method taught me to observe more closely the PIP participants' sounds, gestures, facial expressions, and voice changes and to link them with countertransference as reported by the therapist. The videos showed three participants' ongoing efforts at establishing and rejecting contact. We could observe a *traffic of rapid interactive behaviours signifying unconscious urges and defences against them*.

The question now arose if the Layered Analysis method could yield information on infantile sexuality. Might even interactions that we studied there elucidate Laplanche's thesis that such sexuality emerges as enigmatic or compromised messages in the traffic between adult and infant? One central question was: If, as Laplanche suggested, the infant's sexuality emerges in the wake of enigmatic messages representing the adult's infantile and repressed sexuality, *do these interchanges manifest in ways that we can discern* through the Layered Analysis method?

I will thus apply the perspective on infantile sexuality as discussed by Laplanche and Pontalis (1968) and developed by Laplanche alone (1989, 1995, 1999a, 1999b, 2007b) and other scholars (Benjamin & Atlas, 2015; Diatkine, 2008; Fonagy, 2008; Saketopoulou, 2020; D. K. Silverman, 2001; Van Haute, 2005; Widlöcher, 2002; Zamanian, 2011). I start with a vignette and then turn to Laplanche's elaboration of Freud's original thoughts of infantile sexuality.

Clinical vignette: mother Flora and baby Fleur, 5 months

When I see parents in postnatal consultations, I always suggest they bring the baby for some sessions. The aim is to get a picture of their relationship and of the baby's state. Meeting mother Flora at the Child Health Centre, I thus asked her to bring her daughter Fleur to the next session. Actually, Flora did not worry about Fleur or their contact. Rather, she sought help because she felt tormented that she had become a mother at a somewhat later age and her pregnancy had been unplanned. This prevented her from thinking or speaking about herself as a "mother", a word that she truly hated. At the same time, she said she was developing a warm and powerful bond with the girl.

The first time I met Fleur, she often avoided looking at me. Later, when Flora spoke more calmly about difficulties in thinking of herself as "a Mum", the girl gave a broad, enchanting, and babbling smile and sought mother's eyes at length. I suggested to Flora that we meet regularly and investigate her issues. We agreed to meet once weekly, the three of us. When I felt we had a reliable alliance, I asked to videorecord sessions. She consented to this and to my later request to use clips for scientific writing and showing them with discretion to professionals in the field.

As PIP treatment proceeded, the eye contact between mother and daughter did not worry me – but there were quite a few moments when *Fleur avoided my eyes*. The session before the one below, I had pointed out this difference to Flora. She had not any noticed gaze avoidance at home and conceded that my comment worried her. "But on the other hand, it's important to point into the sun", she said, meaning to speak frankly about embarrassing matters.

A clip from the eighth session

The seven-minute clip is the same as sketched in Chapter 9. It begins two minutes into the eighth PIP session, some weeks before Christmas. I had selected it for discussion in the Layered Analysis group because I had been appalled and bewildered by mother's comment comparing Fleur's night-time diaper changes to "an assault", which in our language unequivocally denotes sexual violence. I had also experienced a rupture in my contact with the two and a heavy fatigue that I attributed to a change in the countertransference. When viewing the clip after the session, I also noted that when Flora said "assault", Fleur whined briefly and I moved my torso abruptly backwards and then leant forward again, but now with a blank face. I refer to the video analysis in Chapter 9.

The group observed that the recoil episode was preceded by four minutes of Flora talking incessantly and cheerfully: they had been at the Child Health Centre yesterday, she made "an instant connection" with their new health visitor, the girl had her vaccination, and so on. The members now noticed that, in the session's beginning, baby Fleur often drooped her head without any eye contact with mother or me. When she avoided my eyes, I responded by nodding, smiling, leaning forward, or humming – whereupon she drooped again. Mother noted this and explained, as if glossing over its emotional impact, "Fleur is morning shy", "she's just hiding", or "she's tired".

Mother: "Actually, we are both tired. We slept badly because she woke up at 2 o'clock and I was suddenly wide awake. I thought of picking up my cell phone, though I knew it wasn't any good. But after an hour, I started reading an e-book and fell asleep. When one – or I should say I – is awake at night, one starts brooding about things that need to be fixed, you know, good and bad stuff."

Then she criticised her husband for not doing his share in the household, thereupon shifting to telling Fleur, "Are you blowing bubbles [of saliva]?" My mounting distress could be noted as I began stroking my index fingers as if soothing myself. To establish contact, I asked Flora, friendly but somewhat abruptly, "How are things between the two of you?" She answered, now in a slightly sad vibrato:

M: "We're good actually, it's always like that, one thinks one understands how babies function and then they change. Yesterday, we tested not changing diapers before bedtime, because she's woken up COMPLETELY inconsolable, as if one were ASSAULTING her"!

This was the moment when I swiftly and unwittingly retracted my torso and then moved it forward again. Later, as the group extended its analysis beyond that reported in Chapter 9, we focused on the runup to the recoil. The girl often sought contact with me, but when I responded with a contacting gesture or word, her head drooped. This pattern was confusing and frustrating, which I had been conscious of in the session. But now, renewed viewings on my own of the passage revealed that as Fleur was cooing gently, *my lips twice made a kissing movement*. Briefer than half a second, it was accompanied once by an even briefer subdued sound of a kiss. I had been totally unaware of all this.

The fact that I discerned these "kisses" only after repeated viewings raised important questions. Smiling and greeting Fleur reflected my conscious aim of making contact. But kissing in the air is, of course, not my way of approaching patients. What were the sources of this unconscious behaviour? Could it reflect my infantile sexuality emerging as a kiss? Why hadn't anyone of us in the group observed it? Was it a defensive avoidance? Before approaching the questions, I will briefly describe a challenge when writing about PIP. How can a text do justice to the simultaneous interactions between all the session participants, let alone what we assume goes on inside each of them?

A note on clinical polyphony

The challenge of writing about PIP clinical process is how to illustrate three persons' communications, especially when one of them does not contribute with words. The challenge becomes even heavier when we bring in the speed of therapy interactions and the therapist's difficulties to register their embodied manifestations. We might come a bit closer to a textual rendition if we conceive of these complex interactions as an ongoing *polyphony* between mother, baby, and therapist. Such a text could be compared to a musical score. In such a "score", each part or voice could be identified, named, and notated individually. A musically educated person can grasp roughly, by reading a score, how the music will sound. Similarly, a psychoanalyst might find it easier to "read the score" if it is summarised as a set of voices. Writing it up would, however, needs amendments to make it a readable and flowing text. Accordingly, I have written the clinical material as a flowing text, hoping one may conceive of it as a rendition of many simultaneous voices.

Let us try this setup on the session with Flora, Fleur, and me. We could then speak of *one voice* expressing mother Flora's cheerful and logical explanations to any head droop, gaze avoidance, or yawns of the girl. Yet, when I listened to the colour of her voice, I noticed a sad and tense vibrato. To put it more accurately, the first voice was thus actually two: one cheerful *word flow* and a second *voice* that I felt was disheartening. A *third voice* expressed my disbelief and discomfort with mother's explanations. The countertransference was blatantly expressed by my recoil. As noted earlier, this voice was only partly discerned by me. I knew I disbelieved her statements, but the video revealed parallel embodied expressions such as my recoil, blank face, and collapsed posture. At the spur of the moment, all this was unconscious to me. A *fourth voice* was my effort at contacting the girl through smiles and words of greeting. Her behaviour constituted the *fifth voice* as she was searching for me and drooping when I responded. Finally, the *sixth voice* occurred beyond my awareness and at variance with my friendly and conscious fourth voice: my "kisses in the air" (Table 10.1).

No voice was leading. It was more like a perpetual flow of voices, some more implicit than explicit, unconscious than conscious, embodied than verbal. At times, some voices were salient; other times, they receded. Sometimes, a voice was not perceived by a participant; other times, he or she seemed to defend against recognising it – or it had simply escaped perception. It was essential to listen to all voices simultaneously, as to an orchestral *tutti*. From that perspective, we discern three persons trying simultaneously to get in contact and to avoid it. The girl looks at Mum and then shuns her. She turns to the analyst, but the mother also moves her away from him. He is annoyed with her verbosity, tries to reach the girl, first consciously by words and looks and then unconsciously by "the kiss". In addition, this trio can be interpreted as an early manifestation of an oedipal triangle, where the mother obstructs a closer therapist-baby contact.

The table below visualises the partition-like structure of the interactions. I hope it helps in understanding the complex interactions that take place simultaneously in such treatments. But the table has its limitations too. In a musical partition, all voices follow the same bar-line and the same tempo. In therapy, each voice may have its own rhythm, especially when rupture is impending or present. Flora's chatting was up-tempo, Fleur's turning to and away from me and mother had a slower rhythm, as did my leaning forwards and backwards when I was contacting her but then gave up. In fact, many ruptures can be viewed as crashes in rhythm, with all the unpleasure and stress that such events evoke. The rhythms I am talking about here refer to

Table 10.1 Clinical polyphony in the first four minutes of the clip

Voice	Main performer	Characteristics
1	Mother	Happy words
2	Mother	Sad tone of voice
3	Therapist	Conscious and unconscious embodied discomfort and disbelief in mother's words
4	Therapist	Seeks contact with baby
5	Baby	Seeks contact/droops, more with therapist than with mother
6	Therapist	"Kisses" in the air to baby

the auditive, the visual, the kinetic, and the proprioceptive spheres, namely how we sounded, gestured, moved, and so on.

I end this section by countering an objection from an imagined reader. I understand if the book's running parallel of astronomy and psychotherapy may seem far-fetched. For someone who does not share my fascination with the night sky or who does not need metaphors to understand the gist of my arguments, the parallel may be redundant. I accept that. But as for the parallel between music and therapy, I am less inclined to yield. Making music and doing psychotherapy have many things in common (Grassi, 2021; Grier, 2019; Markman, 2006; Salomonsson, 2011), one of which is that they emerge in the course of *time*. Unlike a painting or a text, they move forward relentlessly, and there is never any stop – delete – remake. At times, in music and therapy, time may *seem* to stand still – but it doesn't. There is a flow in both activities, and it is the difficulty in transferring this flow that I have tried to capture with the simile of the musical score. Of course, I accept if you don't need it to grasp what goes on in a therapy session, but you would need hefty arguments to persuade me that a musical and a psychotherapy experience have nothing to do with each other (Salomonsson, 2011).

Countertransference and the kiss

Why did I play the "sixth voice" of "kisses in the air", and why had I not perceived it earlier? I will link the two questions with a discussion of countertransference, whereas ensuing sections will connect them with the concept of infantile sexuality. As for countertransference, I was conscious of my vexation with mother's first voice. Her chatty words conveyed that she was the main person, I should listen to her, and she did not allow the girl to enter the scene as a person in her own right. Besides, the girl was "all right". Her first voice conflicted with my fourth voice of seeking contact with Fleur. I communicated, "I am interested in you, Fleur", while the mother conveyed, "See to my needs, I don't trust you enough, and I'm not keen on you getting in deeper contact with my girl".

Countertransference was thus imbued with all sorts of affects. Many were conscious to me, whereas their embodied expressions were not. In the session, I was aware of feeling shocked by the diaper change-assault comparison but not of my recoil and still-face. True, an alternative interpretation could be that, unconsciously, I wanted to show her that I, as a man, did not intend to assault her. However, my reflections on the countertransference have not supported that interpretation. I rather emphasise the gap between my conscious feelings and unconscious actions; at her word "assault", I sensed I was stunned and found her connection unpleasant. In contrast, my recoil and ensuing blank face were unconscious. I was thus *more aware of the countertransference's ideational and emotional content than of its embodied manifestations*.

As for the "kisses", I was aware neither of them nor of any sexual excitation. Yet which kind of sexuality are we talking about? Did I yearn for bodily intimacy with the girl or her mother? The answer is no. I liked Fleur but did not find her unusually charming. Paedophilia is impossible for me to connect with my own sexuality. As for the mother, I liked her, and I was concerned as well as frustrated with her. But I felt no erotic attraction. It seems more probable that the "kisses" reflected my efforts at getting in a more emotionally intimate contact with Fleur. Yet a kiss is an improper, clumsy, and inefficient way of seeking contact with an avoidant baby. The more incomprehensible I viewed my behaviour, the more I was inclined to think that it was also governed by impulses of which I was completely unconscious. At this point, the concept of infantile sexuality demands our attention. Before heeding this appeal, we must investigate the concept's heuristic value. This is important, not the least since modern infant research has used and prioritised other explanatory models.

Infantile sexuality or match/mismatch?

One might claim that Laplanche's ideas are redundant in this context since we already have well-defined behavioural categories emanating from meticulous observations by researchers of adult-infant interactions. For example, infant researcher Ed Tronick (Tronick & Beeghly, 2011) might speak of an ongoing *match and mismatch* between me and Fleur. A typical adult-infant interaction is "messy: It moves from matching (coordinated, synchronous) states of shared meanings and intentionality to mismatched (miscoordinated, dyssynchronous) states and back to matching intentional states via an active, jointly carried out reparatory process" (7). In these terms, Fleur and I tried to "match", though with repeated mismatches and renewed matching efforts.

Or we could focus on parent-infant *synchrony*, as studied by Ruth Feldman (2007). She describes the intricate dance

> During short, intense, playful interactions; [it] builds on familiarity with the partner's behavioral repertoire and interaction rhythms; and depicts the underlying temporal structure of highly aroused moments of interpersonal exchange that are clearly separated from the stream of daily life.
> (329)

Clearly, Fleur's and my contact efforts were not in sync.

These and other researchers' observations are succinct and fascinating, especially their emphasis on the role of interactive rhythm. But, in my view, they do not go deep enough beneath observable data to address what goes on unconsciously in the participants. This is where videorecorded sessions in conjunction with analysis of the countertransference can help us. Like the cited researchers, a PIP therapist observes interactions between baby, mother, and himself/herself. In addition, understanding of the countertransference can add psychoanalytic interpretations of observable behaviours which, in turn, can be linked with unconscious levels in all three participants.

Analysing the clip in retrospect, I detected nothing new in my counter-transference at first. But when I at last perceived the kiss, it opened an unexpected window to my *embodied expressed wish* for a more intimate contact with Fleur and to the level of my despair when this was thwarted. Her apprehension that I did something beyond the ordinary was also mirrored by her body: the second my lips formed a kiss, she looked aside. We could translate this into Fleur's question, *"What do his lips want from me? I'm unsettled!"* This paraphrases Laplanche (1989) as he describes the baby's unconscious question when confronted by mother's enigmatic messages: "What does the breast want from me?". In this view, I unconsciously produced a message signifying pleasurable human contact but also a riddle or an excess (R. Stein, 2008) that she must avoid. To conclude, infant research observations, though meticulous and skilled, do not cover the unconscious strata that Laplanche addressed and thus his concept of infantile sexuality is far from redundant.

Infantile sexuality from Freud to Laplanche

To investigate if the concept of infantile sexuality can be used in a clinical parent-infant context, we need first to comprehend Freud's views on its origin and manifestations. It may start from internal or external sources, and these "germs of sexual impulses" (1950b, 176) will lean on (*anlehnen*) the instinct of survival then to become an autonomous sexual drive with a specified trajectory via erotic zones. Freud observed it in the newborn's thumb-sucking (180), but he also stated that it becomes "accessible to observation round about the third or fourth year of life" (177). To summarise Freud, infantile sexuality is an innate propensity, it is unclear to which extent it is observable at birth, and it involves an adult who provides the infant with "an unending source of sexual excitation and satisfaction from his eroto-genic zones... the mother regards him with feelings that are derived from her own sexual life... [she] treats him as a substitute for a complete sexual object" (223).

At this point, an essential question appears: When Freud coined the concept, did he refer to the sexuality of adults or babies? The simplest answer is "to both". The previous paragraph summarises his developmental take on the concept, namely that a baby is born with a sexual drive that develops over the years. However, he also linked it to parts of adult sexuality whose behavioural aspects are overt (kisses, looks, smelling, caressing, etc.) but which contain unconscious fantasies and memories as well. These latter aspects refer to *infantile sexuality in the adult*. To Freud, they lay behind neuroses, such as when repressed anal sexuality underlies an obsessional neurosis. Returning to the clip, the kiss reflected my unconscious oral, namely infantile sexuality. Thus, in this discussion, I am mainly addressing infantile sexuality *in the adult*. This being said, one cannot study such an interaction *only* from the adult's perspective. One must also include the baby's perspective. In my view, when Fleur turned away from my kissing lips, she indicated that her infantile sexuality was stirred by my enigmatic message – precisely because she was not yet able to sustain and integrate such signals.

Laplanche (1999b) reformulated Freud's concept into a residue of interactions where the parent emits "enigmatic messages" stemming from his or her unconscious infantile sexuality. In the very young baby, "certain representations are underlined, delimited, offered up, implanted... by the adult world [via enigmatic signifiers]. The first, the most important... is clearly the breast" (64). The breast can be a sweet-smelling, warm, nourishing – or frustrating and empty – part of the mother's body. Or it can be a bottle that offers – or refuses – the baby the desired nourishment. The baby will experience satisfaction or frustration but something else as well: the interchange with mother also has constituents that he can "*sense* but not *make sense* of" (Scarfone & Saketopoulou, 2023, 115, italics in the original). This refers to how a mother's compromised messages are received by her child. We could thus add to the quote above (S. Freud, 1905a, 223) – about the mother providing the baby with an unending source of sexual excitation of his erotogenic zones – that this also results in the baby's continuous efforts to make sense of what goes on in this traffic and how it feels to him/her, whether pleasant or unpleasant.

Freud's (1905b) nonjudgemental suggestion – that the mother should "spare herself any self-reproaches" (223) when she unconsciously connects her daily care of the infant with her sex life – perhaps prevented him from probing deeper into the source of many clinical baby worries. I refer to the psychic conflict between a mother's conscious wish to care for the infant and her unconscious sexual connotations of such care. Such conflicts may emerge as she offers the child "verbal, non-verbal and even behavioural signifiers which are pregnant with unconscious sexual significations" (Laplanche, 1989, 126). In my view, they are the roots of quite a few postpartum disorders that also contain distressed mother-infant interactions.

True, the baby may also harbour seeds of conflicts or – if that term indicates too much of advanced psychic functioning – of contradictory and stressful representations of the adults around. Fleur looked at and then avoided me as if thinking, "This guy is interesting, no, he's frightening so I look away". These divergent attitudes arose consequent upon her interactions with me and mother. One could object that it was *her* innate sexuality that generated the aversive behaviour. PIP therapists Thomson-Salo and Paul (2017) criticise Laplanche for overlooking that infants do have an "innate biologically preexisting sexuality" (322). They invoke biological and interaction research supporting such an innate drive, like Freud did. They argue that Laplanche "exaggerates the infant's passivity" since "the infant's activity can be seen in the 1st hour of life, when newborns placed on the mother's belly creep up to the breast and, before latching on, turn first to look at the mother's eyes" (224).

Such behaviours at the breast in newborn babies have been demonstrated in videos (Widström, Ransjö-Arvidsson, & Christensson, 2007) and articles (Widström et al., 2011). Yet which metapsychological model do their findings attest to? To an innate sexual *drive* in the baby which pushes him or her to crawl to mother's breast? Or to *instinct*-driven behaviours (creeping, licking, latching on, sucking for milk) which the mother interprets *consciously* by means of her attachment system to feed the baby – but which she also interprets, *unconsciously*, through the prism of her infantile sexuality? Or are both alternatives applicable? To me, Thomson Salo's and Paul's critique of Laplanche is interesting and relevant, but from a metapsychological perspective it is as impossible to refute or endorse as is Freud's idea of an innate infantile sexuality. We can thus neither reject nor support that Fleur's avoidance of me and turning to mother also mirrored her innate but now conflicted infantile sexuality.

As Fleur saw my kisses, she must metabolise them by her nascent ego and relegate them to her Unconscious. We can name this "transport" *primal repression* (S. Freud, 1915a) to describe how babies signify affects and impulses in "an archaic mode" (Salomonsson, 2014a, 123). Like in an undeveloped celluloid film, all information has been perceived and registered. But whereas a photographer will use chemicals to develop the film into a photo, an infant cannot make her registrations accessible to mental processing. One difficulty is probably that "the psychic apparatus registers the traces of affective experiences before it is prepared to establish mnemic traces of perceptions" (Green, 1995, 211). Such traces are both stirring and incomprehensible, which make them frightening, exciting, and confusing. Fleur turned away from my kisses because they conveyed something which she, owing to her lack of necessary life experiences, could not process and even less comprehend. They were consigned to her Unconscious as incomprehensible and "undeveloped" registrations coupled with negative affects without any coherent ideational counterparts. The charge of metabolising this experience was too heavy for her. Hence, she avoided me, the source of such befuddling communications.

When Laplanche focused on the adult's rather than the baby's contributions, he underlined, as said previously, that the adult's messages are enigmatic to the sender as well. Thus, the kisses remained unperceived by me for a long time, and even as I saw them, their full import was beyond my comprehension. Probably, this "blindness" sprang from similar situations in my childhood when my parents exposed their infantile sexuality through kisses and otherwise. Or to put it in a behaviourally less exact – but conceptually more precise – formulation: as a child I had "no way of responding in any appropriate way to what [affected me] in the sexually enigmatic or compromised part of [my parents'] communication" (Scarfone, 2014, 339).

Laplanche emphasised that the deep or enigmatic meanings of the messages that are transferred to the child in daily interactions escape recognition and understanding. Would this force us to conclude that no specific and observable adult behaviours exist that represent infantile sexuality more closely than do other demeanours and actions? This is difficult to answer via Laplanche's texts since he "presented his theoretical position extensively but never provided clinical examples" (D. K. Silverman, 2022, 5). According to Vaughan (2017), today's psychoanalytic discourse tends to overuse Laplanche's idea of the enigmatic message and to take "theoretical discussions on the subject into the ether of overabstraction at the expense of real life" (345).

Scarfone and Saketopoulou (2023) are aware of this problem and try to bring the concept of enigmatic (or, as they say, compromised) messages into modern attachment discourse. For example, a parent's neglect can be seen both as an enigmatic message and as his or her "difficulties with attachment" (111). Flora's verbosity could be viewed as containing an enigmatic message of "I can't connect with you because I'm overwhelmed with my own bewilderment". It could also be described in attachment terms as an instance of her insensitive behaviour (Ainsworth, Blehar, Waters, & Wall, 1978) vis-à-vis her daughter. This highlights a point that is often overlooked: infantile sexuality and the compromised messages it may generate refer not solely to the sensuous and pleasant but also to resentment, awe, threat, grief, and so on. Flora's word stream showed her concern of Fleur but, probably, also her ambivalence that was hard for her to integrate.

Do enigmatic messages have behavioural characteristics?

To show a real-life connection between Laplanche's theory and observable infant-adult behaviour, I have used the kisses in the video to exemplify an enigmatic message because (1) a kiss is an ambiguous signifier, ranging from the childish and innocent to the adult and seductive, (2) I was completely unaware of it, (3) it occurred beyond my explicit therapeutic technique, and (4) when I sought contact with mother and Fleur, countertransference was charged with unpleasure rather than those affects we normally link with a kiss, such as pleasure or excitement.

An alternate position would be that we can say nothing about how enigmatic messages are expressed – because they are unobservable. If this be true, the kisses would say nothing of relevance about enigmatic messages. But in my view, such a stance is unreasonably restrictive. Indeed, if the Unconscious were completely occluded to observations, intuitions, and conjectures, psychoanalysis would be impracticable. My argument thus works under the assumption that some behaviours, gestures, tone inflections, scents, glances, and so on are more likely than others to express – or, to put it more cautiously, to be interpreted – as enigmatic messages.

This study adds to papers by authors post Laplanche who have applied his concepts to clinical relations, countertransference dilemmas, and the undercurrent of infantile sexuality in daily life. In contrast, PIP therapists, apart from Thomson-Salo and Paul (2017) as quoted, have not written much on these topics. But is it true that Laplanche gave no clinical illustrations of the traffic of enigmatic messages? Did he actually mean that they are indeed unobservable? This can hardly have been the case. Let us recall that he spoke of enigmatic, not invisible, messages. He did refer to attachment research and infant observation, in line with a movement among some French analysts at the time (Golse, 2001; Lebovici, 1991).

Since the advent of attachment theory and the works by Brazelton and Daniel Stern, many other researchers have demonstrated that the idea of a baby, at first enclosed in himself or closed to the mother-baby dyad and who, nobody knows how, should individuate, this is a myth. In this sense, attachment theory fills a void that Freud left aside to what he called the autoconservative instincts.

(Laplanche, Danon, & Lauru, 2002, 16)

Laplanche also cautioned against an over-reliance on attachment theory:

The negative aspect [of attachment theory] is that one does not see any further. It prevents us from seeing the sexual aspect and how (because that requires a more detailed observation) the mother – child dialogue when approaching perfection is parasitized from the start by the maternal unconscious.

(Laplanche et al., 2002, 16)

Laplanche's project was essentially theoretical: to integrate his conception of infantile sexuality with the corpus of Freud's psychoanalytic theory. As cited above, he was also influenced by empirical observations by attachment researchers at the time. Scarfone (2014) has noted that Laplanche gave few concrete descriptions of mother-child dialogues exemplifying the traffic of enigmatic messages. He clarifies that, to Laplanche, "attachment is a normal biological or ethological phenomenon, [and] also serves as the carrier wave for what emanates from the adult's unconscious desires and fantasies" (337). The latter ingredient Laplanche called *noise*, which "comes to disturb and compromise the preconscious-conscious message" (Laplanche, 2007a, 215). Scarfone (2014) uses the same metaphor plus another one: infantile sexuality is "so omnipresent that one loses awareness that it infiltrates everything human"; indeed, it is "like the *air* we breathe" (342, italics added).

"Noise" and "air", two metaphors of the traffic of infantile sexuality, evoke a main question. To me, the metaphors are dissimilar. As I listen to conversations in an airplane, I might hear nothing but noise. Yet, by intense listening, I might discern a tone, a word, or a scream. In contrast, when I inhale, I can discern nothing but air that is basically alike everywhere. Noise as a metaphor of the sexual traffic is, as I therefore argue, more apt because it may contain concealed but discernible information. Similarly, human interaction contains behavioural details that we can distinguish as being derivatives of the infantile sexual. This is where the video kisses enter the scene.

But can we really claim that there are *unequivocal* behavioural signs of unconscious impulses in a mother, which are implanted as enigmatic messages in the baby? Of course not, because such a claim would be contrary to ordinary psychoanalytic practice. As analysts, we perceive signifiers in the clinical situation, process them, add our subjective associations and emotions, and then conceive of an interpretation. We search for *meaning* more than for *behavioural details*, which highlights that the analyst contributes to forming an interpretation. To emphasise, any semiotic undertaking (da Rocha Barros & da Rocha Barros, 2011; Olds, 2000) – that is, linking a sign with an interpretant – involves a *creative* act. Since such acts may yield different results, we cannot say that enigmatic messages have fixed and well-defined signifiers or expressive forms, such as that kissing lip movements always signify the subject's infantile sexuality. However, *this cautionary remark should not prevent us from asking if certain signifiers are more indicative of infantile sexuality compared with others.*

A Laplancheian perspective on the video clip

The question now is if the referred sighs, smiles, recoils, and kisses exemplify Laplanche's enigmatic signifiers. There is no doubt that, to him, infantile sexuality manifested in real-life communications within primal object-relations:

> The realm of reality specific to the message includes the following features: (1) the message is not necessarily verbal, nor even integrated into a semiotic system, but it is always inscribed in a (signifying) materiality; (2) the message, before representing something (a signified), always represents an other for someone: it is communication, address; and (3) the message, by virtue of its materiality, is dedicated to polysemy.
>
> (Laplanche, 2017, 199)

The preconscious – conscious messages run in everyday parent-infant attachment behaviours, such as a diaper change or a chat with the baby. What makes it also comprise an enigmatic message? Would it have some discernible manifestation? Here, Laplanche is not clear.

We do not have to look far to find concrete examples of what I call enigmatic signifiers. Can analytic theory afford to go ignoring the extent to which women unconsciously and sexually cathect the breast, which appears to be a natural organ for lactation. It is inconceivable that the infant does not notice this sexual cathexis... It is impossible to imagine that the infant does not suspect that this cathexis is the source of a nagging question: what does the breast want from me, apart from wanting to suckle me and, come to that, why does it want to suckle me?

(Laplanche, 1989, 126)

The quotation is problematic. First of all, feelings about breastfeeding are extremely varied (Friedman, 1996) and may swing between idealisation and contempt (Miller, 1987). A mother's attitudes therefore need psychoanalytic investigation to determine how she cathects breastfeeding. In other words, her *experiences* of feeding the baby rather than "her actual feeding style" – for example, by breast or bottle – influence how she bonds with her infant (Bar Emet Gradman & Shai, 2023, 1). Furthermore, the quote by Laplanche contains many negative expressions: "we do not have to look", "cannot afford ignoring", and "inconceivable that the infant does not notice the sexual cathexis". It would be more helpful to formulate in positive phrases how enigmatic messages look, smell, sound, or feel. Finally, we should recall from earlier in the chapter that fantasies embedded in primal seduction may also contain aggressive, rejecting, and confusing messages. We thus need to deprive the term of any unequivocal blissful atmosphere and comprehend that it can also be felt by the baby as threatening, alienating, saddening, and upsetting.

Do all these arguments lead us to surrender, stating that there are no perceptible differences between situations that mother and/or baby may interpret as seductive or not? Yet such an argument would clarify little and raise the question of the phenomenology of primal seduction. According to Scarfone and Saketopoulou (2023, 112), Laplanche claimed there is "no direct communication from unconscious to unconscious". Here, his carrier wave concept may help us: enigmatic messages are transmitted in preconscious – conscious communications which, in Fleur's case, contained "noise", namely features that were incomprehensible to her and evoked affects of anxiety or unpleasure. Another feature made the kiss an even more bungled message: it was also "enigmatic for the sender" (Laplanche, 1996, 11), namely for me.

A message is thus enigmatic when it *leaks behavioural details that contradict intentions that are conscious to the sender and/or conceal or skew intentions that are unconscious to him/her*. These details may occur as a facial or bodily movement, tonus change, stillness, voice change, silence, and use of words that are equivocal, harsh, or affectionate, and so on. I reached out to Fleur, she avoided me, I was frustrated and added, unbeknownst, a kissing movement. Later, I was shocked by the comparison of diaper change and sexual assault and said nothing. Meanwhile, my body "spoke" by recoiling from mother's violent comparison. Much of this was understood only retrospectively since, in the session, my self-reflection was hampered by our complex interactions. This limitation could, however, be turned into a deeper understanding of the enigmatic messages in the session. This can be achieved via an analyst's self-reflection in session and analysis of video clips afterwards.

We expect therapists to work towards accessing their unconscious reactions in- and out-side of sessions to deepen their insight of mother and baby and to share it. To illustrate, later in the session, Flora and I had a more vital contact, and I asked why she thought the girl was gaze-avoidant in sessions but not at home. She answered, "I think it has to do with how I feel *here*". She unfolded events that yielded a deeper understanding of the assault theme. She had mentioned a delivery phobia before, but only now did she become explicit about it. She had thought of delivering alone in a parking lot or killing herself. She then visited the emergency room due to her panic attacks, and an obstetrician arranged a caesarean section in due time.

When I told her that she might have experienced my comment about gaze avoidance prior to the reported session as coming from a "surgeon ripping up old wounds", I signalled that she was free to speak about her mistrust of me. She replied that she did trust me, but only now did she understand that she could also *talk* with me about her mistrust. This led her to viewing me more as someone ready to empathise with whatever she might think of me. It also led her to become more unrestrained and tolerant towards herself. She revealed that when I had mentioned the difference between Fleur's looking into Mum's eyes but avoiding mine, it was tough to hear "that something isn't OK with Fleur. I often feel criticized by the nurses at the Centre as well".

She added that before our sessions, she had tummy aches and Fleur got fussy. "I think I've infected Fleur with my own fears when we're coming to you. That's why she's avoiding your eyes. That's tough to realise". She thus formulated her understanding of what I conceived as Fleur's import of mother's transference to me. To Fleur, I was a threat because I spoke with the mother about things that made Mum anxious – which, of course, unsettled the baby. Yet, as suggested earlier, when Fleur avoided my eyes right after the "kiss", this probably occurred because she got bewildered by it. Having already been affected by mother's apprehension of me, the kiss made her conceive of me as an even more incomprehensible person.

Final questions

The clinical material suggests that some gestures of mine in a PIP session could be conceived of as enigmatic messages. They arose in an entangled situation between me, the baby, and the mother. Although I was aware that we were in an impasse, its embodied forms in my lips and torso were unconscious. Precisely therefore, they affected mother and child. The mother turned her baby away from me, and the baby avoided looking at me. I have used the sequence to substantiate Laplanche's concepts and to show how my embodied and unconscious communication affected the dyad.

Before concluding, three final questions need to be approached. *The first* is if enigmatic messages are inherently and invariably counterproductive for a baby's development. The question is warranted in view of Fleur's distress when I made the kissing movements. I will answer via another example (Salomonsson, 2022). A mother, Edna, and her 5-week-old son Leonard were in PIP with me. One session, she reported that Leonard had got a thrush infection in the mouth. She must give him a bitter medication and wash her breasts with an anti-mycotic solution before breastfeeding. This impoverished their relationship during the weekend, but now their contact was "much better" again. Yet she looked sad, and the boy was staring between the two of us, a bit fussy. Here is an excerpt from a videorecorded session as I tried to establish emotional contact with him.

Analyst to the boy:	You've really got into trouble, the two of you (trying to capture his gaze, and after a while he looks at me). Hello, Leonard, oh, what a fine gaze you've got!... You had a bad start, you and Mum. You came on the slant/glide from each other (my two palms gliding against each other. He peers at my hands and gets a bit sleepy).
Mother smiling to the boy:	You thought that was funny, eh?
Analyst:	You've been gliding from each other (My hands are still gliding and he is still sleepy). Mum is so sad, she really longed to have a baby, but then you've been gliding away from each other. (The boy gets more alert, smiles while looking at my hands).

In retrospect, I conceive of the expression "on the glide" plus the hand movements as a bungled message. It was a spontaneous and conscious gesture depicting mother and son gliding apart. The video reveals my smile as I recognised some concealed connotations of "on the glide". In our language, it is used for a youngster who has embarked on a risky or promiscuous lifestyle. A lubricant is called "glide-agent". My gliding palms signified loss of contact. It is also probable that his ensuing sleepiness and smile could be explained by the lulling effect of my hands' motions, while the words' sexual references, unintended and unconscious at first, could not be grasped by him. I did subject him to an enigmatic message, but the result, his "falling asleep with flushed cheeks and a blissful smile" (S. Freud, 1905b, 182), shows that such messages can also be productive and helpful. Accordingly, Freud suggested that a mother who allows her baby care to also be influenced by her infantile sexuality "is only fulfilling her task in teaching the child to love" (223).

The second question concerns if these observations are confined to my personal PIP technique. To answer, I will bring a videorecorded PIP case from a colleague. A mother of a seven-month-old girl speaks in agitation about her mother-in-law. Having the girl in her lap, she describes her relative as intrusive, self-centred, and without empathy when her grandchild rejects her clumsy contact efforts. The mother handles the girl similarly by tucking her hand under the girl's sweater and kissing her neck insensitively. The girl avoids mother's face and turns to the therapist. As mother continues disparaging her relative, she smiles furtively with a touch of triumph.

The mother's conscious and verbal messages indicate concern for her baby and critique of her mother-in-law. However, her ways of handling the child, and her peculiar smile, contradict her words. Not only does she mimic her mother-in-law, but she also shows excitation or pleasure. This, too, could be labelled an enigmatic message, leaving the baby confused about what is a loving caress and a clumsy attack. The therapist reports that she sensed this confusion but found no other way of handling her countertransference distress than by moving her torso backwards with a strained smile, as seen in her video. This shows that incidents such as in Fleur's and Flora's case are not idiosyncratic but also occur in PIP treatments with other therapists.

The *third and final* question is if Jean Laplanche would have found these examples and conclusions relevant to his theory. As mentioned earlier, he joined the attachment concept with that of "unilateral sexuality" (2007a, 2007b, 100) in the so-called fundamental anthropologic situation. He thus sought to dismantle what I call the spurious transmission gap between classic psychoanalysis and attachment and behavioural research. I conclude that he would have welcomed PIP vignettes to investigate his ideas about the enigmatic messages in the banal day-to-day traffic between adult and baby. Perhaps, he would even have agreed that my kisses to Fleur exemplified such messages. In 2023, I discussed the clip with Laplanche scholar Dominique Scarfone in terms of enigmatic messages. Earlier, in 2011, I had asked Jean Laplanche if we could look together at some of my videos to hear his opinions on the topics discussed in this paper. He readily agreed and we set up a meeting. Sadly, it was cancelled at the last minute due to his illness. Sometime later, he passed away. With this chapter, I salute an innovative and courageous thinker.

The Infantile and infantile sexuality

I have used the vignette to investigate the concept of *infantile sexuality*. It is time to ask if it is connected to *the Infantile*. In brief, *infantile sexuality is part of the Infantile – but not the other way around*. Infantile sexuality emerges in interactions with parents whom we depend on, desire, fear, love, and enjoy being with. Even if they were perfectly committed to and in tune with the child, they would be unable to comprehend and still every need, pang, or desire in the baby. In addition, parents do not entirely comprehend themselves either. In other words, they have an Unconscious. When they do not discern and understand what it urges them to do, feel, and fantasise, it has free rein to penetrate their Conscious. This creates the muddled messages Laplanche talked about.

To illustrate, I suggest that when I kissed Fleur in the air trying to make contact, I was overcome by my Infantile. It could be formulated as, "I'm trying to reach you, but I feel so frustrated. Come closer". At this point, I believe I unconsciously identified with her infantile helplessness. I shifted from an adult's ordinary ways of making contact with a baby, such as by smiling, to a concrete extending my lips towards her. I have argued that this motion also expressed a desire stemming from my infantile sexuality. But she could not understand my motions because our states of mind were very different. This was confusing and must be repressed to form kernels of *her* infantile sexuality. In this, I do not mean that the event was detrimental to her. All babies sometimes misunderstand and are misunderstood. But if her experiences were to be repeated in many interactions, they might build up a portion of an Infantile that one day interfered with her basic trust and attachment in intimate relationships.

Source

This chapter is a reworked version of a published paper (Salomonsson, 2025). I thank the publisher for giving permission to quote it in the book.

Chapter 11

Metaphors as traces of the Infantile

Chapters 8–10 focused mainly on the impact of *nonverbal* communication such as gestures, frowns, and tone of voice. We will now highlight how words in psychotherapy sessions impact on the participants and on the course on the therapy, specifically *metaphors* that occur spontaneously to the analyst and which he then shares with the patient. This may happen notably when he is confronted with a complicated and frustrating situation. A previous paper (Salomonsson, 2022) included a vignette of a parent-infant psychotherapy (PIP) case, in which I was frustrated by not getting in deeper emotional contact with the mother of a three-week-old boy, Leonard, who was also mentioned briefly in Chapter 10. His mother Edna could not put words to her visible disappointment at the lack of cordial and calm contact with her son. Metaphors began to emerge in me like "You're so tense, Leonard, like *cramping*... Maybe Mum's got a cramp in her head, too, so she cannot speak or think". Another metaphor was that of a little *girl cowering behind a wall*, portraying the defences against her emotions and her son as well.

At first, the mother, with her fears of diving into the world of feelings, objected that my metaphors did not tell her much. Later, they evolved into tools, images, or toys that we could "play" with in sessions. For example, she slowly realised that her "wall" was not a very good thing – which she had claimed initially. She came to understand how it prevented her from letting loose feelings of love, care, worries, and vexation about the boy. The metaphors helped her catch up with a primary maternal preoccupation (Winnicott, 1956) that had been slow to start during pregnancy.

I have argued that PIP contains certain characteristics that promote this metaphorical thinking in the analyst. Other child analysts have also written about expressing their spontaneous metaphors. The ones presented by Serge Lebovici and colleagues (Lebovici et al., 2002; Lebovici & Stoléru, 2003) often had an embodied connotation that they voiced as "metaphorizing interventions" in parent-infant work. They helped the analyst understand, contain, and interpret what the dyad was enacting. Johan Norman (1989) described "visual images" in analyses with adults and children. Some derived

DOI: 10.4324/9781003640363-11

from his personal experiences and were clinically useful in that they revealed aspects of the patient's unconscious dilemmas and increased his empathy.

In my paper (Salomonsson, 2022), I asked why metaphors seem to emerge more frequently in PIP than in other settings. I concluded that it is related to (a) the countertransference, which awakens infantile strata in the analyst and pushes him or her to concrete thinking; (b) the rapid oscillations between verbal and non-verbal communication in sessions, which makes all the participants use body language, such as gestures and facial expressions; (c) the setting's affinity to psychodrama and couple therapy; and (d) the kinship between how a tiny baby produces simple concepts (Mandler, 2004) based on their perceptions and how adults create metaphors from their basic infantile experiences (Lakoff & Johnson, 1980/2003). The common denominator of the baby's concepts and the adult's metaphors is their embodied nature. To exemplify, when a frightened baby crouches under her bed cover – and when I suggested to Leonard's mother the imagery of a frightened girl by the wall – both are embodied expressions of fear.

The PIP setting thus has many ingredients that can push the therapist towards metaphorical functioning. It may also create a certain laxity or proximity to primary process functioning in the therapist. A PIP session is often a visual, audible, smelly, and emotional drama. I believe that an analyst familiar with such drama with babies tends to translate more often, unwittingly and spontaneously, scenes with adult analysands in a similar manner. What goes on in the consulting room's scant interior and dampened sensorial input may be experienced in the form of more vivid imaginaries or metaphorical scenarios emerging in the therapist. I will get back to the link between PIP experiences and metaphors, but for now I will stick to the book's main clinical group, that of adult patients.

Thomas in analysis: the snail

Thomas is in his mid-forties when he seeks psychoanalysis. Earlier, he lived with Irene for some years, but now he is a bachelor. Irene recently suggested that his father's suicide when he was eleven years old must have affected him deeply. He did not dismiss her idea but does not understand *how* it would affect him today. An office employee, he dreams of a future as an artist. In the interviews, he keeps emotions in check while telling me that he suffers from a paralyzing sadness and lack of intimate contact. He has many friends and is a womanizer but can never stay in a relationship for long. They end with Thomas feeling bitter, resentful, and that something is wrong with him.

Analysis starts with four sessions a week. They often tend to be monotonous, intellectual, and dull. He has a sarcastic touch, as when I say it is difficult for me to concretely hear his comments and he responds, "That's your problem". He is aloof and haughty – and extremely sensitive to rejection. If he sends an SMS without receiving a quick answer, he conjures up scenarios proving that the receiver doesn't care about him. This sensitivity almost reaches paranoid levels.

Sometimes, the question of becoming a father emerges. If I show any interest in that issue, he withdraws. When he is dating a woman, they soon end up in bed, but it does not take long until he interprets "her lack of response" as the forthcoming end of their relationship. To avoid this slight, he breaks up in advance. I discover that I try to stay close to him while he repeatedly pulls out. I recognize the similarity between my position and that of Nellie, another previous lover. At times, when he has withdrawn from her, she has nonetheless remained friends with him, for which he is very thankful. She and I seem to share the experience of being fobbed off by Thomas. At this point, I share a metaphorical image that comes to my mind.

Analyst: "I'm thinking of a snail. It's inside the shell but cautiously sticking out its antennae. As soon as it senses danger or rejection from outside, it quickly retreats. Maybe something similar is going on between you and me, and between you and Nellie."

Thomas: "A funny thing about snails, the contrast between their hard shell and their moist, disgusting entrails."

Analyst: "I was thinking of when the snail withdraws. You are underlining its disgusting interior. It's a tricky situation: Reaching out for contact is risky, you withdraw when you feel fobbed off, but then you are alone with your repugnant self."

Thomas: "Nellie is a snail, too. She says she is fond of me but doesn't want a relationship. I accept it and withdraw, but I feel lousy."

The snail metaphor is fanning out into many meanings. Consciously, I had intended it only as an image of a creature that reaches out for contact but gets scared and pulls back. In retrospect, I think it also expressed my vexation of not getting beneath Thomas's narcissistic shell. It was as if I were knocking on it and begging him in vain to peep out. His comment about him and Nellie as two snails added an interactive meaning to the metaphor; their cautious advances and retreats, with hopes of union and fears of dismissal, could also be applied to our interaction. He often felt snubbed by me, whereas I could feel it was hopeless to stay in contact and so I lost focus on him. Hearing him speak about the snail's disgusting entrails, which I thought represented his grim self-esteem, made me empathize with the tangled interchanges with people he yearns for.

Some weeks later, he is walking around town when a terror attack is perpetrated nearby. He hears the sirens and sees the commotion but keeps on walking, feeling that it is not his business. Listening to his hardboiled account is taxing for me, and the snail comes to my mind but now from another angle. I think of its glassy, intricate, and beautiful shell, which I interpret as an idealized version of his isolation as he prides himself on remaining unperturbed by the upheaval in town. The snail's exterior and interior thus communicate pride and self-disgust interchange as well as isolation and contact-seeking. For example, when a new lover calls him on the phone, he hesitates to answer, fearing that she will dismiss him in the end. It is safer to get back inside the shell and marvel at its hard and shiny surface protecting his solitude. Alone is strong, as the saying goes.

The snail – psychodynamics of a metaphorical image

It seems a common occurrence in psychoanalytic therapy that the analyst's metaphors pop up in taxing countertransference situations. I refer to feelings of powerlessness, vexation, blockage of contact, and difficulties in understanding the dynamics and the content of the dialogue. If the analyst acknowledges the countertransference in such an impasse, it may happen that he converts it, spontaneously and without conscious effort, to a metaphor. This process applies to the genesis and evolution of the snail image. Initially, I saw before my inner eye a snail from behind, its head warily peeping outside, on the alert if danger should strike. I was taken by the contrast between the shell and the slimy and sensitive antennae. Already at this point, it illustrated the fragile to-and-fro motions between the snail and the outer world. Translating the metaphor to the world of object relations, the snail's motions resemble the ones that take place between Thomas and the object he desires. He reaches out to his lover or to me and then retracts. When he added the disgusting entrails, he revealed his fear that any object he is longing for will view his desire as repugnant and reject him.

Let us now follow the evolution of the snail metaphor. One day as he is speaking of his complicated relationship with Irene, Thomas says:

Thomas: "I'll give you some psychoanalytic candy. My mother told me I was born with teeth, so she couldn't breastfeed me."

Analyst: "What's the candy about it?"

Thomas: "That you'd relish this info, just like you did with my father's suicide, that you'd consider it crucial for why I developed into the guy I am today. You'd be right and I'd end at the bottom of the ladder."

Analyst: "So there'd be no discussion or interchange between us, just that I'd be right and you'd be wrong, like a one-way relationship. You'd give pieces of information and I'd respond in triumph, 'What did I tell you!?'"

Thomas: "A one-way relationship… I certainly recognize that with many women I met."

Thomas thus views our relationship, not as a potentially interesting play of give-and-take but as a dictate issued by me. Supported by this view, he manages to avoid the serious questions concealed in his mother's story. Was he really born with teeth? What did she feel about her newborn and about breastfeeding? How did she look at him when putting him to the breast? We might imagine a mixture of fear, disgust, tenderness, and withdrawal. She told him his precocious teething was the problem. But maybe it would be more fertile to apply an interactive perspective: to focus on an unhappy match between an infant – with or without teeth – wanting to suckle and his mother fearing, for whatever reason, that he would bite her nipple. The snail baby and the mother holding him could then be seen as a metaphor of two persons' emotional communication: on the one side, a baby wanting Mum's nipple while noting that she rejects him; on the other side, her wish to feed him but fearing his bite. This might create a feeling in Thomas of being undesired and undesirable, leaving him with an intense unstilled emotional hunger. As for the mother, we could think of her as despairing about how to decipher and approach her baby. From an analytic perspective, it is of course impossible to settle if newborn Thomas actually had teeth or not. What we, in contrast, are entitled to conceive of is a clash of two participants' self-representations: her helplessness and lack of enjoyment and pride in adjusting to her baby and his needs – and his confusion when he's hungry and smells the breast but then something obstructs the interaction.

To sum up, the meaning of the snail metaphor evolved in at least three steps. At first, its main import emerged from *my* perspective: "Thomas, you are inaccessible to me, like a snail in its shell". It pointed to his isolation tendency but also to my unresolved countertransference vexation. Its second import was born out of *his* snail perspective: "When I reach out for contact, I risk feeling disgusting and then being dismissed". Now, my countertransference changed into an empathic stance towards his predicament. The third meaning was

> We are snails, Thomas, both you and me. I reach out for you, and you retract into your shell. This makes me feel rejected and entices me to recoil. Then you'll peep out after a while, looking for contact with me, but you wonder if I'll peep out again or remain in bitter but splendid isolation.

In this interpretation, there would not be one perpetrator and one victim but two people locked in an unhappy relationship.

Metaphor theory

We have learnt about a tricky clinical situation with contact effort and avoidance between Thomas and me. As I was reflecting on our present relation, the snail metaphor appeared. This event raises interesting theoretical questions. To understand how metaphors are born and what roles they play in psychoanalytic therapy, we first need to summarize some aspects of linguistic metaphor theory. Later, we will link the genesis of metaphor with infant development in particular. In what have become classical works, George Lakoff and Mark Johnson (1980/2003, 1999) extend the meaning of metaphor. They dispute it is a mere figure of speech or literary embellishment. They see it as an *overarching mode of concept-making* that permeates almost every human thought and sentence.

According to the classical view, metaphor is "'detachable' from language, a device that may be imported into language in order to achieve specific, prejudged effects" (Arlow, 1979, 368). Lakoff's and Johnson's (1980/2003) idea is that *language is "metaphorically structured"* (12), as demonstrated in many everyday words and expressions. To exemplify, the word "symbol" is "a communication element intended to simply represent or stand for a complex of person, object, group, or idea" (www.britannica.com). Its etymology joins two Greek words meaning "together" and "throw". A symbol helps us "throw together" an object and its representation, or representamen in Peirce's terminology. At bottom, to "throw together" is an embodied, physical act. Likewise, the word "metaphor" itself stems from two roots: "across" and "bear, carry". The snail metaphor "carries across" Thomas's emotional and relational isolation to a mollusc that is adroit in retracting and peeping out. The examples show the concrete and embodied roots of abstract words. The theory of Lakoff and Johnson has impacted philosophy and linguistics, but criticism has also been voiced (Kövecses, 2008; Wilson & Golonka, 2013), also from the psychoanalytic domain (Simpson, 2007).

To illustrate with metaphors in clinical practice, an analyst might suggest to a sad patient, "After the summer break, you feel there's a wall between us. Nothing comes to your mind, it's like a big cramp inside". "Wall" is an *embodied* metaphor for what the analyst assumes is the patient's experience of lack of contact, and "cramp" refers to fruitless efforts at thinking about his feelings. The metaphors extend sensorimotor experiences of physical restraint to an emotional experience. True, "summer break" is also such a metaphor in that "break" compares separation to a fracture. Evidently, human beings use metaphor "effortlessly, and mostly unremarked, in ordinary language... It is... an inevitable, intrinsic aspect of human thought, reasoning, and speech" (Wallerstein, 2011, 90).

What do I mean when suggesting that wall, cramp, and snail are *embodied* metaphors? The point is that all three refer to experiences that can be related to the body. A wall prevents me from concretely reaching somebody or something I yearn for. A cramp makes my movements clumsy and inefficient. Finally, a snail peeping out of its shell and then retracting in danger situations relates to a child cautiously reaching out to touch and then pulling back when being scared. To my knowledge, Lakoff and Johnson had no clinical experiences of infants. It was a stroke of genius when they claimed that many *primary metaphors* emerge from basic bodily *infantile* experiences. For example, infants strive for physical proximity with the primary object and get anguished if they are separated. In a concrete sense, a wall and a cramp imply blocked access, confinement, or blockage in general. The snail brings to mind a peek-a-boo game with its fear of separation and joy of return.

These metaphors arise when the *source*'s concrete meaning (here, blocked muscular motion) is coupled or conflated with a *target* domain (here, a faltering emotional contact). As used here, the shared source of "wall" and "cramp" is muscular inhibition, whereas their target is frustration at the poor emotional contact. As for the snail, its source might be situations when I held a snail in my hand and was surprised and disappointed by its sudden retreat when I knocked on the shell.

These linguists do not claim that first there is a bodily event (source), which then links with an emotional experience (target). Actually, source and target are conflated to create the metaphor. This is one reason that the two terms are a bit cumbersome. Being metaphors themselves, they seem to indicate that the source relates to the target as a launch pad to a missile. But in the session, the snail imagery was not born prior to functioning as a metaphor of our emotional contact. It would be closer to the truth to say that source and target – or "launch pad" and "missile" – occurred *simultaneously as a creative stroke*, namely when *mind and body cooperated*. We can speak of a *psychosomatic act* where body and soul, motion and emotion, worked in unison. Could we even suggest that such acts are not polarities but phenomena that are fused into one entity? This idea was broached in Chapter 9 when I used the term "soulbody" to depict how babies communicate.

Situations that engender such conflations are called *primary scenes* (Grady, 1997). For example, "wall" exemplifies "emotional intimacy is proximity" (293) – as when we say, "my cousin and I are close". This scene applies in an inverted form, "emotional alienation is distance", to the snail. In my imagery, it retracted when I tried to get close to it, namely to Thomas. Later, it also referred to the obverse of another primary scene by Grady, "appealing is tasty", namely "unappealing is yucky" like its slimy and unpleasant body. Such primary scenes are "minimal (temporally delimited) episodes of subjective experience, characterized by tight correlations between physical circumstance and cognitive response" (24). To understand what a metaphor actually means, one must also have acquired an ability to *de-conflate* source and target (Lakoff & Johnson, 1999, 49). Thus, one must understand that a snail's retracting antenna and my frustration when not reaching Thomas emotionally are not identical. His comment about the contrast between its hard shell and disgusting entrails showed that he did understand the metaphor and was ready to play with it. Later I will return to the *aspect of play* in the clinical use of metaphors.

Primary scenes can yield metaphors only if we have become able to form concepts of what we perceive. If I had no concepts of snails and my encounters with them, the metaphor would never have been born. But when do we begin to form concepts? As for a snail metaphor, no such concept is born until the child has seen or heard about it. But note that Grady's primary scenes are formulated in vague and abstract forms. This helps us understand why the traffic between various "sources" can flow quite easily. For example, a child may experience something as disgusting – let us say, his baby puree – and may later connect this feeling with a slimy snail he sees on the ground. Both objects are felt to be "yucky".

Jean Mandler (2004), a cognitive scientist, assumes that "conceptual interpretation of what one perceives happens at least crudely from birth... What is innate is a mechanism that operates on perceptual information" (66). Mandler calls this device *perceptual meaning analysis*. Infants thus ascribe "meaning to what they perceive, and those meanings form concepts" (67). Thus, the baby puree and the snail may combine into a concept like "disgusting, slippery, I don't like it" – with all the necessary reservations when we put words to a baby's world of experiences. In sum, perceptual meaning analysis is a "concept-making engine, transforming perceptual information into another form" (70). Before the advent of language, it is the only way we can form concepts.

Mandler (2004) illustrates the process by way of a primary scene: the baby "sees an object nearby, she cries, the object begins to move, approaches, looms, and she is picked up" (72). The fact that such scenes can be accompanied by strong emotions seems rarely emphasized by linguist authors – in contrast to psychoanalytic writers. One early example is Freud's (1895/1950) description of a screaming baby fed by the mother who is "simultaneously the [baby's] first satisfying object and further his first hostile object, as well as his sole helping power" (331). The baby's meaning analysis creates a concept of a mother or of a part-object-mother, and this process is accompanied by strong and varying affects, as seen in any screaming baby.

Mandler (2004) suggests that the infant abstracts sensory information through *image-schemas*. These representations are spatial, dynamic, fluid, but not necessarily visual. They derive from the baby's perceptual meaning analysis. To Mandler, "they are not conscious and can neither be attended to nor ignored" (81). Clausner and Croft (1999) add that such schemas are "more than elements of linguistic theory: they have *psychological reality*" (13, italics added). They show the increasing interest among linguists to also consider emotional components in these meaning-making processes. Think of the image schema UP-DOWN, which Martínez, Español, and Pérez (2018) exemplify with a mother playfully lifting and sinking a pillow above her baby's head while his arms move up and down. Her voice ascends and descends, which supports the idea that image-schemas are often multi-modal; in this example, vision, proprioception, and hearing operate in unison. It also shows that long before the child learns to link the word "up" to things above, he forms an up-concept, which can be formulated as "up is where Mum's pillow is" or "where the clouds are". This process coexists with strong affects – in this case, joy, thrill, and affection in baby and mother.

Let us now investigate if the snail imagery fits into our conceptual analysis of metaphors. True, it is not a succinct, conventional metaphor but a mental imagery, but Lakoff and Johnson (1999) stress that "not all conceptual metaphors are manifested in the words of a language. Some are manifested in grammar, others in gesture, art, or ritual. These nonlinguistic metaphors may, however, be secondarily expressed through language and other symbolic means" (57). This makes our snail qualify as such a metaphor. Is it constructed through a conflation of source and target domains? The answer is yes. It inverts Grady's primary metaphor "emotional intimacy is proximity" into "lack of emotional contact is distance". I had a source experience of not reaching desired objects that hide inside their casings, here the snail retreating into its shell. This was conflated with my frustrating target experience of not reaching Thomas's "inside", namely his suffering self. Another conflation was concealed in the image's second meaning of the snail's body representing something disgusting and Thomas feeling similarly. To conclude, this snail metaphor is indeed structured according to Lakoff and Johnson's conflation of source and target domains.

The snail raises the question if the use of metaphors in analysis relates to the search for traces of the Infantile in my patients. I will return to this question at the end of this chapter. Do I use metaphors with adult patients as well? The answer is yes, as seen, for example, in my work with Thomas and Bess. We recall Bess with her partner and his proposal of an outing in the park followed by her flat rejection. She and I felt quite differently about the event. She was enraged while I thought she had smashed a comfy idea. This led to my two metaphorical images: the first about a furious toddler who doesn't have it her way and the second about a baby fretting at mother's breast. They expressed emotional conflicts between Bess and him and, by extension, her and me. Also, they can be seen as my efforts at curbing my frustration. I thus suggest there is a particular link between metaphors created by the analyst and his or her countertransference displeasure.

Psychoanalysts writing on the clinical use of metaphors

We have followed the metaphor of the snail with Thomas and of the fretting baby with Bess. This leads to the question how other analysts view work with metaphors. A more positive attitude, which relates to a change in our views of psychoanalytic practice, has emerged in recent decades. It is moving

From the model of an applied science of discerning and interpreting unconscious meaning to methods of promoting new products of mental activity.... Rather than deciphering or translating a disguised text, the *analyst participates in a process that creates a text.*

(Kirshner, 2015, 67, italics added)

This shift also affects how we conceive of our interventions. Otto Kernberg (1997, 99) speaks of an "antiauthoritarian attitude" evolving in psychoanalysis, which questions "the privileged nature of the analyst's subjectivity". We are less inclined today to enunciate to the patient what went on in his childhood and to profess what his issues and symptoms "actually mean". We are more into a joint project whose aim is that the patient becomes more agile and variegated when reflecting on his feelings, attitudes, and actions. By *facilitating* such a development in the patient, we hope to provide him or her with means to achieve it alone in the future.

In what Kirshner calls the analyst's authoritative position, metaphors are merely valued as "arrows" pointing to the patient's "real" history. In an alternative "deconstructive" position, they are seen as tools for helping the patient express and reflect on anxieties. Arlow (1979, 381) formulates this as a series of "approximate objectications of the patient's unconscious thought processes, [in which the analyst] supplies the appropriate metaphors". Another analyst, Modell (2009) suggests we use a metaphor to "unconsciously interpret our affective world" and that it is "an organizing template that establishes the categories of emotional memory" (8). Similar views were expressed further back in time (Lindén, 1985; Shengold, 1981).

It is not evident if these analysts sanction *voicing* their metaphors to the patient. Ogden (1997), however, often elaborates a metaphor that he or the patient has introduced "usually unself-consciously" (723). He sees metaphor as "an integral part of the attempt of two people to convey to one another a sense of what each is feeling (like) in the present moment and what one's past experience felt like in the past" (722). Already, Reider (1972) suggested that a metaphor

> Enables both patient and therapist to maintain sufficient discontinuity between primary and secondary process, and permits insights that can be tolerated... [It] serves the defensive function of allowing the patient to keep a necessary distance from conscious awareness, while serving the function of reducing the distance between therapist and patient.
>
> (468)

Civitarese and Ferro (2013) describe metaphors as "a reverie produced on the spot" (203) in the analytic field. They link them with pictograms (Aulagnier, 2001) that capture "proto-emotional states" and thus help the analyst in "naming something which was previously unnamed" (Ferro, 2006). Such states often emerge in a constricted clinical situation. I thus believe it is mostly when the *therapeutic process is thwarted that the analyst tends to use metaphoric interventions*. To sum up, the more we see therapy as a continuous dialogue between the patient and us – both with clearly defined roles – and where we test different versions of truth that make the patient's suffering more comprehensible to him or her, the more metaphors can emerge as a useful instrument. This position is not at all restricted to analysts coming from object relations or intersubjectivity traditions.

Metaphors in psychoanalysis: their validity and clinical utility

We now need to probe if I am prescribing an unrestricted "pro-metaphor" stance. Do I suggest that an analyst's metaphor can reveal as much as the dream (S. Freud, 1900) about the patient's Unconscious? First, a qualification of this question is needed: Freud was clear that it is not the dream itself but *the interpretations* of it that is "the royal road to a knowledge of the unconscious activities of the mind" (608). Consequently, the analyst's subjective perspective always contributes to dream interpretations. Though they provide pieces of knowledge about the analysand's Unconscious, they do not reveal the Truth about it. The royal road is thus not a smooth highway to a predetermined yet unknown destination.

Similarly, clinical metaphors also need to be interpreted, and, of course, other analysts' subjectivities might have yielded divergent interpretations of "cramp", "snail", or "fretting baby". Wallerstein (2011) is thus right that though metaphor has been "central to the fabric of psychoanalysis from its very beginning", we must also clarify its "limitations, and its possibility for obfuscation" (93). I would express it in this way: *the usefulness of the analyst's metaphor is limited by his or her narcissism – in both its libidinal and epistemological sense.* As for the libidinal sense, an analyst may become enchanted by a metaphor, which prevents him from probing if it is an overvalued idea about what goes on in the patient. He may think it is evocative, while the patient feels it is dull or insignificant. We must charter such risks by scrutinizing how the patient responds to the metaphor: Does it facilitate the clinical process or block it? I will soon return to this point.

The epistemological limitation concerns the validity of metaphor – and here, the comparison with the dream comes to a halt. A patient's dream is created by him or her at night without any direct influence by the analyst. In contrast, the metaphors presented here were initiated by me in session. Thus, we don't know to what extent they capture the fantasy world of the patient or the analyst – or of both. Thus, a focus on psychoanalysis as dialogue should not blur that it is *the analysand* who requests alternative perspectives on himself that he cannot perceive. After all, Thomas did not seek analysis to learn about *my* internal world. We are thus uncertain to what extent a clinician's metaphor illuminates – or dims – insight into the patient's internal world.

This validity problem is, however, not restricted to metaphors. As soon as we apply a hermeneutic perspective to another human being's experience, we are fettered by this problem: to what extent is our understanding governed by our personal world of ideas – and to what extent does it say something that is meaningful to the patient? This challenge applies when we interpret an analysand's dreams, slips, questions, comments, non-verbal signals, and so on. Yet the analyst's metaphors are special in two senses:

1 They express a psychological assumption in the form of an imagery. Instead of using the snail metaphor, I could have told Thomas: "You long for intimacy with your lover, but as soon as it happens, you distance yourself from her". It is difficult to claim that my snail metaphor has a greater heuristic value than such a conventional interpretation. Rather, its potential value lies in enabling Thomas to "play" with it and to do so more easily than if I had voiced the traditional interpretation. This was substantiated by his comment about the "funny thing about snails", namely the contrast between their hard shell and their soft entrails – followed by our play about his feeling disgusting like a slimy snail and my feeling disgusted by it or him.

   This sequence shows that the metaphor remained not as a performance piece of mine but as a means of probing deeper into Thomas's deep-seated problems with intimate relationships. In other words, a metaphor is no panacea to fixing the patient. But if it has been presented and then becomes broadened and deepens our understanding of his struggles, then it can be a fine toy to play with together. Such play is, needless to say, more difficult to establish with patients who are hard to reach. On the other hand, it is precisely when I work with such patients that metaphors tend to come up – and may evolve into valuable "toys".

2 If the validity of an analyst's metaphor is not evident, a sensible approach is to take it to the next step and elaborate an interpretation, which can be tested in the analyst-patient interaction. We can describe this in Peirce's philosophical terms (Kloesel & Houser, 1998; Misak, 2018; J. Muller & Brent, 2000; Rennie, 2012). A metaphor is a kind of inductive statement about inner reality. Its form is skewed, displaced, and indirect. The patient and I must then rely on abductions and deductions to establish to what extent it is credible and useful and if we wish to further refine it or discard it.

A penultimate point: metaphors in psychoanalysis are not specific in their linguistic structure. They are like any other metaphor or visual image: they yield new perspectives that can be more vivid, playful, and conducive to further elaboration. Their specificity rather lies in the circumstances that engender them. They arise from a combination of the analyst's wish to convey a tentative understanding of the patient's predicament, his or her inability or hesitation to transmit it through more conventional interpretations, and his access to a creative act that leads up to the metaphor. This emotional charge differentiates the clinical metaphor from many others used in everyday life. We must also recall that clinical metaphors are not a new "trick" to capture the Unconscious. As Ogden (1997) suggests, they are part of Bion's grand concept of *reverie*. I guess every analyst now and then comes up with metaphors in words or images. The difference between us perhaps lies in the extent to which we have them and convey them to the patient.

The analyst's metaphors and the Infantile

The final point reverts to my question if metaphors suggested by the analyst relate to the search for traces of the Infantile in the patient. My affirmative response needs some qualifications. It is not only the patient's Infantile that gives rise to the metaphor in the analyst. Importantly, *the analyst's* Infantile is also taking part. Had I never experienced feeling snubbed, hungry, and misunderstood, I could not have used Bess's rage with her partner as an inspirational source for the imagery of the fretting baby. Had I never desired someone yet feeling that I hit upon a hard shell, and had I then not blamed myself that I was the reason for being rejected, I could not have come up with the snail metaphor with Thomas. Thus, though the analyst comes up with the metaphor, two Infantiles join in creating it: the analysand's and the analyst's. True, we are looking for the analysand's Infantile, but the outcome depends on whether I am prepared to allow *my* Infantile to help him with the quest.

The metaphors in this chapter are unsophisticated, simple, and retrieved from everyday life. A slimy snail – what could be more mundane? If I had suggested to Thomas, as sketched earlier, "you long for intimacy with your lover" and so on, I would have expressed myself more precisely. But as an imagery, it would be far less evocative. Would it lead him to a kind of thinking that was creative and emotionally anchored? I doubt it. In contrast, the snail's slime versus its shell and its motions outwards and inwards all mirror a child's world of imagination. Thomas at first refuses such "primitive comparisons" and snaps ironically with another metaphor: he will give me a piece of "psychoanalytic candy". This imagery is as childish, concrete, and emotional as the snail, but it reveals a painful memory: according to the family myth, he was born with teeth. Now we have touched a trace of his Infantile. Maybe he was born that way, maybe not. Maybe his mother expressed her ambivalence about him through this saga, maybe not. What is not "maybe", however, is that Thomas has great difficulties in coming close to someone he desires. He fears being rejected, and to prevent it from happening, he snubs the one he desires.

This leads me to repeat that experiences with PIP can help us conceive of what goes on in sessions, also with adult patients, in simple, figurative, and embodied terms. Mothers and babies tend to enact, in a most evocative and graphic way, what they are feeling at the moment. Of course, mothers speak about their anguish, but their language is at times unclear and contradictory. Their faces – in particular, the eyes – say all the more. And babies are all nonverbal but bodily very expressive when they smile, fret, avoid mothers' eyes, or are just happy.

True, this scenic quality exists in any psychotherapy setting. Let us, however, recall the powerful embodied trilogues in PIP. They make PIP sessions "superscenic" in ways that Bernard Golse (2006) has compared to an opera. Think of Verdi's *Rigoletto* when the crippled father discovers that his daughter has been abducted. He could have articulated his humiliation and rage in a merely verbal cue. But his broken-hearted, pulsating, and stormy aria, "*Cortigiani vil razza dannata*" (Courtiers, vile cursed race, for what price did you sell my beloved?), makes our empathy with him all the deeper. Similarly, I think such an influx of impressions in their various modalities explains why PIP, especially, induces in the analyst a propensity to use metaphors such as the ones described here. This "opera" brings us nearer to the world of emotions.

Source

This chapter is a reworked version of a published paper (Salomonsson, 2022). I thank the publisher for giving permission to quote it in the book.

Chapter 12

What is the Infantile

And what is it not?

This book has dealt with the concept "the Infantile". Chapter 1 started by applying it to two clinical cases: one bygone and one present. In Chapter 2, I went on to define it and to suggest it as a useful concept in psychotherapies with adults. I hope the ensuing chapters added theoretical and clinical substance. The present chapter summarises how I regard the position of the Infantile in psychoanalytic metapsychology. For anyone who is unfamiliar with texts on such subjects, this chapter may seem abstruse and hard to digest. My argument is that if I investigate a clinical phenomenon emerging in a certain treatment method – and in this book it is psychoanalysis – I am obliged to find out if it aligns with the theories of that practice. Therefore, we will now focus on psychoanalytic metapsychology. But please stay on board since, to make the discussion accessible, I will illustrate it with the book's cases and an example from the world of opera. This will be a long discourse since both phenomena and concepts are hard to grasp and define in words. Now, is the Infantile…

- a new or even novel concept?
- a synonym for infantile trauma?
- an adjective or a noun?
- a psychological structure, a developmental period, a cluster of experiences, or what?
- anchored in psychoanalytic clinical theory and metapsychology?
- relevant to psychoanalytic therapies with adults as well as with parents and infants?

A new concept?

The word "infantile" is of course not new in psychoanalysis. But an essential question is whether my way of applying it as a *concept, the Infantile*, is new. We know it is an elaboration of Guignard's (2021, 2022) concept. But is

DOI: 10.4324/9781003640363-12

that usage novel or "old wine in new bottles", an iteration of established psychoanalytic theory? In their review of analytic metapsychology, Laplanche and Pontalis (1973) caution

> The function of specific concepts or groups of concepts [tend to] re-emerge at a later stage, transferred on to other components of the system. Only by offering an interpretation can we hope to trace certain constant structures of psycho-analytical thought and experience as they pass through transformations of this kind.
>
> (xii)

I heed this warning and will suggest my answer presently. Here, I only repeat that when we explore the infant's mind, we are treading on familiar psychoanalytic ground. Freud made many conjectures about little babies' experiences when he built metapsychological theories and interpreted clinical passages. For example, in his dream theory, he imagined that a hungry baby hallucinates the satisfying breast. This mental creation is a precursor of what later emerges as the dream work, which creates "a substitute for an infantile scene modified by being transferred on to a recent experience" (S. Freud, 1900, 546). He uses the word "infantile" hundreds of times as a descriptor like infantile sexuality and infantile neurosis. He certainly believed that infantile experiences could promote pathology later in life, as in the cases of Wolfman (S. Freud, 1918) and Little Hans (S. Freud, 1909). Is our "Infantile" concept in the book but an effort to elevate into an abstract noun what he had already used as a prefix? In the Little Hans case, he said the boy's anxiety was

> like every infantile anxiety, without an object to begin with: it was still anxiety and not yet fear. The child cannot tell [at first] what he is afraid of... simply because he himself did not yet know... in the street he missed his mother, whom he could coax with, and that he did not want to be away from her.
>
> (S. Freud, 1909, 25)

This depicts vividly the boy's separation anxiety linked with his infantile sexuality. As Freud suggested in the Wolfman's case, disturbances in these domains during early childhood can have severe consequences later in life. After him, other analysts continued writing about how early development links with psychopathology in older children and adults. I will focus on Melanie Klein, Wilfred Bion, and D.W. Winnicott.

Klein (1935, 1940) expanded Freud's (1917) theory of depression by clarifying how an infant may suffer from a sense of guilt due to aggressive impulses towards the loved object. Later in life, this unsolved conflict may lead to clinical depression. In Chapter 7, Laura exemplified this development of a girl ridden by ambivalence towards her mother, who seemed poorly equipped to respond adequately and with empathy to her emotional needs. Yet, though Klein often spoke of the links between infant mental life and adult psychological disorders, she based her conclusions on analyses with *verbal* children and only rarely on observations, let alone treatments, of real *babies*.

As for Winnicott, he always emphasised the links between infantile experiences and adult disorders. To exemplify, a False Self (1960) can emerge when a baby adapts to an unresponsive or intrusive parent through "compliance" (145). Later in life, this can lead to the adult's sense of leading a quasi-life and feeling disconnected from one's True self. As for his concept "fear of breakdown" (1974), he argues that psychotic illness is "a defence organization relative to a primitive agony" (104), a state that he joins with a baby's horrendous experiences. An adult may thus fear "a breakdown that has already been experienced [in infancy]" (104). Laura's adult life has been a consistent but vain flight from such infantile agony. She has sought to ward off experiences of being an after-thought daughter of a depressed, ambivalent, and non-responsive mother. Winnicott was asking himself which perspective is the richest informant on infant experience: analysis of psychotic adults or observations of infants. I shall presently return to this topic and his position.

Bion (1962) devised the theory of containment relying on work with psychotic adults. It is deeply anchored in his notions of – but not his systematic observations of – the mother-infant interaction. When he assumes that the alpha-function "makes available to the infant what would otherwise remain unavailable for any purpose other than evacuation as beta-elements" (36), I would illustrate with Bianca in Chapter 4. There was a fine line between her receiving my address as emanating from my alpha-function and intending to help her – or as a gunfire of my beta-elements from a defective contact-barrier, where the unconscious design was to rid myself of grave displeasure.

Had the referred authors read this book, I guess they might agree: "Your clinical examples coincide with our notions of the infancy-adulthood link. If you want to subsume them under 'the Infantile', OK, but is that concept really novel?" We are back to Laplanche's and Pontalis' warning above. An alternative candidate from established analytic theory could be *the Id*, one of the structures that Freud introduced in 1923. According to his definition, in this part of the mind "we are lived by unknown and uncontrollable forces" (23). In his figure below, the Id has a larger territory than the Ego and consists of repressed content plus something else not clearly stated Figure 12.1.

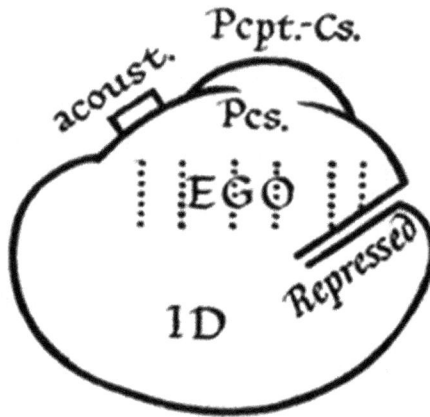

Figure 12.1 From *The Ego and the Id* (S. Freud, 1923).

The major part of the Id consists of something else than repressed material. It has an unruly and ungovernable character, for which Freud (1933) once again used a metaphorical image:

> We call [the Id] a chaos, a cauldron full of seething excitations. We picture it as being open at its end to somatic influences, and as there taking up into itself instinctual needs which find their psychical expression in it... It is filled with energy reaching it from the instincts, but it has no organization, produces no collective will, but only a striving to bring about the satisfaction of the instinctual needs subject to the observance of the pleasure principle.
>
> (73)

Freud defined the Ego more clearly than the Id. As seen in the picture above, it lies above the Id, "as the germinal disc rests upon the ovum" (1923, 24). It develops from the system Pcpt (Perception, sometimes Consciousness is added), from what the child perceives in the external and the internal worlds.

> Internal perceptions yield sensations of processes arising in the most diverse and certainly also in the deepest strata of the mental apparatus. Very little is known about these sensations and feelings; those belonging to the pleasure-unpleasure series may still be regarded as the best examples of them. They are more primordial, more elementary, than perceptions arising externally and they can come about even when consciousness is clouded.
>
> (Freud, 1923, 21–22)

Freud speaks of sensations, feelings, primordial, and elementary when describing the Id. Though the word "infantile" is absent, we are clearly into primeval times. Returning to the Id in *New Introductory Lectures* (1933), he mentions somatic influences, no organisation, no collective will, only a striving for satisfaction. But here, too, the word infantile is absent.

To sum up, Freud describes the Id as full of infantile urges but does not mention that this would link it to babies' ordinary or traumatic experiences. It is unclear why, because in other works, he provided many models of infants' experiences. Perhaps the figure above can give a cue. There is a big blank area in the Id and between it and the Ego. Is it really empty, or is it trafficked by some other psychic process? We will soon return to this question when we study primal repressions.

I am bringing out real babies to show why I disagree that "the Infantile" is a mere *façon de parler* or synonymous to the Id. My use of the term relies on experiences of parent-infant psychotherapy (PIP), infant observation, as well as adult psychotherapy. One way of meeting claims that the Infantile is identical to the Id is to say that Freud would certainly have agreed that the Id has many infantile characteristics, but as I apply the Infantile, it is more firmly rooted in our life history. Guignard calls it (2022, 5) "a historical/ahistorical conglomerate" (2022, 5). In my usage, *the historical aspect gets more emphasis than the ahistorical.*

The reason that neither Freud, Klein, Winnicott nor Bion mentioned PIP is, of course, that it did not exist at the time. Bion did not work clinically with infants. Winnicott did it extensively, and his writings show a profound understanding of infants interacting with their mothers. However, he did not involve himself in the painstaking relationships that emerge once we take on board mother and baby in PIP. In the spatula game, (1941) he observed babies – but he did not engage in therapeutic relationships with them. When striving to conceive of infant life, he relied more on psychotic patients. "Dependent or deeply regressed patients can teach the analyst more about early infancy than can be learned from direct observation of infants, and more than can be learned from contact with mothers who are involved with infants" (1960, 141).

I disagree with Winnicott's surprising conclusion that deeply distressed adults can teach us more about infancy than infants themselves. I have shown that direct contacts with babies and mothers in agonizing PIP interactions add substance and concretion to our conjectures about the infant's emotional life. I have then drawn lines to psychotherapies with adults to add further support to my conjectures about their emotional lives. When these patients become overwhelmed by past and present experiences, and I experience certain countertransference phenomena, I may ask myself, "Maybe I could interpret this from the perspective of the patient's and/or my Infantile". To resolve this section's caption, using the word "infantile" in psychoanalysis is, as said, not new. But a more important question remains: is the concept of *"the Infantile" novel in that it would help us comprehend better clinical situations in adults, like distress, depression, somatic symptoms, and negative therapeutic reactions – and perhaps their anchorage in the patients' prehistories?* We will approach this question in the next section.

The Infantile: structure, developmental period, cluster of experiences, or what?

On which metapsychological level should we place the Infantile? Now that we know that we cannot put it on the same level as the Id, could we subsume it under Freud's topographical model and say it is identical to the Unconscious? But like the Id, the Ucs. is a broader concept than the Infantile. Freud repeats (1900, 1915b, 1923, and the figure above) that the Ucs. consists of much more than repressed psychic material. When Guignard (2022) says the Infantile is a "basic structure" (5), she refers neither to the Ucs. nor to the Id in Freud's topographical and structural models. She rather includes it among "*'concepts of the third type'*, which aim at describing 'the-links-between-the-links'; they are fit to deal with dynamic situations that develop in various and often recurrent time-and-space [clinical circumstances]. They are altogether complex and mouldable concepts" (1). Guignard places the Infantile on par with, for example, Winnicott's False Self (1960) and transitional object (1953), Kohut's Self (1971) and the French term *le sujet*. Several such concepts exist in psychoanalytic clinical theory, such as the claustrum (Meltzer, 1992), character armour (Reich, 1933), the analytic third (Ogden, 1994), and the dead mother configuration (Green, 1986).

Every one of the referred concepts was invented by an analyst who perceived a clinical phenomenon that other colleagues perhaps had intuited as well. But they had not paid enough attention, or lacked interest or creative courage, to focus on them and devise fitting analytic concepts. In contrast, when Winnicott, Meltzer, Ogden, Guignard and others met with a phenomenon in session, they coined a concept to cover it and investigated it in their practice and writings. Other analysts found it valuable and emblematic of their clinical experiences, and thus it gradually became part of the analytic canon.

Inspired by Guignard, I have used the Infantile concept for phenomena and events in the reports of the book's patients. Working with them, I began conceiving their enactments and experiences of pain, shame, anxiety, and despair as manifestations of the Infantile. This was because their symptoms, behaviours, and values had some baby-like qualities, or they spoke of factual infancy traumas, and I noted countertransference experiences that pointed to my identifications with an imaginary baby. Here, we find another reason why the Infantile and the Id are not identical concepts: Guignard emphasises that we discern the Infantile through our interactions with the patient (2022, 4). In contrast, when Freud explored concepts like the Id or the Unconscious, he did not mention countertransference. His writing was more that of an objective researcher and theoretician than of a human subject involved or entangled in an intersubjective traffic with his patients.

Could we anchor the Infantile in psychoanalytic metapsychology beyond saying it is a "third-type" or "mouldable concept"? I think so, and I start by quoting Guignard again: The Infantile is the "locus of primary fantasies and *mnesic traces* of our *first* sensorial and motor experiences. It is also the most acute point of the *non-verbal* emotions and feelings" (2021, 1, italics added). The italicised words underscore her references to infancy: the *first* period of life when we communicate in a *nonverbal* mode and later have only *mnesic traces* of it. To some extent, her Infantile thus relates to infants' experiences. This book makes such connections even more clearly. However, though we add that this "third-type" concept is firmly anchored to the baby's experiences, we still don't know which of this caption's alternatives is most apt: is the Infantile a structure, period, cluster, or "what"? Clearly, we need to understand better how the infant handles its first memories and feeling traces.

How do we handle our "mnesic traces"?

When Guignard mentions mnesic (memory) traces in connection with the Infantile, she brings us to another question. What happens to these traces later in life? And, whether they overwhelmed us or not, they needed to be handled by being stowed away, transformed, or maybe deleted altogether. Freud mentioned a few mechanisms, and I will focus on *repression proper* and *primal repression*. I will illustrate the first term with Bess and her partner Fred in Chapter 2. Let us imagine that when he suggested the outing, she replied, "John, what a lovely idea!" If she then noticed that she was replacing Fred's name with that of her ex-boyfriend, she might realise this was because she was angry at Fred. Her unconscious ire worried her and was kept in check by "repression proper". As a result, she made a slip of the tongue.

But in reality, Bess got mad at Fred because she lost control over their dinner plans. When I spoke of the whining baby, she mentioned events that had been resting in her Preconscious: facts about a premature birth and separation from mother. Her face softened, her eyes became moist, her voice broke, and she spoke of her experiences of – yes, of what? I would say her reactions to my baby imagery had two sources: one factual and one emotional. One was her explicit recall and address of the parents' accounts of her delivery. The other was her emotional reactions to her knowledge that she was born prematurely into an immigrant family, separated from Mum, and had food problems and now she was enraged by Fred's "change of plans" or – as it emerged – his spontaneous and tempting idea.

Where had these emotions been hiding all these years? What emerged was *not* that certain events in Bess's life, hitherto subjected to repression proper, now got de-repressed and "popped up". The pristine experiences had been kept at bay by another function: primal repression. In this conception, we are focusing on what occurred then inside little Bess, and how she was affected by the parents' worries about her. This makes it hard to differentiate what went on inside mother and baby, respectively. Mother could handle her distress through repression proper, but this mechanism was not at hand for baby Bess, and we will soon learn why. What remained for her was to develop a crust, a living fossil, a primal repression. It had been dormant until she felt deceived by Fred, heard my baby imagery, and captured a trace of her Infantile: a set of emotionally charged experiences rooted very early in her life. These emotions were now seeping through the crust.

The previous caption asked about the theoretical status of the Infantile. Is it a structure, developmental period, cluster of experiences, or "what"? The time has come to clarify this "what". I suggest *the Infantile corresponds to those parts of the Unconscious that have been primally repressed.* I will presently clarify the latter term, but for now I use it to refer to those unconscious representations that are the furthest from, and least accessible to, the Conscious. They are opaque and obscure and demand a psychoanalytic clinical method to become discernible. As the analyst's own Infantile is stirred up, he may intuit that he is close to a primally repressed object in the patient. He may feel uncomfortable, anxious, excited, or elated. There may emerge an idea, hunch, dream, or a metaphor, which he uses to grasp the patient's Infantile. This occurs in an emotional link with the patient. The analyst places himself as a containing mother who discerns her baby's agony and strives to communicate with him. This follows Bion's model of the container – contained relation. At fortunate moments, the patient's and the analyst's Infantile go together to reach a deeper understanding of the patient, as when Bess and I grasped her aversion to the good things that Fred offered her.

Primal repression: Tristan as model

The Infantile covers how we *may have felt* in our earliest days – but we must clarify that we neither remember these events explicitly nor can ascertain that they were ever registered at all. This is also supported by neuroscientific findings of infant memory functioning (Josselyn & Frankland, 2012; Li, Callaghan, & Richardson, 2014; Madsen & Kim, 2016). The protracted postnatal development of brain regions, especially the hippocampus, prevent babies from forming stable memories. Since the metapsychology of primal repressions is so convoluted, we are easily tempted to leave it aside and settle for neurodevelopmental explanations instead. Yet they merely emphasise that we cannot *explicitly* recall events in our infancy. Then what about *implicit* and *procedural* memories? Neonates quickly learn to adapt and develop their reflexes, and they will forever recall a myriad of other aptitudes. But are these capacities relevant to a discussion of primal repression? As we will see, I do not think so.

The question takes us to an epistemological divide, also broached in the preface. The way we gain knowledge differs between the natural and the human sciences. The concept of primal repression belongs to the latter, where an analyst seeks to understand (*verstehen*) the patient's experiential world. The concept was thus devised from clinical encounters with patients and analysts, not from observational lab research. Further, it deals not with common skills like walking or talking but with idiosyncratic and highly subjective experiences, which are also influenced by what parents and others told us over the years – as we know from Bess's case. Finally, they cannot be "discovered" by the analyst but *intuited* and *interpreted* in dialogue with the patient.

One of the first characters to ignite my interest in primal repression was Tristan in Richard Wagner's opera *Tristan und Isolde* (Salomonsson, 2014a), a man who lost his parents in infancy and was weighed down by a love story ending with suicide. (For intriguing links between the opera and Wagner's personal early trauma, I refer to Oberhoff (2016)). Tristan was sent by King Marke, his nephew and foster father, to escort Isolde to Cornwall to become Marke's queen. Tristan and Isolde had a bitter prehistory together, but when they drank a magic potion, they fell heedlessly in love. Isolde married Marke but one night, she and Tristan fathomed and expressed the depth of their love. They were disclosed, a fight ensued, and the wounded Tristan was brought to his birthplace.

Waiting for Isolde, Tristan embarks on an exasperated self-analysis. He realises that his yearning for her is a sequel of an infantile trauma: he lost his father before birth and his mother immediately thereafter. His childless uncle Marke raised him as his son. Tristan sings of the losses that made him depressed and yearning for salvation, which he concludes is possible only by dying with Isolde. This also means reuniting with his dead mother, as when he asks Isolde to follow him to "the dark land of Night, out of which my mother sent me."

Some passages in Tristan's soliloquy point to his intuitions about phenomena that we will subsume under the concept of primal repression (*Urverdrängung*). He sings:

I was where I had been before I was,
and where I am destined to go:
in the wide realm of the Night of the world.
But one certain knowledge is ours there:
divine, eternal, utter oblivion (Urvergessen).

Tristan addresses his *sehnsüchtige Mahnung*, yearning exhortation, that Isolde will soon return. Where is that place where he once was and is destined to go? The word *Urvergessen* suggests it as a metaphor of a primordial and now forgotten state of mind. He yearns for it but can only dimly recognise it. When hearing a shepherd's mournful tune, he comes to think of the death of his parents. He now links his present longing for Isolde with the early losses of his parents. When she finally returns to him, their love could have been consummated. But his yearning for Isolde to bring him peace of mind actually means death. When the two reunite, he cries that he will now pursue her as he once pursued her former betrothed. He sees her approaching and in an ecstasy of redemption, rage, infatuation and despair, he collapses in what I conceive of as a suicidal act.

Tristan illustrates how primal repression works and what its consequences may be. His acts are incomprehensible to him and coupled with immense emotions. When he and Isolde drink the potion, her previous rage at Tristan and his guilt towards her are "fully cleansed". They fall in love helplessly, but Tristan turns into depressive brooding. Our understanding of his anguish increases as we learn about the losses in infancy. But for Tristan, only to touch on what he learnt about these events is insufferable. He is in the throes of primal repressions and becomes overwhelmed by their emotions of agitation, infatuation, fury, guilt, yearning, and helplessness.

These tempestuous emotions can indeed be called the traces of Tristan's Infantile. But is his *Ur-trauma*, as he claims, really the loss of his parents? After all, he can recall neither his father's death before he was born nor the loss of his mother. Then why does he sing that he prepared the potion "from my father's distress and mother's anguish"? Why these projective identifications onto parents he never knew? He highlights memory traces that contributed to his misery, but they cannot pertain to the factual loss of his parents because such traces do not exist. Instead, they must refer to him as a child who experienced sorrow and helplessness in the faces of the people around. This family milieu might have elicited projective identifications in him, though not onto his real parents but onto the ones that he imagined.

Tristan illustrates central components of primal repressions. They concern events or affects that are profoundly unconscious and impossible to explicitly recall. When a stressful situation occurs, affects that have been dormant for decades may emerge. His despair illustrates such a resurgence. Overwhelmed by affects, he does not answer the King's question why he wounded him: "O King, I cannot tell you that; what you ask you can never know". In fact, Tristan does not know the answer himself.

Nonetheless, the *beginning* of such understanding appears in the last act's "self-analysis". That moment corresponds to what may emerge in psychoanalysis when a patient begins to have hunches or *Ahnungen* about the deeper roots of her incomprehensible behaviour or feeling state. Think of Bess's *Ahnung* of what lay beneath her violent reaction to Fred's proposal. Yet there is an important difference between her and Tristan: she has an analyst who helps her connect events of then and now. Tristan was surrounded by kindhearted people, but they did not grasp how his infatuation and history were linked. His silence and restraint also contributed to the catastrophe.

Metapsychology of primal repressions

The section on Tristan illustrated his struggle to understand his disaster and his inability to avert it. I mentioned the concept of primal repression, and now we need to expound on it theoretically. Freud introduced primal repression or *die Urverdrängung* in 1915b:

> There is a first phase of repression, which consists in the psychical (ideational) representative of the instinct being denied entrance into the conscious. With this a fixation is established; the representative in question persists unaltered from then onwards and the instinct remains attached to it.
>
> (1915a, 148)

Freud states that mental content can be buried so deeply and irretrievably that one can neither recall, comprehend, nor formulate it in words. Already in *The Interpretation of Dreams* (1900), he had suggested that "the core of our being, consisting of unconscious wishful impulses, remains inaccessible to the understanding and inhibition of the preconscious" (603). Later, Freud (1911) made a threefold division of the repression process, where the first phase of fixation is "the precursor and necessary condition of every repression". One instinct or instinctual component "is left behind at a more infantile stage... fixation appears in fact to be a passive lagging behind" (67). Whereas the 1915 quote above describes primal repression as an *active* process ("being denied entrance"), those of 1900 and 1911 depict it more as *passive*.

The question of viewing primal repression as a *passive* or *active* process is important (Akhtar, 2020; Beratis, 2020; Frank & Muslin, 1967). In the *passive* sense, it might be taken to support that everything that we cannot recall has in fact been repressed. But let's say we don't remember the colour of our baby clothes. Now, is that due to repression? Or did we simply forget it? Or did we even register it? Impossible to state, but if we apply passive primal repression to such phenomena, we'd lift the concept out of the domain where it belongs: to the Unconscious in the psychoanalytic sense and to experiences with an emotional charge. In contrast, the term *active* primal repression is apt in connection with my patients' distress in the sense of a response to trauma. For example, Bess's rage against Fred expresses such an active primal repression. Freud's vision of the active process is expressed in his later writings:

> It is highly probable that the immediate precipitating causes of primal repressions are quantitative factors such as an excessive degree of excitation and the breaking through of the protective shield against stimuli.
>
> (Freud, 1925–1926, 94)

Too much excitation, or "a situation analogous to the trauma of birth" (Freud, 1925–1926, 140), will yield a primal repression. Bess's trauma was indeed the separation from her mother after birth but also how the family came to handle it. Tristan's trauma was the loss of his parents – but only if we include the effects on his family environment. Frank and Muslin (1967) ask if Freud, when using the concept in the active meaning implies, was actually discarding the passive variant. They answer in the negative:

> At first glance it would seem that Freud has discarded his earlier theory of the primally repressed as occurring passively. Only a close examination of his later writings demonstrates that he now presupposes the existence of this phenomenon and that the newer theory represents an addition.
>
> (Frank & Muslin, 1967, 73)

If we were to ask if active or passive primal repressions are *clinically* the most relevant, I would vote for the active form. I will soon return to this position, but first we need to approach another problem with primal repression. Freud's 1915b formulation, that an instinct is denied entrance into the Conscious, seems to implicate that the subject never knew anything about it. But how can one recall and process something that one never registered? Maze and Henry (1996) criticise the "logical impossibility" (1087) of the clause that "the repressed must be known in order to remain unknown". Yet in my view, they build an argument on a logic that applies only to verbal representations. They do provide a counterargument: maybe a beginning of an impulse was allowed to enter consciousness, which then enabled it to become primally repressed? But no, they argue that this does not work because "although the infant had imagined a situation that would gratify some specific instinctual impulse, it had never *admitted to itself* that it had had such an image" (1092, italics added). But using the verb "to admit" in connection with a baby is, in my view, adultomorphic and misplaced. It pre-supposes a verbal and intellectual capacity way beyond that of an infant.

Since primal repressions fundamentally emerge in infancy, namely within the preverbal sphere, we must apply another logic to understand their workings. To exemplify, baby Bess's separation from mother and then returning to a more distressed version of her were probably traumatic. It had long since been subjected to active primal repression. Comparing Bess and Tristan, we could say that prior to her therapy session, she was lagging behind him in understanding her distress. She did not connect her irritation at Fred with her infancy, while Tristan began connecting, namely in the opera's final act, his hunger for Isolde with the loss of his parents. But when I suggested to Bess the imagery of the whining baby, she started catching up with Tristan by telling me about traumatic events in infancy. She also intuited that they had perturbed her mother and their relationship. Finally, she expressed a hunch or an *Ahnung* that all this was linked with her recent squabble with Fred.

Bess also came to understand that the trauma continued beyond the separation from her mother as it affected her childhood milieu: her food issues, mother's overly concern, and Bess's gaze avoidance. We can say that primal repressions were co-constructed (Beebe & Lachmann, 2002) by mother and baby. Thanks to our clinical dialogue, we could now de-construct them – in the sense not of her recalling the original events but of grasping how they sneaked into her squabble with Fred and other men.

We now return to what goes on in the baby's mind when it establishes primal repressions. My enquiry has many inspirational sources. First, there is Freud's struggle with the concept. Second, findings from PIP did not exist in his time, and they can now help us in understanding primal repressions better. Third, I have argued that we need a theory of signs to account for the "primal representations" (Salomonsson, 2014a, 32) that the infant mind produces and which are then remade into primal repressions. Here, C.S. Peirce's (Kloesel & Houser, 1992, 1998) semiotic theory has proven valuable for my understanding. Fourth, an important source is Laplanche's (2007b) theory of the traffic of enigmatic messages between mother and baby and how they may sediment into the "*inconscient enclavé*" or the enclosed Unconscious. A fifth source is Green's (1995) theory of primitive affect registrations. Finally, I also rely on authors investigating the metapsychology of primal repression (Akhtar, 2020, Beratis, 2020, Cohen & Kinston, 1986; Frank & Muslin, 1967; Kinston & Cohen, 1986; Mangini & Graham, 2010).

The concept of primal repression is difficult to comprehend because the phenomena it covers are opaque and abstruse. Another challenge is how to put words to phenomena that are distinctly nonverbal. My first take on this task was to turn to semiotic theory (Salomonsson, 2007a, 2007b, 2014a) since I felt that discussions of primal repressions leaned too heavily on a logic that pertained to the verbal experiential domain. It was a bit like trying to explain why music affects us to someone who "hath no music in himself, nor is not moved with concord of sweet sounds" (Shakespeare, *The Merchant of Venice*, V:1).

The association to music also indicates that our mind toils with many more forms of signification than words. For example, music is just one of many *sign systems*. When using the term "sign", I refer to Peirce's point of departure that signs are obligatory for the mind to function. A stimulus may reach the infant but not until his or her mind has created an internal sign can it work with the perception (Kloesel & Houser, 1998, 10) or, in Mandler's (2004) words, perform a perceptual meaning analysis (see Chapter 11 here). This work is accompanied by experiences that Peirce sorts in three universal categories: Firstness, Secondness, and Thirdness. Firstness is an immediate experience unrelated to other experiences. "Assert it and it has already lost its characteristic innocence" (Kloesel & Houser, 1992, 248). Secondness is related or juxtaposed to other experiences. Thirdness applies to laws, conventions, and regularities.

Peirce's theory, which was also discussed in Chapter 8, comprises how all human experiencing is signified. Since we are focusing on the infant mind, we will stay with Firstness and Secondness and the two sign forms that infants work with: icon and index. Firstness refers to the potential or the raw "suchness" of things before they are actualised or connected to other entities. A clinical example is Laura's mother's "dead eyes" in Chapter 7 as they evoke her nameless horror. In terms of signs, they are icons that "convey ideas of the things they represent simply by imitating them" (Kloesel & Houser, 1992, 1998). Secondness experiences are juxtaposed to other experiences. The type of sign that most often conveys them – the index – urges us to act, oppose, react, and compare. Laura struggles with this aspect when she needs a phone and sees mine. At first, my eyes are a scary Icon of Scare to her, and she cannot ask me to borrow it. Then, she can change into viewing them as a friendly index of "Yes, you may use it". One sign, here my eyes, can thus be interpreted in both its iconical and indexical aspects and evoke varying and clashing interpretants.

Applying a semiotic perspective on primal repressions helps us abandon Freud's quantitative ("excessive degree of excitation") and concrete ("denied entrance into the conscious" and "breaking through of the protective shield") conceptions. Instead, I suggest that such repressions inscribe original sense perceptions as mental signs of an icon kind and entail more of a Firstness experience. They thus *do not delete the initial perceptions but transform how they are signified*. Our earliest perceptions and experiences may have been perceived and registered and then been transcribed into other significatory forms. The fact that the original will never reappear does not invalidate the claim that there was once a terrifying first registration which, to illustrate with Laura, could be written as "black eyes, sinister look, tummy ache", words that, of course, should be read as my imaginations.

Can primal repressions lead to creativity and joy?

I have spoken of primal repression as a mechanism that re-signifies negative experiences. But can it also promote the individual's development? Here is a response:

> Free excitation can also be directed and transformed in a representative sense precisely by the action of primal repression following on from inevitable [but] not catastrophic traumatic stimuli.
>
> (Mangini & Graham, 2010, 54)

This would correspond to Freud's first view of primal repression: an instinctual component has remained passively at a more infantile stage. Such fixations can exist "in a state different from that in the other regions of the mind, far more mobile and capable of discharge" (S. Freud, 1933, 74). As primal repression starts working on them, they are subjected to what Winnicott (1988, 19) calls "imaginative elaboration". Mangini and Graham (2010, 57) suggests that primal repression "determines the birth and development of the symbolizing process in every phase or moment of psychic life". This would answer our question: yes, *primal repressions also help establish healthy and creative psychic functioning*. But note the words "not catastrophic traumatic stimuli" above. If that condition is unfulfilled, the psychic apparatus cannot avail primal repression, it becomes "anchored to the somatic, cluttered with repetitive, operative, oversaturated and immobile sensations and thoughts" (57). The individual cannot face up to desires as they emerge. Conversely, in "not catastrophic" situations, primal repression can deal with them harmoniously. There develops a "good gymnasium for thought, and primal repression [has functioned as] the architect of the Unconscious" (57).

We will soon get to the object's role in assisting the person to create primal repressions. First, we need to return to the term *fixation*. As said, Freud (1911, 67) suggested that the first phase of repression "consists in fixation, which is the precursor and necessary condition of every 'repression'". This "lagging behind" should not be read as a mere negative process. To exemplify, Freud (1905b) speaks of kissing as moulded on our experiences of sucking at mother's breasts (181). The pleasure is then transferred to another body part or to an external object like a pacifier. Later, we seek "the corresponding part – the lips – of another person" (182). When two adults embrace in a kiss, we can suggest that they share a play with each other's primal repressions of previous lustful interchanges with the breast. If we had offered them this interpretation on the spot, they would no doubt be unimpressed since their repressions were successful: their delight showed that they had succeeded in creating the "vital humus" (Mangini, 57) indispensable for sensual pleasure and good psychic functioning.

Fixations are thus important for interactive pleasure and for "creating the premises that lead to the formation of the representation and of thought" (Mangini, 61). In breastfeeding, there is a "link between the glance of the baby and that of its mother". This yields a somatic, sensorial, and sexual base "along which the excitement is magnetized". The outcome can go two ways. If "the experience of contact with the object is not too intrusive and does not occupy all the psychic space of thought" (62), a wholesome primal repression is working. In the future, the adult will recall not the breastfeeding per se but sharing emotional contact and understanding with someone else. To this is added all the playful and sensuous ways that we enjoy and develop with the one we love.

In other situations, the mother or other caretakers cannot provide adequate containment for the child. To speculate, the bereaved King Marke is such a case. Among the book's case examples we can choose Bianca's mother, described as insensitive to her children's emotional needs. This plus baby Bianca's abandonment and exposure to sweating and itching in the swaddle prevented her from developing the "humus" for passive primal repressions. As an adult, she could neither play, joke, relax, nor have sex in a tender and mutual way. In other terms, her infantile sexuality had not been transformed into primal repressions of pleasure, calm, and lust.

Bianca was often edgy and agitated, but it was different with Colin and Simone. When kissing, they were ecstatic but when it was over there was nothing more to be discovered in the lover or in themselves. The lover was like a drug they must have, now and now and now. Probably, early breaches of proximity and trust with the mother had disturbed the settling of primal repressions that could have helped them enjoy kissing, though not as love's sole pleasure. The lover's lips and smell were icons which, as long as they were worshipped, offered bliss and exemption from anxiety. As with every icon, they were static, one-dimensional, and closed to being probed in a sincere dialogue.

To re-approach and conclude our question about the status of the Infantile concept, it is not identical to the Id as a structure, to the Unconscious as a system, or to a certain developmental period. It comprises a cluster of experiences and behaviours in line with how babies encounter the world. Its metapsychological position is that of a concept of the third type (Guignard, 2022), on par with the False Self and others. As I have suggested, it comprises *the primal repressions of the Unconscious* and refers to the infant's experiences that were once signified as icons and indices. Clinically, the most important experiences are those that occurred when affects and perceptions overflowed and were signified in ways that blocked further elaboration. Thus, the book has spoken of eczema, swaddling, and a mother who is depressed, or another who is afraid of breastfeeding her toothless son; the experiences of Colin, Bianca, Laura, and Thomas impacted their budding Unconscious. They were primally repressed, could not be reached explicitly, and seized a major position in their Infantile and in their agony.

Infantile trauma

After struggling with all these complex metapsychological issues, we face one final question. Does the Infantile actually mean "infantile trauma"? After all, the book's cases might have created impressions that it simply refers to adverse events in infancy. My response is no and yes. Infantile trauma refers to events that we know, with reasonable certainty, happened in the patient's early life. Colin, young Eric, and Bianca are good examples. But in Bess's case, calling her brief neonatal care an infantile trauma would be overblown. We can answer the question in a simple and brief way: "infantile trauma" refers to extraordinary events that really happened, whereas "the Infantile" – whether it issues from trauma or not – has characteristics that *remind us* of how babies may experience the world. There is indeed a historical dimension to the Infantile, but more importantly, it describes a person's psychological functioning and emotions. To sum up, we can paraphrase a point made in Chapter 10 on infantile sexuality: infantile trauma is part of the Infantile – but *not the other way around*.

The time has come to bid farewell to the Infantile and to our astronomical metaphor. On a clear and dark autumn night in the Northern Hemisphere, we see two neighbouring constellations shimmer in the sky: Andromeda and Cassiopeia. They are named after two Greek mythological characters in a tangle of tragic family relations.[1] Cassiopeia, the "mother", is actually a handful of stars some hundred light years afar, which we perceive as one group. Andromeda, the "daughter", is a galaxy of a trillion stars, 2½ million of light years away. These celestial bodies are above us in tonight's sky – and they were also there eons ago. Everything we observe today in the sky reaches us from the past. It is the same with the Infantile, *a concept about now and then, the present and the past.*

In the centre of the Andromeda, as in many other galaxies, there is a black hole. It might be tempting to extend the metaphor and suggest that the Infantile corresponds to such a hole. This needs a clarification, however. At first, the term "black hole" is a misnomer. It is actually a celestial body packed with an enormous amount of matter. The known laws of physics break down at its core, implying that "nothing, not even light, can escape, because gravity is so strong" (Hawking, 1988, 232). In contrast, the theory of the Infantile argues that some "particles", *Ahnungen*, or traces can – and sometimes do – escape from their state of primal repression. To exemplify, Colin had just become a father but now felt and acted like the forlorn baby he had likely been decades ago. As for young Eric, the family did not grasp that his present unruly behaviour was linked with his neonatal surgery.

We could say that the Infantile consists of "psychological matter" which, however, behaves differently from matter inside a black hole. Our term comprises the primal repressions of the Unconscious. These traces of meaning, primal representations, or whichever term we apply to them can indeed be splintered and condensed similarly to matter inside a black hole. But unlike the entrapped matter inside such holes in the Universe, traces of the Infantile may sometimes break free as a shimmer of an affect, a symptom, or a sudden incomprehensible behaviour. Such phenomena cannot be observed in the way an astronomer observes his celestial objects with a telescope. But they can be inferred with the help of another tool, the psychoanalytic instrument.

At this point, we see why I have insisted on speaking of "the Infantile" rather than its equivalent, "the primal repressions of the Unconscious". True, "the Infantile" sounds more compelling and is easier to pronounce. But there is a much more significant reason for keeping it. As said above, "the Infantile" weighs the balance more in favour of the historical aspects of mental functioning. In other words, it expresses more clearly the connections between a person's present emotional state and his or her earliest experiences in life. We also realise why I have persisted in using the Infantile as a noun and not as an adjective. We can use "infantile" as an adjective when we join it with nouns like anxiety, trauma, sexuality, and period. But as a noun, "Infantile" becomes a term that helps us gather our clinical impressions and shape them into conceptions that link the patient's present and past experiences. In this way, it may inspire us to reverie, thoughts, metaphors, and so forth, which we can transform into suitable communications to the patient. I thus suggest that the Infantile concept gives meaning to certain passages in psychotherapy. I have also taken care to show that it is anchored in psychoanalytic clinical theory, metapsychology, and infant research. Of course, any new concept in a discipline may become reified, diluted, idealised, or rejected. The fate of this concept will be decided by future analysts. I hope its heuristic value and clinical usefulness will be explored by therapists who work with adults only as well as those who also work with parent-infant therapy.

Note

1 Princess Andromeda's mother, Queen Cassiopeia, boasted of being more beautiful than the sea nymphs. Poseidon's punishment for this insult was to place a terrible sea monster by the shores of the kingdom. Her spouse, King Cepheus was told that chaining their beautiful daughter Andromeda onto a rock by the sea would appease the sea god and save his kingdom. Andromeda thus had to bear the cost of her mother's vanity and her father's callousness.

Clinical epilogue

Harry, a man now in his seventies, was in a lengthy analysis with me three decades ago, long before I had seen any infants and mothers in therapy. In the analysis, we talked much about his earliest years – but not about his Infantile to the extent and depth that I have described in this book. When he recently contacted me in a severe crisis, I noted that I contained him in a different way – I got "into the crib" with him, as expressed in Chapter 4 about Bianca.

When Harry started his analysis, he was full of wrath, especially with women and society. With women, he could be verbally aggressive, sneering and disparaging. When he talked about society, his critique could be well substantiated but also full of scathing resentment. These traits had begun to scare him, and he sought analysis. The analysis focused much on the extremely infected relationship with his mother and the death of his father when he was about three years old. Harry deeply mourns that he has no explicit memories of his father, whereas the analysis was filled with accounts of his and mother's bickering and fighting. The climate between the two was alternately tempestuous and calm, friendly and hostile and, very often, on a hysterical note. The mother could be playful and charming. But she could also scream hysterically at Harry when they were fighting, "I wish I were dead. Then you can come to the cemetery and pee on my tombstone!" As a boy, Harry was sometimes rude and belligerent. Other times, he was "the little Professor", compulsively ordering the carpet fringes at home. The boy aroused great concern in his environment, and he was in a lengthy child therapy. His male therapist became an important father figure who helped Harry keep on track in life, stay in school, and earn a university degree.

Our analytic sessions could be belligerent and snappy, but he was also an interested participant with a witty sense of humour. His arrogant attacks in the transference were often followed by shame and remorse. They resembled the quarrels he used to have with his mother. On the other hand, Harry's humour explained why he had many friends who appreciated him for his frankness and acumen. When we ended the analysis, both he and I felt it had been meaningful and beneficial.

DOI: 10.4324/9781003640363-13

Thirty years later, Harry calls me because his anxiety is "over the top". He says he fears he has a neurological disease. (To uphold anonymity, I will say only that it gives minor or major handicaps, and that many patients live with it for many years.) We set up an appointment, and in the interview some days later, I strongly suspect he is right about the diagnosis. I tell him, "It is worth checking out if you're right. If you wish, I can refer you to a neurologist I trust." Harry is grateful and gets an appointment with the neurologist, while he and I set up another hour. Next session, he is enraged that I told him what I thought about his misgivings. "You could have told me in a gentler way! I'm so damned anxious, I don't know what to do." Later, he calms down, and I ask if he wants to see me again and he readily consents.

The neurologist confirms Harry's misgivings about the disease, prescribes medications, and refers him to a specialist team. Meanwhile, he decides to stop seeing me since he feels that I am "loveless" and that psychoanalysis is as well. He is grateful that I referred him to the neurologist but cannot forgive me for having confirmed his suspicions about the disease. I am surprised at his sudden decision to terminate our contact. I also feel sad and concerned since he is in a very brittle emotional situation. Also, I like working with Harry. But I realise that his feelings about a loveless analysis say something central about our collaboration, and I wonder what this "something" could be.

Harry returns after some months and says he wants to see me regularly to help him curb and understand his panic. We start a twice-weekly therapy. "I don't know if it's the disease or something psychological that is haunting me". He has lived alone for many years and manages his life pretty well, though the disease can interfere with his daily chores. He is neat, well dressed, and completely lucid. Harry has retained his usual bite, which sometimes escalates into arguments with me. Another pattern from before is when he gets stormy and dramatising. "I'm going to die any day, do something, I can't go on! People laugh in the streets, I want to scream that they're laughing while I'm dying." He feels like a wretched old-timer just about to stumble and fall at any moment. Moments of such panic and self-pity alternate with angry outbursts. "You're sitting here with your smart comments and making money out of my suffering!" As in my early work with Bianca in Chapter 4, I focus on how he switches into projective accusations of me, women, or society. I feel very sad and empathic with his vulnerable situation. Yet my comments can lead to old patterns re-emerging; he gets annoyed, claims that I misquote him, or misquotes what I've said to him. Tension rises, there follows some squabbling between us, and then the gust soon abates.

Various themes arise and disappear quickly. He can lash out that "nobody wants to see a wreck like me, nobody's calling to see me… The other day, as I had lunch with Jim, he said I looked better. But my friend Sue says I look worse". When I point out that he swings between speaking about his isolation and meeting his friends, he sees the inconsistency but mutters, "Well, that's how I am". He says every friend has left him "because I'm just talking about my disease". In fact, all his real friends are still around, and they do care for him.

One day Harry suddenly says, "I don't need our fussing, it doesn't help me, I have quarrelled all my life, with Mum, you, women, and God knows whom. You must handle me in a different way! I'm having such a panic." Without any consideration beforehand, I answer calmly and look straight into his eyes, "There, there, I know. There, there, it's hard". The words come to my mind like when a parent is comforting a crying little child. Harry looks at me in surprise, then turns silent and calm.

> This is just what I need. I need you to lull and shush me, I can't do it myself. I roam about in my flat, inventing all sorts of catastrophes in my head, and with a hell lot of anxiety. We must find this lull together!

These sequences emerge repeatedly in sessions. He starts with panic about dying and accuses me, his neighbours, and the world. We identify, more and more in a joint insight, that such interchanges are "more of the same". Instead, we need to find a common rhythm as I look at him silently or say to him, "So... so, yes... this is terrible, there, there". He calms down, looks at me, and now and then I can see a light-hearted smile on his face. He says, "They have prescribed SSRI [selective serotonin reuptake inhibitor] medications, but they don't curb my panic. This does it, the thing that we're doing right now."

One day, Harry rushes into the consulting room:

> I know what it's all about! I must learn to die as a man. I saw a TV documentary about Mohammad Ali, the boxer. Everybody hated him for his provocative behaviour. Later, he got some disease. In the film, he seemed to be a conscientious and concerned person. He explained that he always acted like a diva and a rogue to inspire ghetto guys to claim their rights and let nobody bully them. He was also very generous. I want to be like him, stop complaining about myself and prepare myself whenever death may come, and feel that I've done good things, too. I know I have, and my children and friends repeat it to me, but I can't feel it, because I'm so bloody preoccupied with myself! This is what I mean with dying as a man. I don't refer to 'dying with their boots on'. This is different! I want to think of others as well.

Some months later, Harry reports that when he wakes up at night, he is agitated and fearful of his future. But he manages to soothe himself by thinking about my "shushing words". Sometimes, while still lying in bed, he discerns puzzle pieces of a man's face, as if they were mounted on the surface of a globe with a lamp inside. He thinks these images refer to me and maybe also to a dim notion of his father.

> It's like I'm alone and panic because you disappear from me. This puzzle, maybe I'm trying to glue together shards of you to feel calmer. I've often longed to recapture at least one memory of my father when I was little, but I doubt it'll ever happen. This globe man helps me to fall asleep again.

I will end this brief epilogue with a point on therapeutic technique. When I report about my "there, there" to Harry, I do not refer to it as a standard therapeutic feat. Of course, an analyst needs to represent reality and formulate concise and comprehensible interpretations. "There, there" emerged on the spot, as I sensed his panic and helplessness and got in contact with similar feelings of my own. This inspired my "music of containment" (Salomonsson, 2011), a term that once emerged as I worked with a mother and baby. One day, the girl was crying incessantly, and I tried to enter in a "dialogue" as I respected and followed the ups and downs in her dynamics and tempo. This "music of containment" resembled my "there, there" with Harry. To me, the emerging globe at night indicates that an internal object, which had always been brittle and was smashed even more by his panic about the disease, was slowly healing.

After ten months of therapy, he says in a deeply earnest tone:

> I saw my physiotherapist the other day. She says my illness hasn't gotten worse. Strange, all the time I've been convinced that I'm dying tomorrow. Maybe it took me a year to grasp that I've a handicap. I hate it, but that's the way it is.

In such a situation, there is no need of my "There, there". This is because he is now closer to a depressive positioning, where he admits the sorrowful fact about his disease, his tendency to accuse everything and everybody for it, and the possibility of looking at it with greater clarity and compassion.

In other situations, Harry panics and then my shushing words are called for. I want to suggest an alternative dialogue to the one he had with his mother. His father's death must have left her devastated and made it hard to contain her son in a tranquil and self-reflective way. I assumed this had paved the way for Harry's histrionic trait and heated interchanges with me and others. True, he contributed to this climate with hostile projections, which we needed to analyse since they meddled with his reality perception and made him lonely and ashamed of himself in the end. But I also felt that this man – with his disease and fears of being crippled and dying – needed me to address him in a shushing and lulling way in his most heartbroken moments. Both he and I understood that we sometimes needed to look at each other in silence, waiting for some thought to emerge in either one of us. In such moments, the atmosphere was calm, serene, and pensive.

I sometimes wonder what would have happened if I had been more open to such an approach with Harry in his analysis many years ago. In other words, if I had I been more sensitive to his Infantile and helped bring out more of such moments, would this have changed the direction and outcome of his analysis? Reflections like these are a major reason for writing this book.

References

Abraham, K. (1923). Contributions to the theory of the anal character. *International Journal of Psychoanalysis*, *4*, 400–418.

Abraham, K. (1927). *Selected papers on psycho-analysis*. London: Maresfield Reprints.

Abraham, N., & Torok, M. (1984). Notes on identification within the crypt. *Psychoanalytic Inquiry*, *4*, 221–242.

Adamson, L. B., & Frick, J. E. (2003). The still face: A history of a shared experimental paradigm. *Infancy*, *4*(4), 451–473.

Aguayo, J., & Salomonsson, B. (2017). The study and treatment of mothers and infants, then and now: Melanie Klein's 'Notes on Baby' (1938/39) in a contemporary psychoanalytic context. *Psychoanalytic Quarterly*, *86*(2), 383–408.

Ainsworth, M. S., Blehar, M. C., Waters, E., & Wall, S. (1978). *Patterns of attachment: A psychological study of the strange situation*. Oxford: Lawrence Erlbaum.

Akhtar, S. (2020). Repression: A critical assessment and update of Freud's 1915 paper. *American Journal of Psychoanalysis*, *80*, 241–258.

Allen, A. (1965). Stealing as a defence. *Psychoanalytic Quarterly*, *34*, 572–583.

Anthony, E. J. (1974). Dominique: The analysis of an adolescent: By Françoise Dolto. (Book review). *Psychoanalytic Quarterly*, *43*, 681–684.

Anzieu, D. (Ed.) (1989). *Psychanalyse et langage. Du corps à la parole (Psychoanalysis and language. From the body to the word)*. Paris: Dunod.

Anzieu, D. (1995). *Le Moi-peau* (2nd ed.) (*The Skin-Ego*, 2019. Translated by Naomi Segal. New York: Routledge). Paris: Dunod.

Anzieu-Premmereur, C. (2017). Using psychoanalytic concepts to inform interpretations and direct interventions with a baby in working with infants and parents. *International Forum of Psychoanalysis*, *26*(1), 54–58.

Anzieu-Premmereur, C., & Pollak-Cornillot, M. (2003). *Les pratiques psychanalytiques auprès des bébés (Psychoanalytic practice with babies)*. Paris: Dunod.

Arlow, J. (1979). Metaphor and the psychoanalytic situation. *Psychoanalytic Quarterly*, *48*, 363–385.

Aulagnier, P. (2001). *The violence of interpretation. From pictogram to statement (La violence de l'interprétation: du pictogramme à l'énoncé*, 1975. Paris: PUF). London: Routledge.

Avdi, E., & Georgaca, E. (2007). Discourse analysis and psychotherapy: A critical review. *European Journal of Psychotherapy and Counselling*, *9*(2), 157–176. https://doi.org/10.1080/13642530701363445

Avdi, E., & Seikkula, J. (2019). Studying the process of psychoanalytic psychotherapy: Discursive and embodied aspects. *British Journal of Psychotherapy*, *35*(2), 217–232.

Avdi, E. et al. (2020). Studying the process of psychoanalytic parent–infant psychotherapy: Embodied and discursive aspects. *Infant Mental Health Journal*, *41*, 589–602. https://doi.org/10.1002/imhj.21888

Axelrad, S. (1960). On some uses of psychoanalysis. *Journal of the American Psychoanalytic Association*, *8*, 175–218.

Bacon, R. (2002). Winnicott revisited: A point of view. *Free Associations*, *9B*, 250–270.

Bacon, R. (2013). Listening to voices, hearing a person: Françoise Dolto and the language of the subject. *British Journal of Psychotherapy*, *29*(4), 519–531. https://doi.org/10.1111/bjp.12046

Balestriere, L. (2003). *Freud et la question des origines* (*Freud and the question of origins*) (2nd ed.). Bruxelles: De Boeck & Larcier.

Balter, L., Lothane, Z., & Spencer, J. H. (1980). On the analyzing instrument. *Psychoanalytic Quarterly*, *49*, 475–503.

Bar Emet Gradman, S., & Shai, D. (2023). What nourishes maternal bonds? Focus on subjective bottle and breastfeeding experiences predicting parental bonding. *Current Psychology*. https://doi.org/10.1007/s12144-023-04322-9

Baradon, T., Avdi, E., Sleed, M., Salomonsson, B., & Amiran, K. (2023). Observing and interpreting clinical process: Methods and findings from 'Layered analysis' of parent–infant psychotherapy. *Infant Mental Health Journal*, *44*(5), 691–704.

Baradon, T., Biseo, M., Broughton, C., James, J., & Joyce, A. (2016). *The practice of psychoanalytic parent-infant psychotherapy – Claiming the baby* (2nd ed.). London: Routledge.

Baranger, M., Baranger, W., & Mom, J. M. (1988). The infantile psychic trauma from us to Freud: Pure trauma, retroactivity and reconstruction. *International Journal of Psychoanalysis*, *69*, 113–128.

Barbosa, M., Beeghly, M., Moreira, J., Tronick, E., & Fuertes, M. (2021). Emerging patterns of infant regulatory behavior in the Still-Face paradigm at 3 and 9 months predict mother-infant attachment at 12 months. *Attachment & Human Development*, *23*(6), 814–830.

Beebe, B. (1982). Micro-timing in mother-infant communication. In *Nonverbal communication today* (Contributions to the sociology of language), edited by M. R. Key (Vol. 33, 169–195). Mouton: De Gruyter.

Beebe, B. (2000). Brief mother-infant treatment using psychoanalytically informed video microanalysis. *Infant Mental Health Journal*, *24*(1), 24–52.

Beebe, B. (2003). Brief mother-infant treatment: Psychoanalytically informed video feedback. *Infant Mental Health Journal*, *24*(1), 24–52.

Beebe, B. (2005). Mother-infant research informs mother-infant treatment. *The Psychoanalytic Study of the Child*, *60*, 7–46.

Beebe, B., & Lachmann, F. (2014). *The origins of attachment. Infant research and adult treatment*. New York: Routledge.

Beebe, B., & Lachmann, F. (2020). Infant research and adult treatment revisited: Cocreating self-and interactive regulation. *Psychoanalytic Psychology*, *37*(4), 313–323.

Beebe, B., & Lachmann, F. M. (2002). *Infant research and adult treatment: Co-constructing interactions*. Hillsdale, NJ: Analytic Press.

Benecke, C., & Krause, R. (2005). Facial affective relationship offers of patients with panic disorder. *Psychotherapy Research*, *15*(3), 178–187.

Benecke, C., Peham, D., & Bänninger-Huber, E. (2005). Nonverbal relationship regulation in psychotherapy. *Psychotherapy Research*, *15*(1–2), 81–90. https://doi.org/10.1080/10503300512331327065

Benjamin, J. (2009). A relational psychoanalysis perspective on the necessity of acknowledging failure in order to restore the facilitating and containing features of the intersubjective relationship (the Shared Third). *International Journal of Psychoanalysis*, *90*, 441–450.

Benjamin, J., & Atlas, G. (2015). The 'too-muchness' of excitement: Sexuality in light of excess, attachment and affect regulation. *International Journal of Psychoanalysis*, *96*(1), 39–63.

Beratis, S. (2020). Thoughts about repression. *International Journal of Psychoanalysis*. *IJP Open*, *7*, 1–22.

Bergelson, E., & Swingley, D. (2012). At 6–9 months, human infants know the meanings of many common nouns. *Proceedings of the National Academy of Sciences of the United States of America*, *109*(9), 3253–3258. https://doi.org/10.1073/pnas.1113380109

Bick, E. (1968/2011). The experience of the skin in early object relations (1968). *The Tavistock Model: Papers on child development and psychoanalytic training* (133–138). London: The Harris Meltzer Trust.

Bion, W. R. (1962). *Learning from experience*. London: Karnac Books.

Bion, W. R. (1965). *Transformations*. London: Karnac Books.

Bion, W. R. (1970). *Attention and interpretation*. London: Karnac Books.

Biringen, Z., Robinson, J. L., & Emde, R. N. (1998). *Emotional availability scales* (3rd ed.). Fort Collins: Colorado State University.

Blandon, A. Y., Calkins, S. D., Keane, S. P., & O'Brien, M. (2008). Individual differences in trajectories of emotion regulation processes: The effects of maternal depressive symptomatology and children's physiological regulation. *Developmental Psychology*, *44*(4), 1110–1123.

Blum, H. P. (2003). Repression, transference and reconstruction. *International Journal of Psychoanalysis*, *84*(3), 497–503.

Bohleber, W. (2010). *Destructiveness, intersubjectivity, and trauma: The identity crisis of modern psychoanalysis*. London: Karnac Books.

Bornstein, M. H., Arterberry, M. E., & Mash, C. (2004). Long-term memory for an emotional interpersonal interaction occurring at 5 months of age. *Infancy*, *6*, 407–416.

Boston Change Process Study Group (2002). Explicating the implicit: The local level and the microprocess of change in the analytic situation. *International Journal of Psychoanalysis*, *83*(5), 1051–1062.

Boston Change Process Study Group (2005). The "something more" than interpretation revisited: Sloppiness and co-creativity in the psychoanalytic encounter. *Journal of the American Psychoanalytic Association*, *53*(3), 693–729.

Boston Change Process Study Group (2007). The foundational level of psychodynamic meaning: The implicit process in relation to conflict, defence and the dynamic unconscious. *International Journal of Psychoanalysis*, *88*(4), 843–860.

Brenman, E. (1980). The value of reconstruction in adult psychoanalysis. *International Journal of Psychoanalysis*, 61, 53–60.

Britton, R. (1989). The missing link: Parental sexuality in the Oedipus complex. In *The Oedipus complex today: Clinical implications*, edited by R. Britton, M. Feldman, & E. O'Shaugnessy (83–101). London: Karnac Books.

Britton, R. (2000). Hyper-subjectivity and hyper-objectivity in narcissistic disorders. *Fort Da*, 6(2), 53–64.

Bronfman, E., Parsons, E., & Lyons-Ruth, K. (1999). *Atypical maternal behavior instrument for assessment and classification (AMBIANCE): Manual for coding disrupted affective communication*. Unpubl. manuscript. Harvard Medical School.

Brown, L. J. (2009). From "disciplined subjectivity" to "taming wild thoughts": Bion's elaboration of the analysing instrument. *International Forum of Psychoanalysis*, 18, 82–85.

Bruner, J. (1990). *Acts of meaning*. Cambridge, MA: Harvard University Press.

Butner, J. E. et al. (2017). A multivariate dynamic systems model for psychotherapy with more than one client. *Journal of Counseling Psychology*, 64(6), 616.

Campos, J. (2014). *An experiment by Joseph Campos: The Visual Cliff*. Retrieved from http://www.youtube.com/watch?v=p6cqNhHrMJA

Campos, J., Walle, E. A., Dahl, A., & Main, A. (2011). Reconceptualizing emotion regulation. *Emotion Review*, 3(1), 26–35.

Canestri, J. (2021). The infantile: Which meaning? *The International Journal of Psychoanalysis*, 102(3), 560–571.

Carver, L. J., & Vaccaro, B. G. (2007). 12-month-old infants allocate increased neural resources to stimuli associated with negative adult emotion. *Developmental Psychology*, 43(1), 54–69.

Cavelzani, A., & Tronick, E. (2016). Dyadically expanded states of consciousness and therapeutic change in the interaction between analyst and adult patient. *Psychoanalytic Dialogues*, 26(5), 599–615.

Chervet, B. (2015). Aux origines de l'irrationnel: le concept de l'infantile (At the origins of the irrational: The concept of the infantile). *Revue Francaise de Psychanalyse*, 79, 1747–1752.

Chinen, A. B. (1987). Symbolic modes in object relations: A semiotic perspective. *Psychoanalysis & Contemporary Thought*, 10, 373–406.

Chronis, A. M. et al. (2007). Maternal depression and early positive parenting predict future conduct problems in young children with attention-deficit/hyperactivity disorder. *Developmental Psychology*, 43(1), 70–82.

Civitarese, G., & Ferro, A. (2013). The meaning and use of metaphor in analytic field theory. *Psychoanalytic Inquiry*, 33(3), 190–209. https://doi.org/10.1080/0735169 0.2013.779887

Clarke, A., Tyler, L. K., & Marslen-Wilson, W. (2024). Hearing what is being said: The distributed neural substrate for early speech interpretation. *Language, Cognition and Neuroscience*, 39(9), 1097–1116. https://doi.org/10.1080/23273798. 2024.2345308

Clausner, T. C., & Croft, W. (1999). Domains and image schemas. *Cognitive Linguistics*, 10(1), 1–31.

Cohen, J. (1985). Trauma and repression. *Psychoanalytic Inquiry*, 5(1), 163–189.

Cohen, J., & Kinston, W. (1986). Repression theory: A new look at the cornerstone. *Revista Catalana de Psicoanalisi*, 3(2), 239–256.

Cohn, J. F., & Tronick, E. (1989). Specificity of infants' response to mothers' affective behavior. *Journal of the American Academy of Child & Adolescent Psychiatry, 28*(2), 242–248.

Conradt, E., & Ablow, J. (2010). Infant physiological response to the still-face paradigm: Contributions of maternal sensitivity and infants' early regulatory behavior *Infant Behavior & Development, 33*(3), 251–265

Cowsill, K. (2000). 'I thought you knew': Some factors affecting a baby's capacity to maintain eye contact. *Infant Observation, 3*(3), 64–83.

Cramer, B., & Palacio Espasa, F. (1993). *La pratique des psychothérapies mères-bébés. Études cliniques et techniques (The practice of mother-infant psychotherapies. Clinical and technical studies).* Paris: PUF.

da Rocha Barros, E. M., & da Rocha Barros, E. L. (2011). Reflections on the clinical implications of symbolism. *International Journal of Psychoanalysis, 92*(4), 879–901.

de Saint-Exupéry, A. (1946). *Le Petit Prince (The Little Prince).* Paris: Gallimard.

DeCasper, A. J., & Fifer, W. P. (1980). Of human bonding: Newborns prefer their mothers' voices. *Science, 208*(4448), 1174–1176.

Decety, J. (2010). The neurodevelopment of empathy in humans. *Developmental Neuroscience, 32,* 257–267.

Diatkine, G. (2008). La disparition de la sexualité infantile dans la psychanalyse contemporaine (The disappearance of infantile sexuality in contemporary psychoanalysis). *Revue Francaise de Psychanalyse, 72*(3), 671–685.

DiCorcia, J. A., Snidman, N., Sravish, A. V., & Tronick, E. (2016). Evaluating the nature of the still-face effect in the double face-to-face still-face paradigm using different comparison groups. *Infancy, 21*(3), 332–352. https://doi.org/10.1111/infa.12123

Dimberg, U., Thunberg, M., & Elmehed, K. (2000). Unconscious facial reactions to emotional facial expressions. *Psychological Science, 11*(1), 86–89.

Dolto, F. (1982). *Séminaires de psychanalyse d'enfant, vol. 1 (Seminars on child psychoanalysis, vol. 1).* Paris: Editions du Seuil.

Dolto, F. (1984). *L'image inconsciente du corps. (The unconscious image of the body).* Paris: Éditions du Seuil.

Dolto, F. (1985). *Séminaires de psychanalyse d'enfant, vol. 2 (Seminars on child psychoanalysis, vol. 2).* Paris: Editions du Seuil.

Dolto, F. (1994a). *Solitude.* Paris: Gallimard.

Dolto, F. (1994b). *Tout est language (Everything is language).* Paris: Gallimard.

Dor, J. (2000). *Introduction to the reading of Lacan.* New York: Other Press.

Downing, G., Bürgin, D., Reck, C., & Ziegenhain, U. (2008). Interfaces between intersubjectivity and attachment: Three perspectives on a mother–infant inpatient case. *Infant Mental Health Journal, 29*(3), 278–295.

Dreher, M., Mengele, U., Krause, R., & Kämmerer, A. (2001). Affective indicators of the psychotherapeutic process: An empirical case study. *Psychotherapy Research, 11*(1), 99–117. https://doi.org/10.1080/713663855

Edhborg, M., Lundh, W., Seimyr, L., & Widström, A. M. (2003). The parent-child relationship in the context of maternal depressive mood. *Archives of Women's Mental Health, 6*(3), 211–216.

Emanuel, L. (2011). Brief interventions with parents, infants, and young children: A framework for thinking. *Infant Mental Health Journal, 32*(6), 673–686.

Emanuel, L., & Bradley, E. (Eds.) (2008). *"What can the matter be?" – Therapeutic interventions with parents, infants, and young children*. London: Karnac Books.

Eshel, O. (1998). "Black holes", deadness and existing analytically. *International Journal of Psychoanalysis, 79*, 1115–1130.

Eubanks, C. F., Muran, J. C., & Safran, J. D. (2018). Alliance rupture repair: A meta-analysis. *Psychotherapy, 55*(4), 508.

Faimberg, H. (2005). *The telescoping of generations: Listening to the narcissistic links between generations*. London: Routledge.

Feldman, M. (1993). The dynamics of reassurance. *International Journal of Psychoanalysis, 74*, 275–285.

Feldman, R. (2007). Parent-infant synchrony and the construction of shared timing; physiological precursors, developmental outcomes, and risk conditions. *Journal of Child Psychology & Psychiatry & Allied Disciplines, 48*(3–4), 329–354.

Feldman, R. et al. (2009). Maternal depression and anxiety across the postpartum year and infant social engagement, fear regulation, and stress reactivity. *Journal of the American Academy of Child & Adolescent Psychiatry, 48*(9), 919–927.

Ferenczi, S. (1949). Confusion of the tongues between the adults and the child (the language of tenderness and of passion). *International Journal of Psychoanalysis, 30*, 225–230.

Fernald, A. (1993). Approval and disapproval: Infant responsiveness to vocal affect in familiar and unfamiliar languages. *Child Development, 64*(3), 657–674. https://doi.org/10.2307/1131209

Fernald, A. (2004). Hearing, listening and understanding: Auditory development in infancy. In *Blackwell handbook of infant development*, edited by G. Bremner & A. Fogel (35–70). Oxford: Blackwell Publishing.

Ferro, A. (2006). Clinical implications of Bion's thought. *International Journal of Psychoanalysis, 87*(4), 989–1003.

Ferry, A. L., Hespos, S. J., & Waxman, S. R. (2010). Categorization in 3- and 4-month-old infants: An advantage of words over tones. *Child Development, 81*, 472–479.

Field, T. (2010). Postpartum depression effects on early interactions, parenting, and safety practices: A review. *Infant Behavior & Development, 33*(1), 1–6.

Field, T., Healy, B., Goldstein, S., & Guthertz, M. (1990). Behavior-state matching and synchrony in mother–infant interactions of nondepressed versus depressed dyads. *Developmental Psychology, 26*, 7–14.

Fonagy, P. (1999). Memory and therapeutic action. *International Journal of Psychoanalysis, 80*(2), 215–223.

Fonagy, P. (2008). A genuinely developmental theory of sexual enjoyment and its implications for psychoanalytic technique. *Journal of the American Psychoanalytic Association, 56*(1), 11–36.

Fonagy, P., Campbell, C., & Luyten, P. (2022). Alliance rupture and repairs in mentalization-based therapy. In *Rupture and repair in psychotherapy: A critical process for change*, edited by C. F. Eubanks, L. W. Samstag, & J. C. Muran (253–276). Washington, DC: American Psychological Association.

Fraiberg, S. (1980). *Clinical studies in infant mental health*. New York: Basic Books.

Fraiberg, S. (1982). Pathological defenses in infancy. *Psychoanalytic Quarterly, 51*(4), 612–635.

Fraiberg, S., Adelson, E., & Shapiro, V. (1975). Ghosts in the nursery. A psychoanalytic approach to the problems of impaired infant-mother relationships. *Journal of the American Academy of Child Psychiatry, 14*(3), 387–421.

Frank, A., & Muslin, H. (1967). The development of Freud's concept of primal repression. *Psychoanalytic Study of the Child, 22*, 55–76.

Freud, H. C. (2011). *Electra vs. Oedipus: The drama of the mother-daughter relationship*. London: Routledge.

Freud, S. (1893–1895). *Studies on hysteria. SE 2*. London: Hogarth Press.

Freud, S. (1895/1950). *Project for a scientific psychology. SE I*. London: Hogarth Press.

Freud, S. (1897). *Letter 69, Extracts from the Fliess Papers SE 1*. London: Hogarth Press.

Freud, S. (1900). *The interpretation of dreams. SE 4-5*. London: Hogarth Press.

Freud, S. (1905a). *Fragment of an analysis of a case of hysteria. SE 7* (1–122). London: Hogarth Press.

Freud, S. (1905b). *Three essays on sexuality. SE 7* (123–246). London: Hogarth Press.

Freud, S. (1908). *Character and anal erotism. SE 9* (167–176). London: Hogarth Press.

Freud, S. (1909). *Analysis of a phobia in a five-year-old boy. SE 10* (1–150). London: Hogarth Press.

Freud, S. (1910). *The future prospects of psycho-analytic therapy. SE 11* (139–152). London: Hogarth Press.

Freud, S. (1911). *Psycho-analytic notes on an autobiographical account … (Schreber). SE 12*. London: Hogarth Press.

Freud, S. (1912). *Recommendations to physicians practising psycho-analysis. SE 12* (109–120). London: Hogarth Press.

Freud, S. (1915a). *Repression. SE 14* (141–158). London: Hogarth Press.

Freud, S. (1915b). *The Unconscious. SE 14* (159–216). London: Hogarth Press.

Freud, S. (1916–1917). *Introductory lectures on psychoanalysis. SE 15–16*. London: Hogarth Press.

Freud, S. (1917). *Mourning and melancholia SE 14* (237–258). London: Hogarth Press.

Freud, S. (1918). *From the history of an infantile neurosis* (Vol. 17, 1–124). London: Hogarth Press.

Freud, S. (1920). *Beyond the pleasure principle. SE 18* (1–64). London: Hogarth Press.

Freud, S. (1923). *The Ego and the Id. SE 19* (3–66). London: Hogarth Press.

Freud, S. (1925–1926). *Inhibitions, symptoms and anxiety. SE 20* (87–178). London: Hogarth Press.

Freud, S. (1927). *The future of an illusion SE* (Vol. 21, 1–56). London: Hogarth Press.

Freud, S. (1933). *New introductory lectures on psychoanalysis. SE 22* (1–182). London: Hogarth Press.

Freud, S. (1937). *Constructions in analysis. SE 23* (255–269). London: Hogarth Press.

Freud, S. (1940). *Splitting of the Ego in the process of defence. SE 23* (271–278). London: Hogarth Press.

Freud, S. (1950 [1892–1899]). *Extracts from the Fliess papers. SE 1* (175–282). London: Hogarth Press.

Frie, R. (2007). The lived body: From Freud to Merleau-Ponty and contemporary psychoanalysis. In *The embodied subject. Minding the body in psychoanalysis,* edited by J. P. Muller & J. G. Tillman (55–66). Lanham, MD: Jason Aronson.

Friedman, M. (1996). Mother's milk. A psychoanalyst looks at breastfeeding. *The Psychoanalytic Study of the Child, 51,* 475–490.

Gabbard, G. O. (2001). A contemporary psychoanalytic model of countertransference. *Journal of Clinical Psychology, 57*(8), 983–991.

Gadamer, H. G. (1975/1989). *Truth and method* (2nd ed.). London: Continuum.

Gaddini, E. (1992). *A psychoanalytic theory of infantile experience.* London: Routledge.

Gammelgaard, J. (1998). Metaphors of listening. *Scandinavian Psychoanalytic Review, 21*(2), 151–167.

Gavin, N. I. et al. (2005). Perinatal depression: A systematic review of prevalence and incidence. *Obstetrics & Gynecology, 106*(5 Pt 1), 1071–1083.

Gentile, J. (2007). Wrestling with matter: Origins of intersubjectivity. *Psychoanalytic Quarterly, 76,* 547–582.

Georgaca, E., & Avdi, E. (2011). Discourse analysis. In *Qualitative research methods in mental health and psychotherapy,* edited by D. J. Harper & E. Thompson (147–162). Chichester: John Wiley.

Gervain, J., Macagno, F., Cogoi, S., Peña, M., & Mehler, J. (2008). The neonate brain detects speech structure. *Proceedings of the National Academy of Sciences of the United States of America, 105,* 14222–14227.

Goetzmann, L., & Schwegler, K. (2004). Semiotic aspects of the countertransference: Some observations on the concepts of the 'immediate object' and the 'interpretant' in the work of Charles S. Peirce. *International Journal of Psychoanalysis, 85*(6), 1423–1438.

Golse, B. (2001). Attachement et psychanalyse: ce que Serge Lebovici nous a transmis à propos de la transmission (Attachment and psychoanalysis. What Serge Lebovici transmitted to us, a propos transmission). *Spirale, 1*(17), 83–86. https://doi.org/10.3917/spi.017.0083, https://www.cairn.info/revue-spirale-2001-1-page-83.htm

Golse, B. (2006). *L'être-bébé (The baby – A being).* Paris: Presses Universitaires de France.

Golse, B. (2015). Le sexuel infantile: Instauration, transmission, actualisation. *Revue Francaise de Psychanalyse, 79*(5), 1687–1694. https://doi.org/10.3917/rfp.795.1687

Gottlieb, R. M. (2017). Reconstruction in a two-person world may be more about the present than the past: Freud and the wolf man, an illustration. *Journal of the American Psychoanalytic Association, 65*(2), 305–316.

Grace, S. L., & Sansom, S. (2003). The effect of postpartum depression on the mother-infant relationship and child growth and development. In *Postpartum depression: Literature review of risk factors and interventions,* edited by D. E. Stewart, E. Robertson, C.-L. Dennis, Grace, S. L., & T. Wallington (199–251). Toronto: University Health Network.

Grady, J. (1997). *Foundations of meaning: Primary metaphors and primary scenes.* Berkeley:University of California.

Grassi, L. (2021). *The sound of the unconscious. Psychoanalysis as music.* Oxon: Routledge.

Green, A. (1986). The dead mother. In *On private madness* (142–173). Madison, CT: International Universities Press.

Green, A. (1995). Summary: Affects versus representations or affects as representations? *British Journal of Psychotherapy, 12,* 208–211.

Green, A. (1998). The primordial mind and the work of the negative. *International Journal of Psychoanalysis, 79,* 649–665.

Green, A. (1999). On discriminating and not discriminating between affect and representation. *International Journal of Psychoanalysis, 80,* 277.

Grier, F. (2019). Musicality in the consulting room. *International Journal of Psychoanalysis, 100*(5), 827–851.

Grier, F. (2021). The music of the drives, and the music of perversion: Reflections on a dream of jealous theft. *International Journal of Psychoanalysis, 102*(3), 448–463.

Grotstein, J. (1980). A proposed revision of the psychoanalytic concept of primitive mental states—part I. Introduction to a newer psychoanalytic metapsychology. *Contemporary Psychoanalysis, 16,* 479–546.

Grotstein, J. (1990). Nothingness, meaninglessness, chaos, and the "black hole" I. *Contemporary Psychoanalysis, 26,* 257–290.

Grotstein, J. (1997). Integrating one-person and two-person psychologies: Autochthony and alterity in counterpoint. *Psychoanal Quarterly, 66,* 403–430.

Grotstein, J. (2008). *A beam of intense darkness. Wilfred Bion's legacy to psychoanalysis.* London: Karnac Books.

Guignard, F. (2021). *The Infantile in psychoanalytic practice today. Talks on Psychoanalysis.* Retrieved from https://docs.google.com/document/d/1UC1QF8 Yirl8CZ5i42rWwTxvD5_qfwc5B/edit

Guignard, F. (2022). *The Infantile in Psychoanalytic Practice Today* (Kindle ed.). Abingdon, Oxon: Routledge. [Original: (1996). Au vif de l'Infantile, Delachaux & Niestlé]. The book's first chapter was published in 1995: The Infantile in the analytical relationship. *International Journal of Psychoanalysis, 76*(6), 1083–1092.

Guignard, F., Levy, R., & Ungar, V. (2021). *Florence Guignard and Ruggiero Levy talk about the infantile.* Vancouver: The International Psychoanalytic Association. https://www.ipa.world/IPA/en/IPA1/Webinars/Florence_Guignard_and_Ruggero_ Levy_talk_about_the_Infantile.aspx

Haritha, S. et al. (2024) Emotion detection using facial expression–A comprehensive review. *Indiana Journal of Multidisciplinary Research, 4*(3), 174–178.

Harris, A. (1997). Aggression, envy, and ambition: Circulating tensions in women's psychic life. *Gender and Psychoanalysis, 2,* 291–325.

Harrison, A. M., & Tronick, E. Z. (2007). Contributions to understanding therapeutic change: Now we have a playground. *Journal of the American Psychoanalytic Association, 55*(3), 853–874.

Hatfield, E. (1982). Passionate love, companionate love, and intimacy. In *Intimacy,* edited by M. Fisher & G. Stricker (267–292). New York: Plenum.

Hawking, S. 1988. *A Brief History of Time. From the Big Bang to black holes.* London: Transworld Publications.

Heimann, P. (1950). On counter-transference. *International Journal of Psychoanalysis, 31,* 81–84.

Hodges, J., Steele, M., Hillman, S., Henderson, K., & Kaniuk, J. (2003). Changes in attachment representations over the first year of adoptive placement: Narratives of maltreated children. *Clinical Child Psychology and Psychiatry, 8*(3), 351–367.

Hoffman, L. (2018). The past in the present, the present in the past: Introduction to panel on reconstruction from today's two-person perspective. *Journal of the American Psychoanalytic Association, 66*(3), 473–478.

Houghton, R., & Beebe, B. (2016). Dance/movement therapy: Learning to look through video microanalysis. *American Journal of Dance Therapy, 38*(2), 334–357.

Houzel, D. (1996). The family envelope and what happens when it is torn. *International Journal of Psychoanalysis, 77*, 901–912.

Hurley, A. (2017). 'Her Majesty the Baby': Narcissistic states in babies and young children. *Journal of Child Psychotherapy, 43*(2), 192–207. https://doi.org/10.1080/0075417X.2017.1323942

Januário, G. C. et al. (2024). Functional near-infrared spectroscopy and language development: An integrative review. *International Journal of Developmental Neuroscience.* https://doi.org/10.1002/jdn.10366

Jones, A. (2006). Levels of change in parent-infant psychotherapy. *Journal of Child Psychotherapy, 32*(3), 295–311.

Joseph, B. (1989). *Psychic equilibrium and psychic change.* London: Tavistock/Routledge.

Josselyn, S. A., & Frankland, P. W. (2012). Infantile amnesia: A neurogenic hypothesis. *Learning & Memory, 19*(9), 423–433.

Karmiloff, K., & Karmiloff-Smith, A. (2001). *Pathways to language.* Cambridge, MA: Harvard University Press.

Keren, M. (2011). An infant who was born with a life-threatening skin disease: Various aspects of triadic psychotherapy. *Infant Mental Health Journal, 32*(6), 617–626.

Keren, M., & Tyano, S. (2006). Depression in infancy. *Child & Adolescent Psychiatric Clinics of North America, 15*(4), 883–897.

Kernberg, O. F. (1997). The nature of interpretation: Intersubjectivity and the third position. *Annual of Psychoanalysis, 57*(4), 297–312.

Kernutt, J. (2007). The I, or the eye, and the other: A mother-infant observation vignette analysed using Winnicott's concept of false self. *Infant Observation, 10*(2), 203–211.

Kinston, W., & Cohen, J. (1986). Primal repression: Clinical and theoretical aspects. *International Journal of Psychoanalysis, 67*, 337–353.

Kirshner, L. (2015). The translational metaphor in psychoanalysis. *The International Journal of Psychoanalysis, 96*(1), 65–81.

Klein, M. (1935). A contribution to the psychogenesis of manic-depressive states. In *The writings of Melanie Klein*, edited by R. Money-Kyrle (Vol. 1, 262–289). London: Hogarth Press.

Klein, M. (1940). *Mourning and its relation to manic-depressive states The Writings of Melanie Klein* (Vol. 1, 344–369). London: Hogarth Press.

Klein, M. (1946). Notes on some schizoid mechanisms. In *Envy and gratitude*, edited by R. Money-Kyrle (1–24). London: Hogarth Press.

Klein, M. (1961). *Narrative of a child analysis: The conduct of the psycho-analysis of children as seen in the treatment of a ten year old boy.* London: Hogarth Press.

Klein, M. (1975). *Envy and gratitude and other works 1946–1963*. London: Hogarth Press.

Kloesel, C., & Houser, N. (Eds.) (1992). *The essential Peirce, vol. 1: 1867–1893*. Bloomington: Indiana University Press.

Kloesel, C., & Houser, N. (Eds.) (1998). *The essential Peirce, vol. 2: 1893–1913*. Bloomington: Indiana University Press.

Kohut, H. (1971). *The analysis of the self*. New York: International Universities Press.

Kövecses, Z. (2008). Conceptual metaphors theory: Some criticisms and alternative proposals. *Annual Review of Cognitive Linguistics*, 6, 168–184. https://doi.org/10.1075/arcl.6.08kov

Krause, R. (2010). An update on primary identification, introjection, and empathy. *International Forum of Psychoanalysis*, 19, 138–143.

Krause, R., & Merten, J. (1999, November). Affects, regulation of relationship, transference and countertransference. *International Forum of Psychoanalysis*, 8(2), 103–114.

Kugiumutzakis, G., Kokkinaki, T., Makrodimitraki, M., & Vitalaki, E. (2005). Emotions in early mimesis. In *Emotional development*, edited by J. Nadel & D. Muir (162–182). Oxford: Oxford University Press.

Lacan, J. (1954–1955). *Le Séminaire. Le Moi dans la théorie de Freud et dans la technique de la psychanalyse* (Vol. 2). (Seminar. The Ego in Freud's theory and in the technique of psychoanalysis) Paris: Ed. Seuil.

Lacan, J. (1966/2006). *Ecrits – The first complete edition in English* (B. Fink, Trans.). New York: W. W. Norton & Company.

Lacan, J. (1975). *Encore: Séminaires (On feminine sexuality, the limits of love and knowledge: The Seminar of Jacques Lacan, Book XX, Encore)* (Vol. 20). Paris: Dunod.

Lacan, J. (1991). *Seminar II: The Ego in Freud's theory and in the technique of psychoanalysis*. New York: W.W. Norton.

Lakoff, G., & Johnson, M. (1980/2003). *Metaphors we live by* (Kindle ed.). Chicago: The University of Chicago.

Lakoff, G., & Johnson, M. (1999). *Philosophy in the flesh*. New York: Basic Books.

Laplanche, J. (1989). *New foundations for psychoanalysis* (Nouveaux fondements pour la psychanalyse, 1987) (D. Macey, Trans.). Oxford: Basil Blackwell.

Laplanche, J. (1995). Seduction, persecution, revelation. *International Journal of Psychoanalysis*, 76, 663–682.

Laplanche, J. (1996). Psychoanalysis as anti-hermeneutics. *Radical Philosophy*, Sept/Oct, 7–12.

Laplanche, J. (1999a). *Essays on otherness*. London: Routledge.

Laplanche, J. (1999b). *The unconscious and the Id*. London: Rebus Press.

Laplanche, J. (2007a). Gender, sex and the sexual. *Studies in Gender and Sexuality*, 8(2), 201–219.

Laplanche, J. (2007b). *Sexual La sexualité élargie au sens Freudien ("Sexual". Sexuality enlarged in the Freudian sense)*. Paris: PUF.

Laplanche, J. (2017). Psychical forces at play in psychical conflict. In *Psychoanalytic perspectives on conflict*, edited by M. N. E. Christopher Christian & David L. Wolitzky (195–209). Oxon: Routledge.

Laplanche, J., Danon, G., & Lauru, D. (2002). Entretien avec Jean Laplanche (Interview with Jean Laplanche). *Enfances & Psy*, 17(1), 9–16.

Laplanche, J., & Pontalis, J. B. (1973). *The language of psychoanalysis*. London: Hogarth Press.

Laplanche, J., & Pontalis, J.-B. (1968). Fantasy and the origins of sexuality. *The International Journal of Psychoanalysis, 49*, 1.

Lebovici, S. (1991). La théorie de l'attachement et la psychanalyse contemporaine (The theory of attachment and contemporary psychoanalysis). *Psychiatrie de l'Enfant, 34*(2), 309–339.

Lebovici, S. (2000). La consultation thérapeutique et les interventions métaphorisantes (The therapeutic consultation and the metaphorizing interventions). In *Alliances autour du bébé. De la recherche à la clinique (Alliances around the baby. From research to clinic)*, edited by M. Maury & M. Lamour (223–243). Paris: Presses Universitaires de France.

Lebovici, S., Barriguete, J. A., & Salinas, J. L. (2002). The therapeutic consultation. In *Infant and toddler mental health*, edited by J. M. Maldonado-Durán (161–186). Washington, DC: American Psychiatric Publishing Inc.

Lebovici, S., & Stoléru, S. (2003). *Le nourisson, sa mère et le psychanalyste. Les interactions précoces (The baby, his mother and the psychoanalyst. Early interactions)*. Paris: Bayard.

Leckman, J. F., Feldman, R., Swain, J. E., & Mayes, L. C. (2007). Primary parental preoccupation: Revisited. In *Developmental science and psychoanalysis. Integration and innovation*, edited by L. C. Mayes, P. Fonagy, & M. Target (89–116). London: Karnac Books.

Ledoux, M. H. (2006). *Dictionnaire raisonné de l'oeuvre de F. Dolto* (A commented dictionnary on the work of F. Dolto). Paris: Payot & Rivages.

Leppänen, J. M., Moulson, M. C., Vogel-Farley, V. K., & Nelson, C. A. (2007). An ERP study of emotional face processing in the adult and infant brain. *Child Development, 78*(1), 232–245.

Lessing, H.-U. (2011). *Wilhelm Dilthey: Eine Einführung (Wilhelm Dilthey: An introduction)*. Amazon Kindle. Köln: Böhlau.

Levenson, E. 2005 (1983). *The fallacy of understanding – The ambiguity of change*. Hillsdale, NJ: The Analytic Press.

Li, S., Callaghan, B. L., & Richardson, R. (2014). Infantile amnesia: Forgotten but not gone. *Learning & Memory, 21*(3), 135–139.

Lieberman, A. F. (1992). Infant-parent psychotherapy with toddlers. *Development and Psychopathology, 4*(4), 559–574.

Lieberman, A. F., & Van Horn, P. (2008). *Psychotherapy with infants and young children – Repairing the effects of stress and trauma on early attachment*. New York: The Guilford Press.

Likierman, M. (2003). Postnatal depression, the mother's conflict and parent-infant psychotherapy. *Journal of Child Psychotherapy, 29*(3), 301–315.

Lindén, J. (1985). Insight through metaphor in psychotherapy and creativity. *Psychoanalysis & Contemporary Thought, 375–406*, 375–406.

Litowitz, B. E. (2011). From dyad to dialogue: Language and the early relationship in American psychoanalytic theory. *Journal of the American Psychoanalytic Association, 59*(3), 483–508.

Litowitz, B. E. (2014). Coming to terms with intersubjectivity: Keeping language in mind. *Journal of the American Psychoanalytic Association, 62*, 295–312.

Litowitz, B. E. (2021). Constructing the infantile. *The International Journal of Psychoanalysis, 102*(3), 588–594.

Lojkasek, M., Cohen, N. J., & Muir, E. (1994). Where is the infant in infant intervention? A review of the literature on changing troubled mother-infant relationships. *Psychotherapy: Theory, Research, Practice, Training, 31*(1), 208–220.

Lyons-Ruth, K. (1998). Implicit relational knowing: Its role in development and psychoanalytic treatment. *Infant Mental Health Journal, 19*(3), 282–289.

Lyons-Ruth, K. (1999). The two-person unconscious: Intersubjective dialogue, enactive relational representation, and the emergence of new forms of relational organization. *Psychoanalytic Inquiry, 19*(4), 576–617.

Machover, K. (1949). *Personality projection in the drawing of the human figure (a method of personality investigation)*. Springfield, IL: Thomas.

Madsen, H. B., & Kim, J. H. (2016). Ontogeny of memory: An update on 40 years of work on infantile amnesia. *Behavioural Brain Research, 298*, 4–14.

Mahler, M., Pine, F., & Bergman, A. (1975). *The psychological birth of the human infant. Symbiosis and individuation*. New York: Basic Books.

Mahmoudzadeh, M. et al. (2013). Syllabic discrimination in premature human infants prior to complete formation of cortical layers. *PNAS, 110*(12), 4846–4851.

Mancia, M. (2004). *Primary experiences, implicit memory and non-repressed unconscious: Their role in mental development and the psychoanalytical process*. Paper at the Congress of the European Psychoanalytic Federation, Helsinki.

Mandler, J. M. (2004). *The foundations of mind: Origins of conceptual thought*. New York:Oxford University Press.

Mangini, E., & Graham, H. (2010). On primal repression. *The Italian Psychoanalytic Annual, 4*, 53–69.

Marcus, G. F., Fernandes, K. J., & Johnson, S. P. (2007). Infant rule learning facilitated by speech. *Psychological Science, 18*(5), 387–391.

Markman, H. (2006). Listening to music, listening to patients: Aesthetic experience in analytic practice. *Fort Da, 12*, 18–29.

Martindale, C. (1975). The grammar of altered states of consciousness: A semiotic reinterpretation of aspects of psychoanalytic theory. *Psychoanalysis and Contemporary Science, 4*, 331–354.

Martínez, I. C., Español, S. A., & Pérez, D. I. (2018). The interactive origin and the aesthetic modelling of image-schemas and primary metaphors. *Integrative Psychological and Behavioral Science, 52*(4), 646–671.

Maze, J. R., & Henry, R. M. (1996). Problems in the concept of repression and proposals for their resolution. *International Journal of Psychoanalysis, 77*(6), 1085–1100.

McWilliams, N. (2021). *Psychoanalytic supervision*. The Guilford Press.

Meltzer, D. (1967). *The psychoanalytic process*. Perthshire, Scotland: Clunie Press.

Meltzer, D. (1992). *The claustrum*. Perthshire, Scotland: Clunie Press.

Meltzer, D., & Harris-Williams, M. (1988). *The apprehension of beauty: The role of aesthetic conflict in development, violence and art*. Strath Tay: Clunie Press.

Meltzer, D., Milana, G., Maiello, S., & Petrelli, D. (1982). The conceptual distinction between projective identification (Klein) and container-contained (Bion). *Journal of Child Psychotherapy, 8*(2), 185–202.

Merleau-Ponty, M. (1962). *Phenomenology of perception*. London: Routledge.

Mesman, J., van IJzendoorn, M. H., & Bakermans-Kranenburg, M. J. (2009). The many faces of the Still-Face Paradigm: A review and meta-analysis. *Developmental Review*, 29(2), 120–162.

Miller, L. (1987). Idealization and contempt: Dual aspects of the process of devaluation of the breast in a feeding relationship. *Journal of Child Psychotherapy*, 13(1), 41–55.

Mills, J. (2002). *Hegel's anticipation of psychoanalysis*. New York: State University of New York Press.

Mills, J. (2005). A critique of relational psychoanalysis. *Psychoanalytic Psychology*, 22, 155–188.

Miltz, S., Pennicott-Banks, E. A. E., & Baradon, T. (2023). Addressing the baby and atypical maternal behaviour in psychoanalytic parent-infant psychotherapy. *Journal of Child Psychotherapy*, 49(2), 179–190.

Misak, C. (2018) *Cambridge pragmatism: From Peirce and James to Ramsey and Wittgenstein*. Oxford: Oxford University Press.

Modell, A. H. (2009). Metaphor—The bridge between feelings and knowledge. *Psychoanalytic Inquiry*, 29(1), 6–11.

Moehler, E. et al. (2007). Childhood behavioral inhibition and maternal symptoms of depression. *Psychopathology*, 40(6), 446–452.

Moon, C., Cooper, R. P., & Fifer, W. P. (1993). Two-day-olds prefer their native language. *Infant Behavior & Development*, 16(4), 495–500.

Moon, C., Lagercrantz, H., & Kuhl, P. K. (2013). Language experienced in utero affects vowel perception after birth: A two-country study. *Acta Paediatrica*, 102(2), 156–160.

Morris, H. (1993). Narrative representation, narrative enactment, and the psychoanalytic construction of history. *International Journal of Psychoanalysis*, 74, 33–54.

Muller, J. (1996). *Beyond the psychoanalytic Dyad*. New York & London: Routledge.

Muller, J., & Brent, J. (2000). *Peirce, semiotics, and psychoanalysis*. Baltimore, MD & London: The John Hopkins University Press.

Murray, L., & Cooper, P. J. (1997). Effects of postnatal depression on infant development. *Archives of Disease in Childhood*, 77(2), 99–101.

Murray, L., & Trevarthen, C. (1985). Emotional regulations of interactions between 2-month-olds and their mothers. In *Social perception in infants*, edited by T. M. Field & N. A. Fox (177–197). Norwood, NJ: Ablex.

Murray, L. et al. (2010). The effects of maternal postnatal depression and child sex on academic performance at age 16 years: A developmental approach. *Journal of Child Psychology & Psychiatry*, 51(10), 1150–1159.

Nadel, J., Carchon, I., Kervella, C., Marcelli, D., & Réserbat-Plantey, D. (1999). Expectancies for social contingency in 2-month-olds. *Developmental Science*, 2(2), 164–173. https://doi.org/10.1111/1467-7687.00065

Nadel, J., & Muir, D. (Eds.) (2005). *Emotional development. Recent research advances*. Oxford: Oxford University Press.

Nelson, E. S. (Ed.) (2019). *Interpreting Dilthey*. Cambridge, UK: Cambridge University Press.

Norman, J. (1989). The analyst's visual images and the child analyst's trap. *Psychoanalytic Study of the Child*, 44, 117–135.

Norman, J. (1994). The psychoanalyst's instrument: A mental space for impressions, affective resonance and thoughts. In *The analyst's mind: From listening to interpretation*, edited by L. Schacht, C. Aslan, & R. Tyson (89–100). London: IPA.

Norman, J. (2001). The psychoanalyst and the baby: A new look at work with infants. *International Journal of Psychoanalysis*, 82(1), 83–100.

Norman, J. (2004). Transformations of early infantile experiences: A 6-month-old in psychoanalysis. *International Journal of Psychoanalysis*, 85(5), 1103–1122.

Norman, J., & Salomonsson, B. (2005). 'Weaving thoughts': A method for presenting and commenting psychoanalytic case material in a peer group. *International Journal of Psychoanalysis*, 86(5), 1281–1298.

O'Shaughnessy, E. (1988). W.R. Bion's theory of thinking and new techniques in child analysis. In *Melanie Klein today. Developments in theory and practice. Volume 2: Mainly practice*, edited by E. Bott Spillius (177–190). London: Tavistock/ Routledge.

Oberhoff, B. 2016. *Richard Wagner inside. Die protagonisten seiner inneren bühne (The Protagonists on his inner scene)*. Books on Demand.

Ody, M. (2015). Jouissance: Lust et/ou Genuss ? *Revue Francaise de Psychanalyse*, 79(5), 1771–1771. https://doi.org/10.3917/rfp.795.1771

Ogden, T. H. (1994). The analytic third: Working with intersubjective clinical facts. *International Journal of Psychoanalysis*, 75(1), 3–19.

Ogden, T. H. (1997). Reverie and metaphor: Some thoughts on how I work as a psychoanalyst. *International Journal of Psychoanalysis*, 78, 719–732.

Ogden, T. H. (2004). On holding and containing, being and dreaming. *The International Journal of Psychoanalysis*, 85(6), 1349–1364.

Olds, D. D. (2000). A semiotic model of mind. *Journal of the American Psychoanalytic Association*, 48, 497–529.

Olson, S. L., Bates, J. E., Sandy, J. M., & Schilling, E. M. (2002). Early developmental precursors of impulsive and inattentive behavior: From infancy to middle childhood. *Journal of Child Psychology & Psychiatry*, 43(4), 435–447.

Ornstein, A. (1998). A developmental perspective on the sense of power, self-esteem, and destructive aggression. *Annual of Psychoanalysis*, 25, 145–154.

Palmer, R. E. (1969). *Hermeneutics: Interpretation theory in Schleiermacher, Dilthey, Heidegger, and Gadamer* (Amazon Kindle). Evanston, IL: Nortwestern University Press.

Parsons, C. E., Young, K. S., Rochat, T. J., Kringelbach, M., & Stein, A. (2012). Postnatal depression and its effects on child development: A review of evidence from low-and middle-income countries. *British Medical Bulletin*, 101(1), 57–79.

Paul, C., & Thomson Salo, F. (Eds.) (2014). *The baby as subject: Clinical studies in infant-parent therapy*. London: Karnac

Paulick, J. et al. (2018). Nonverbal synchrony: A new approach to better understand psychotherapeutic processes and drop-out. *Journal of Psychotherapy Integration*, 28(3), 367.

Peluso, P. R., & Freund, R. R. (2018). Therapist and client emotional expression and psychotherapy outcomes: A meta-analysis. *Psychotherapy*, 55(4), 461–472.

Petersen, I., Peltola, T., Kaski, S., Walters, K. R., & Hardoon, S. (2018). Depression, depressive symptoms and treatments in women who have recently given birth: UK cohort study. *BMJ Open*, 8(10). https://doi.org/10.1136/bmjopen-2018-022152

Pines, D. (1993). *A woman's unconscious use of her body. A psychoanalytical perspective* (2010 Kindle ed.). East Sussex: Routledge.

Porter, R., & Winberg, J. (1999). Unique salience of maternal breast odors for new-born infants. *Neuroscience & Biobehavioral Reviews*, 23(3), 439–449. https://doi.org/10.1016/S0149-7634(98)00044-X

Pozzi-Monzo, M. E., & Tydeman, B. (Eds.) (2007). *Innovations in parent-infant psychotherapy*. London: Karnac Books.

Racker, H. (1968). *Transference and countertransference*. London: Karnac Books.

Reck, C. et al. (2004). Interactive regulation of affect in postpartum depressed mothers and their infants: An overview. *Psychopathology*, 37(6), 272–280.

Reddy, V. (2008). *How infants know minds*. Cambridge, MA: Harvard University Press.

Reich, W. (1933). *Character analysis*. New York: Orgone Institute Press.

Reider, N. (1972). Metaphor as interpretation. *International Journal of Psychoanalysis*, 53, 463–469.

Renik, O., & Spillius, E. B. 2004. Intersubjectivity in psychoanalysis. *International Journal of Psychoanalysis*, 85, 1053–1064.

Rennie, D. L. (2012). Qualitative research as methodical hermeneutics. *Psychological Methods*, 17(3), 385.

Rosenfeld, H. (1971). A clinical approach to the psychoanalytic theory of the life and death instincts: An investigation into the aggressive aspects of narcissism. *International Journal of Psychoanalysis*, 52, 169–178.

Rosenfeld, H. (1987). *Impasse and interpretation: Therapeutic and anti-therapeutic factors in the psychoanalytic treatment of psychotic, borderline, and neurotic patients*. London: Tavistock.

Rosolato, G. (1978). Symbol formation. *International Journal of Psychoanalysis*, 59, 303–313.

Rosolato, G. (1985). *Éléments de l'interprétation (Elements of interpretation)*. Paris: Gallimard.

Rucker, N. G. & Mermelstein, C. B. (1979). Unconscious communication in the mother-child dyad. *American Journal of Psychoanalysis*, 39, 147–151.

Safran, J. D., & Muran, J. C. (2000). *Negotiating the therapeutic alliance: A relational treatment guide*. New York: Guilford Press.

Saketopoulou, A. (2020). The infantile erotic countertransference: The analyst's infantile sexual, ethics, and the role of the psychoanalytic collective. *Psychoanalytic Inquiry*, 40(8), 659–677.

Salberg, J. (2015). The texture of traumatic attachment: Presence and ghostly absence in transgenerational transmission. *Psychoanalytic Quarterly*, 84(1), 21–46.

Salberg, J. (2022). Maternal envy as legacy: Search for the unknown lost maternal object. *The International Journal of Psychoanalysis*, 103(5), 726–743. https://doi.org/10.1080/00207578.2022.2043157

Salomonsson, B. (1998). Between listening and expression: On desire, resonance and containment. *Scandinavian Psychoanalytic Review*, 21, 168–182.

Salomonsson, B. (2007a). Semiotic transformations in psychoanalysis with infants and adults. *International Journal of Psychoanalysis*, 88(5), 1201–1221.

Salomonsson, B. (2007b). "Talk to me baby, tell me what's the matter now". Semiotic and developmental perspectives on communication in psychoanalytic infant treatment. *International Journal of Psychoanalysis*, 88(1), 127–146.

Salomonsson, B. (2011). The music of containment. Addressing the participants in mother-infant psychoanalytic treatment. *Infant Mental Health Journal*, 32(6), 599–612.

Salomonsson, B. (2012a). Has infantile sexuality anything to do with infants? *International Journal of Psychoanalysis, 93*(3), 631–647.

Salomonsson, B. (2012b). Psychoanalytic case presentations in a Weaving Thoughts group. On countertransference and group dynamics. *International Journal of Psychoanalysis, 93*(4), 917–937.

Salomonsson, B. (2013a). An infant's experience of postnatal depression: Towards a psychoanalytic model. *Journal of Child Psychotherapy, 39*(2), 137–155.

Salomonsson, B. (2013b). Transferences in parent-infant psychoanalytic treatments. *International Journal of Psychoanalysis, 94*(4), 767–792.

Salomonsson, B. (2014a). *Psychoanalytic therapy with infants and parents: Practice, theory and results.* London: Routledge.

Salomonsson, B. (2014b). Therapeutic action in psychoanalytic therapy with toddlers and parents. *Journal of Child Psychotherapy, 41*(2), 112–130.

Salomonsson, B. (2015a). Extending the field: Parent-toddler psychotherapy inspired by mother-infant work. *Journal of Child Psychotherapy, 41*(1), 3–21. https://doi.org/10.1080/0075417X.2015.1005383

Salomonsson, B. (2015b). Infantile defences in parent-infant psychotherapy: The example of gaze avoidance. *International Journal of Psychoanalysis, 97*(1), 65–88.

Salomonsson, B. (2017). The function of language in parent-infant psychotherapy. *International Journal of Psychoanalysis, 98*(6), 1597–1618.

Salomonsson, B. (2018). *Psychodynamic interventions in pregnancy and infancy.* Oxon: Routledge.

Salomonsson, B. (2020). Psychoanalysis with adults inspired by parent–infant therapy: Reconstructing infantile trauma. *International Journal of Psychoanalysis, 101*(2), 320–339. https://doi.org/10.1080/00207578.2020.1726714

Salomonsson, B. (2021). Gaze avoidance in parent–infant psychotherapy: Manifestations and technical suggestions. *The international Journal of Psychoanalysis, 102*(6), 1138–1157. https://doi.org/10.1080/00207578.2021.1953384

Salomonsson, B. (2022). Psychoanalysis with adults inspired by parent–infant psychotherapy: The analyst's metaphoric function. *The International Journal of Psychoanalysis, 103*(4), 601–618. https://doi.org/10.1080/00207578.2021.2010560

Salomonsson, B. (2023). Patient(s) in parent-infant psychotherapy. In *Child and adolescent psychoanalysis in a changing world*, edited by C. Bronstein & S. Flanders (50–66). London: Routledge.

Salomonsson, B. (2025). What do his lips want from me? Infantile sexuality and enigmatic messages in psychoanalytic parent-infant psychotherapy. *International Journal of Psychoanalysis*, Acc. for publ. May 13, 2024.

Salomonsson, B., & Sandell, R. (2011a). A randomized controlled trial of mother-infant psychoanalytic treatment. 1. Outcomes on self-report questionnaires and external ratings. *Infant Mental Health Journal, 32*(2), 207–231.

Salomonsson, B., & Sandell, R. (2011b). A randomized controlled trial of mother-infant psychoanalytic treatment. 2. Predictive and moderating influences of quantitative treatment and patient factors. *Infant Mental Health Journal, 32*(3), 377–404.

Salomonsson, B., & Winberg Salomonsson, M. (2015). *Dialogues with children and adolescents: A psychoanalytic guide.* London: Routledge.

Salomonsson, B., & Winberg Salomonsson, M. (2017). Intimacy thwarted and established: Following a girl from infancy to child psychotherapy. *International Journal of Psychoanalysis*, 98(3), 861–875.

Sass, L. A., & Woolfolk, R. L. (1988). Psychoanalysis and the hermeneutic turn: A critique of narrative truth and historical truth. *Journal of the American Psychoanalytic Association*, 36, 429–454.

Sato, H. et al. 2012). Cerebral hemodynamics in newborn infants exposed to speech sounds: A whole-head optical topography study. *Human Brain Mapping*, 33(9), 2092–2103. https://doi.org/10.1002/hbm.21350

Scarfone, D. (2014). The three essays and the meaning of the infantile sexual in psychoanalysis. *The Psychoanalytic Quarterly*, 83(2), 327–344.

Scarfone, D., & Saketopoulou, A. (2023). *The reality of the message*. New York: The Unconscious in Translation.

Seligman, S. D. M. H. (1999). Integrating Kleinian theory and intersubjective infant research: Observing projective identification. *Psychoanalytic Dialogues*, 9(2), 129–159.

Shaffer, D. et al. (1983). A Children's Global Assessment Scale (CGAS). *Archives of General Psychiatry*, 40(11), 1228–1231.

Shapiro, E. R. 1996. Grief in Freud's life: Reconceptualizing bereavement in psychoanalytic theory. *Psychoanalytic Psychology*, 13, 547.

Shengold, L. (1981). Insight as metaphor. *Psychoanalytic Study of the Child*, 36, 289–306.

Silverman, D. K. (2001). Sexuality and attachment: A passionate relationship or a marriage of convenience? *The Psychoanalytic Quarterly*, 70(2), 325–358. https://doi.org/10.1002/j.2167-4086.2001.tb00603.x

Silverman, D. K. (2022). Otherness and our sexuality: Laplanche clinically. *Studies in Gender and Sexuality*, 23(1), 5–14.

Silverman, R., & Lieberman, A. (1999). Negative maternal attributions, projective identification, and the intergenerational transmission of violent relational patterns. *Psychoanalytic Dialogues*, 9(2), 161–186.

Simpson, R. B. (2007). That subtle knot: The body and metaphor. In *The embodied subject. Minding the body in psychoanalysis* edited by J. P. Muller & J. G. Tillman (17–28). Lanham, MD: Jason Aronson.

Sletvold, J. (2016). The analyst's body: A relational perspective from the body. *Psychoanalytic Perspectives*, 13(2), 186–200.

Sorce, J. F., Emde, R. N., Campos, J. J., & Klinnert, M. D. (1985). Maternal emotional signaling: Its effect on the visual cliff behavior of 1-year-olds. *Developmental Psychology*, 21(1), 195–200.

Spence, D. P. (1982). Narrative truth and theoretical truth. *Psychoanalytic Q.uarterly*, 51, 43–69.

Spence, D. P. (1986). When interpretation masquerades as explanation. *Journal of the American Psychoanalytic Association*, 34(1), 3–22. https://doi.org/10.1177/000306518603400101

Spence, D. P. (1989). Narrative appeal vs. historical validity. *Contemporary Psychoanalysis*, 25, 517–523.

Spence, D. P. (2000). Remembrances of things past. *Journal of Clinical Psychoanalysis*, 9(1), 149–162.

Spitz, R. (1965). *The first year of life*. New York: IUP Inc.

Stein, A. et al. (2014). Effects of perinatal mental disorders on the fetus and child. *The Lancet, 384*(9956), 1800–1819.

Stein, R. (2008). The otherness of sexuality: Excess. *Journal of the American Psychoanalytic Association, 56*(1), 43–71.

Steiner, J. (1993). *Psychic retreats*. London: Routledge.

Steiner, J. (2018). The trauma and disillusionment of Oedipus. *International Journal of Psychoanalysis, 99*(555–568).

Stern, D. N. (1971). A microanalysis of mother-infant interaction. *Journal of the American Academy of Child Psychology, 10*, 501–517. https://doi.org/10.1016/s0002-7138(09)61752-0

Stern, D. N. (1985). *The interpersonal world of the infant*. New York: Basic Books.

Stern, D. N. (1990). *Diary of a baby* (Kindle ed.). New York: Basic Books.

Stern, D. N. (2004). *The present moment in psychotherapy and in everyday life*. New York: W.W. Norton and Company Ltd.

Stern, D. N. et al. (1998). The process of therapeutic change involving implicit knowledge: Some implications of developmental observations for adult psychotherapy. *Infant Mental Health Journal, 19*(3), 300–308.

Stone, M. (2006). The analyst's body as tuning fork: Embodied resonance in countertransference. *Journal of Analytical Psychology, 51*(1), 109–124. https://doi.org/10.1111/j.1465-5922.2006.575_1.x

Suvini, F. M. (2019). The application of improvisational music therapy in autism. *Life, 2*(2), 53.

Tanis, B. (2021). The infantile: Its multiple dimensions. *The International Journal of Psychoanalysis, 102*(3), 572–587.

Teinonen, T., Fellman, V., Näätänen, R., Alku, P., & Huotilainen, M. (2009). Statistical language learning in neonates revealed by event-related brain potentials. *BMC Neuroscience, 10*, 1–8.

Thomson Salo, F. (2007). Recognizing the infant as subject in infant-parent psychotherapy. *International Journal of Psychoanalysis, 88*(4), 961–979.

Thomson-Salo, F., & Paul, C. (2017). Understanding the sexuality of infants within caregiving relationships in the first year. *Psychoanalytic Dialogues, 27*(3), 320–337.

Toth, S. L., Rogosch, F. A., Sturge-Apple, M., & Cicchetti, D. (2009). Maternal depression, children's attachment security, and representational development: An organizational perspective. *Child Development, 80*(1), 192–208.

Trevarthen, C. (1979). Communication and cooperation in early infancy: A description of primary intersubjectivity. In *Before speech: The beginnings of human communication*, edited by M. Bullowa (321–347). Cambridge: Cambridge University Press.

Tronick, E. (1989). Emotions and emotional communication in infants. *American Psychologist, 44*(2), 112–119.

Tronick, E. (2005). Why is connection with others so critical? The formation of dyadic states of consciousness and the expansion of individuals' states of consciousness. In *Emotional development*, edited by J. Nadel & D. Muir (293–315). Oxford: Oxford University Press.

Tronick, E. (2007a). Infant moods and the chronicity of depressive symptoms: The cocreation of unique ways of being together for good or ill, Paper 2: The formation of negative moods in infants and children of depressed mothers. In *The *neurobehavioral and social-emotional development of infants and children*, edited by E. Tronick (362–377). New York: W. W. Norton.

Tronick, E. (2007b). *The neurobehavioral and social-emotional development of infants and children*. New York: W. W. Norton.

Tronick, E., Als, H., Adamson, L., Wise, S., & Brazelton, T. B. (1978). The infant's response to entrapment between contradictory messages in face-to-face interaction. *Journal of the American Academy of Child and Adolescent Psychiatry, 17*, 1–13.

Tronick, E., & Beeghly, M. (2011). Infants' meaning-making and the development of mental health problems. *American Psychologist, 66*(2), 107–119. https://doi.org/10.1037/a0021631

Tustin, F. (1986). *Autistic barriers in neurotic patients*. London: Tavistock.

Tuters, E., Doulis, S., & Yabsley, S. (2011). Challenges working with infants and their families: Symptoms and meanings—two approaches of infant–parent psychotherapy. *Infant Mental Health Journal, 32*(6), 632–649.

Van Buren, J. (1993). Mother-infant semiotics: Intuition and the development of human subjectivity--Klein/Lacan: Fantasy and meaning. *Journal of the American Academy of Psychoanalysis & Dynamic Psychiatry, 21*(4), 567–580.

Van Haute, P. (2005). Infantile sexuality, primary object-love and the anthropological significance of the Oedipus complex: Re-reading Freud's 'Female sexuality'. *International Journal of Psychoanalysis, 86*(6), 1661–1678.

Vaughan, S. C. (2017). In the Night Kitchen: What are the ingredients of infantile sexuality? *Psychoanalytic Dialogues, 27*, 344–348.

Vivona, J. M. (2019). The interpersonal words of the infant: Implications of current infant language research for psychoanalytic theories of infant development, language, and therapeutic action. *The Psychoanalytic Quarterly, 88*(4), 685–725. https://doi.org/10.1080/00332828.2019.1652048

von Klitzing, K. (2003). From interactions to mental representations: Psychodynamic parent-infant therapy in a case of severe eating and sleep disorders. *Journal of Child Psychotherapy, 29*(3), 317–333.

Vouloumanos, A., & Werker, J. F. (2004). Tuned to the signal: The privileged status of speech for young infants. *Developmental Science, 7*(3), 270–276.

Vouloumanos, A., & Werker, J. F. (2007). Why voice melody alone cannot explain neonates' preference for speech. *Developmental Science, 10*(2), 169–171.

Wachholz, S., & Stuhr, U. (1999). The concept of ideal types in psychoanalytic follow-up research. *Psychotherapy Research, 9*(3), 327–341.

Walle, E., & Campos, J. (2014). The development of infant detection of inauthentic emotion. *Emotion, 14*(3), 488–503.

Wallerstein, R. S. (2011). Metaphor in psychoanalysis: Bane or blessing? *Psychoanalytic Inquiry, 31*(2), 90–106.

Watillon, A. (1993). The dynamics of psychoanalytic therapies of the early parent–child relationship. *International Journal of Psychoanalysis, 74*, 1037–1048.

Wechsler, D. (2005). *WPPSI–III. Manual, del 1. Svensk version*. Stockholm: Psykologiförlaget.

Whitebook, J. (2017). *FREUD – An intellectual biography*. Cambridge: Cambridge University Press.

Widlöcher, D. (2002). *Infantile sexuality and attachment*. New York: Other Press.

Widström, A. et al. (2011). Newborn behaviour to locate the breast when skin-to-skin: A possible method for enabling early self-regulation. *Acta Paediatrica, 100*(1), 79–85.

Widström, A.-M., Ransjö-Arvidsson, A.-B., & Christensson, K. (2007). *Breastfeeding – Baby's choice*. Stockholm: Liber Utbildning.

Wilson, A., & Golonka, S. (2013). Embodied cognition is not what you think it is. *Frontiers in Psychology*, 4(58). https://doi.org/10.3389/fpsyg.2013.00058

Winberg Salomonsson, M., Sorjonen, K., & Salomonsson, B. (2015a). A long-term follow-up of a randomized controlled trial of mother–infant psychoanalytic treatment: Outcomes on the children. *Infant Mental Health Journal*, 36(1), 12–29.

Winberg Salomonsson, M., Sorjonen, K., & Salomonsson, B. (2015b). A long-term follow-up study of a randomized controlled trial of mother-infant psychoanalytic treatment: Outcomes on mothers and interactions. *Infant Mental Health Journal*, 36(6), 542–555.

Winnicott, D. W. (1941). The observation of infants in a set situation. In *Through paediatrics to psycho-analysis* (52–69). London: Hogarth Press.

Winnicott, D. W. (1949). Mind and its relation to the psyche-soma. In *Through paediatrics to psychoanalysis* (243–254). London: Hogarth Press.

Winnicott, D. W. (1953). Transitional objects and transitional phenomena – A study of the first not-me possession. *International Journal of psychoanalysis*, 34, 89–97.

Winnicott, D. W. (1956). Primary maternal preoccupation. In *Through paediatrics to psycho-analysis* (300–305). London: Hogarth Press.

Winnicott, D. W. (1960). Ego distortion in terms of true and false self. In *The maturational processes and the facilitating environment: Studies in the theory of emotional development*, edited by M. M. R. Khan (140–152). London: Hogarth Press.

Winnicott, D. W. (1962). Ego Integration in Child Development. In *The maturational processes and the facilitating environment*, edited by M. M. Khan (56–63). London: Hogarth Press.

Winnicott, D. W. (1971). *Playing and reality*. London: Tavistock Publications.

Winnicott, D. W. (1974). Fear of breakdown. *International Review of Psychoanalysis*, 1, 103–107.

Winnicott, D. W. (1975). *Through paediatrics to psycho-analysis*. London: Hogarth Press.

Winnicott, D. W. (1988). *Human nature*. London: Free Associations Book.

Yerushalmi, H. (2019). Negative capability, heuristics and supervision. *British Journal of Psychotherapy*, 35(2), 290–304.

Zamanian, K. (2011). Attachment theory as defense: What happened to infantile sexuality? *Psychoanalytic Psychology*, 28(1), 33–47.

Zeanah, C., Benoit, D., & Hirshberg, L. (1996). *Working model of the child interview coding manual*. New Orleans: Unpublished manual.

Index

Note that page numbers in *italics* represent figures.

For Product Safety Concerns and Information please contact our EU
representative GPSR@taylorandfrancis.com
Taylor & Francis Verlag GmbH, Kaufingerstraße 24, 80331 München, Germany